Clinical Veterinary Science: Anatomy and Physiology

Clinical Veterinary Science: Anatomy and Physiology

Editor: Herbert Dundas

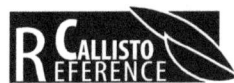

R CALLISTO
REFERENCE

www.callistoreference.com

Callisto Reference,
118-35 Queens Blvd., Suite 400,
Forest Hills, NY 11375, USA

Visit us on the World Wide Web at:
www.callistoreference.com

ISBN: 978-1-63239-962-5 (Hardback)

Trademark Notice: Registered trademark of products or corporate names are used only for explanation and identification without intent to infringe.

Cataloging-in-Publication Data

Clinical veterinary science : anatomy and physiology / edited by Herbert Dundas.
    p. cm.
Includes bibliographical references and index.
ISBN 978-1-63239-962-5
1. Veterinary medicine. 2. Veterinary anatomy. 3. Veterinary physiology. 4. Clinical medicine.
I. Dundas, Herbert.
SF745 .C55 2018
636.089--dc23

Table of Contents

Preface

The main aim of this book is to educate learners and enhance their research focus by presenting diverse topics covering this vast field. This is an advanced book which compiles significant studies by distinguished experts in the area of analysis. This book addresses successive solutions to the challenges arising in the area of application, along with it; the book provides scope for future developments.

The branch of science which helps in the diagnosis and treatment of diseases in animals is known as veterinary science. Different species of domesticated as well as wild animals are treated under this field. Veterinary science also helps in monitoring animals to prevent zoonotic diseases such as anthrax, cat-scratch disease, Chagas disease, Ebola virus disease, etc. This book includes some of the vital pieces of work being conducted across the world, on various topics related to veterinary science. With its detailed analyses and data, it will prove immensely beneficial to professionals and students involved in this area at various levels.

It was a great honour to edit this book, though there were challenges, as it involved a lot of communication and networking between me and the editorial team. However, the end result was this all-inclusive book covering diverse themes in the field.

Finally, it is important to acknowledge the efforts of the contributors for their excellent chapters, through which a wide variety of issues have been addressed. I would also like to thank my colleagues for their valuable feedback during the making of this book.

Editor

Important hemoprotozoan diseases of livestock: Challenges in current diagnostics and therapeutics

Biswa Ranjan Maharana[1], Anup Kumar Tewari[2], Buddhi Chandrasekaran Saravanan[2] and Naduvanahalli Rajanna Sudhakar[2]

1. Department of Veterinary Parasitology, College of Veterinary Science and Animal Husbandry, Junagadh Agricultural University, Junagadh, Gujarat, India; 2. Division of Parasitology, Indian Veterinary Research Institute, Izatnagar, Uttar Pradesh, India.
Corresponding author: Biswa Ranjan Maharana, e-mail: drbiswaranjanmaharana@gmail.com,
AKT: tewarianup@gmail.com, BCS: drbcsaravanan@gmail.com, NRS: sudhi463@gmail.com

Abstract

Hemoprotozoan parasites pose a serious threat to the livestock population in terms of mortality, reduced milk yield and lowered draft power. Diagnosis of these diseases often poses a challenging task. Needless to say that impact of disease in health and productivity is huge though a fair economic assessment on the quantum of economic loss associated is yet to be worked out from India. The diagnosis of hemoprotozoan infections largely depends on various laboratory-based diagnostic methods as the clinical manifestations are often inconspicuous and non-specific. Traditional diagnostic methods rely on microscopical demonstration of infective stages in blood or tissue fluids. However, it is laborious, lesser sensitive, and cannot differentiate between morphologically similar organisms. Recent development in the technologies has opened new avenues for improvement in the accurate diagnosis of parasitic infections. Serological tests are simple, fast but lack specificity. With advent of molecular techniques, as DNA hybridization assays, polymerase chain reaction and its modifications ensure the detection of infection in the latent phase of the disease. Nucleic acid-based assays are highly sensitive, free from immunocompetence and can differentiate between morphologically similar parasites. With the advent of newer diagnostics complemented with traditional ones will be of huge help for targeted selective treatment with better chemotherapeutic agents.

Keywords: *Anaplasma*, *Babesia*, chemotherapy, hemoprotozoa, molecular diagnosis, *Theileria*, *Trypanosoma*.

Introduction

Protozoan parasites are responsible for causing severe infections both in humans and animals worldwide. The infection is mainly transmitted by arthropod vectors, or through blood transfusion [1]. The important hemoprotozoan diseases of veterinary importance are trypanosomosis, theileriosis, babesiosis, and anaplasmosis, which are caused by several species of *Trypanosoma* [2], *Theileria*, *Babesia* [3-5], and *Anaplasma*, respectively, in several species of livestock. The impact of diseases caused by these organisms on health and productivity of farm animals and human beings is huge, though a fair economic assessment on the quantum of incidental economic loss is yet to be worked out from India [6]. The clinical manifestation of the disease varies from fever, anorexia, anemia, threatened abortion, and death in the acute form of infections [7]. Conventional diagnostic methods for most of the infections rely on microscopical demonstration of infective stages in blood or tissue fluids. Diagnosing hemoprotozoan infections by light microscopy examination of invasively acquired specimens at chronic stage of infection is a challenging task. Serological tests developed and designed for indirect antibody-based diagnosis of the infectious parasitic diseases during the year 1970s had wide acceptance globally though a specific serological reference test for many of the infections are still to come. The major difficulty associated with standardization of such test is the paucity of specific non-cross-reactive test reagents [8]. Most popular serologic assays used to detect antibodies to most of the hemoparasitic infections in test sera from animals and humans include immunofluorescence, enzyme-linked immunosorbent assay (ELISA) and its variants and Western blot. The sensitivity and specificity of these tests for detecting infection specific antibody are not known because few comparative evaluations have been published. Detecting some pathogens in infected cell cultures may be possible, but isolating the organisms in cell culture as a means of diagnosing infection is laborious and lengthy and is prone to failure with specimens from non-sterile sites. Therefore, the cell culture is not recommended as a routine laboratory technique for diagnosing most of the hemoparasites hence, though animal inoculation test is ethically prohibitive, still a dependable diagnostic strategy for blood-borne parasites such as trypanosomes. Keeping these in mind, nowadays, molecular diagnosis is the method of choice for identification of parasites. Commonly used molecular tools are polymerase chain reaction (PCR), real-time PCR, loop-mediated isothermal amplification (LAMP), etc. [9]. The nucleic acid-based techniques have the advantage of ensuring the detection of infection in the latent phase of the disease when the level of parasitemia is often below the detection limit of conventional methods as well as in the assessment of the success of the specific chemotherapeutic intervention, besides its epidemiological applications [10]. Although total eradication of the protozoan infections may be impossible, strategies for effective control of the infections in many tropical countries like India can be a feasible goal. To ensure this goal, application of techniques with proven impact needs to be applied especially for identifying the carrier animals. Ironically, diagnostic decisions still rely on microscopy ostensibly for economic reasons. Compared to the microscope and serology-based techniques, the molecular methods offer more sensitivity and specificity, which greatly increase the probability of specific detection in test samples. The molecular detection techniques are useful even in dealing with a large number of samples at a much higher sensitivity and have the required flexibility of automation and up gradation [10]. Therefore, the techniques can be applied for the prevalence studies of a disease of veterinary and zoonotic importance.

Trypanosomosis

Trypanosomosis popularly known as surra is one of the most important hemoprotozoan diseases affecting human and animal health in the tropics [11,12] especially in the South East Asia [13]. The prevalence of surra peaks around the monsoon when the animals are under maximum work-stress owing to agricultural plantations, besides other contributing factors, *viz.*, concurrent disease, poor nutrition, innate and acquired resistance, parasite pathogenicity, and strain of parasite. Effective surveillance for *Trypanosoma evansi* is constrained by a lack of sensitive diagnostic tests and information on *T. evansi* distribution in India. Although the level of awareness in veterinarians and diagnostic laboratories with regard to *T. evansi* is almost adequate, lack of diagnostic techniques of high sensitivity hinders quick identification. Microscopy is the only diagnostic tool besides animal inoculation with virtues of high specificity, ease of use, lack of cold chain [14]. However, its low sensitivity (approximately 100,000 parasites/ml for wet blood film examination, leads to an erroneous judgment of false negativity which often results in even death of the infected individual in the absence of treatment [15]. Only with concentration methods such as microhematocrit centrifugation [16], quantitative buffy coat technique [17], and mini-anion-exchange centrifugation technique [18,19] can detect parasitemia as low as 50 parasites/ml. This limits the utility of microscopy in resource-poor settings.

Immunodiagnostic techniques are useful for diagnosis of trypanosomosis, but most of them have been retrospective surveys so ineffective in controlling the ailment. However, the complement fixation test was used successfully in the control and eradication of dourine in North America [20] and the diagnosis of surra in buffalo in the Philippines [21]. The indirect fluorescent antibody test (IFAT) is both specific and sensitive for detection of trypanosome antibodies in animals and humans [22]. However, a major problem associated with IFAT is the cross reactivity between different species of *Tryponosoma* and requirement of the sophisticated microscope. Other immunodiagnostics followed very often are ELISA [23], card agglutination test (CATT), etc. [24]. CATT can detect early infections as it can detect immunoglobulin IgM. On the contrary, ELISA used to detect immunoglobulin IgG in established infections. A monoclonal antibody-based latex agglutination test has been claimed effective in the diagnosis of surra in domesticated animals under field conditions, which have been reported to be simple, rapid, and cost effective in field conditions [25-27].

A range of nucleic acid amplification-based molecular techniques has been developed to improve the detection of pathogenic trypanosomes. Among them, PCR has the maximum application [28,29]. Several PCR-based diagnostic assays have been developed which include the use of species-specific primers, single and nested PCRs [30], and real-time PCR [31]. Tandem repeat domain of GM6 (cytoskeletal protein) has diagnostic value and its usefulness as seroepidemiological studies of surra has been evaluated among water buffaloes [32]. PCR based on invariant surface glycoprotein 75 gene can be useful in the detection of carrier status of surra in animals [33]. With the use of generic primers in semi-nested PCR targeting variable region of 18s rDNA gene followed by the restriction fragment length polymorphism (RFLP) approach, it is possible to differentiate between important trypanosome species infecting bovines with mixed infections [34]. However, requirements for trained manpower and sophisticated equipment have restricted its use for wide application in the endemic areas. Isothermal reactions, such as LAMP [35] and nucleic acid sequence-based amplification (NASBA) [36,37], have recently been developed for the diagnosis of trypanosomosis; however, the techniques have increased application only for detection of human cases. These diagnostic tests have advantages that they do not need expensive equipment, post-amplification handling requirements and also are highly sensitive in terms of detection of pathogen [38]. However, the importance of PCR in the control of trypanosomosis in screening samples from serologically positive field samples in a specialized reference laboratory and the high accuracy would ease early detection and epidemiological mapping of trypanosomosis. More recently, proteome (i.e., the whole parasite content) and secretome (i.e. naturally excreted/secreted molecules) analysis providing valuable clues for identification of immunodominant antigens of *T. evansi* for detection and control of chronic trypanosomosis [39].

Chemotherapy

Diminazene aceturate (DA) is the most extensively used curative trypanocide against surra in ruminants followed by isometamidium chloride (IMC) (both curative and preventive), cymelarsan (for curative treatment of camels), suramin, and quinapyramine (curative and/or preventive). Its use in horses and dogs is limited due to poor efficacy and tolerance in these species. IMC, a member of phenanthridine family, can be used for curative (0.5 mg/kg bw) and preventive (1 mg/kg bw) treatment of surra in ruminants and horses *via* intramuscular or subcutaneous injection [23]. Further, DA and IMC constitute a "sanative pair," which means that once resistance develops to one of the drugs and another drug can be used to control the infection. Melarsominedihydrochloride (cymelarsan) is the latest trypanocide to be discovered. It is used to control surra at a dose rate of 0.25, 0.25-0.5, 0.5, and 0.75 mg/kg bw in camels, horses, cattle, and buffaloes, respectively. Quinapyramine methyl-sulfate, a member of aminoquinaldine derivatives, can be used to treat the infection by subcutaneous injection at a dose of 5 mg/kg bw. A more effective mixture of quinapyramine chloride and quinapyramine sulfate (triquin) can be used as a curative/preventive drug against *T. evansi* in horses and camels administered by subcutaneous injection at a dose of 8 mg/kg bw. The drug has chemoprophylactic effect which can last up to 4 months. Its use should be restricted to horses and camels only. Quinapyramine is not recommended in cattle because it may induce cross resistance to both IMC and DA [23].

The 50% inhibitory concentrations of the four existing agents were reported as 87.6, 12.5, 1.1, and 0.1 ng/ml for suramin, diminazene, cymelarsan, and quinapyramine, respectively. The diamidine diminazene reported to have the least efficacy among all of the standard drugs currently available in the market. In contrast, cymelarsan demonstrated the best efficacy, yet the costs of this drug, which is higher than those of other trypanocidal drugs, coupled with its limited availability throughout the world (it is available only in the Middle East and Africa), overshadow its beneficial properties. Variation of the glycoprotein between and within *Trypanosoma* spp. is a major stumbling block for vaccine development against this parasite. Hence, researchers are in the process of identifying non-variant regions such as PFR protein, which is universally present in the kinetoplastid flagellum as potential drug and vaccine target [40-44]. Against the backdrop of failed attempts to develop a protective vaccine using native or recombinant proteins of trypanosome origin, development of a live attenuated vaccine using ionizing radiation is believed to be impressive and practical. We are presently working in this area to explore the immunoprophylactic potential of irradiated *T. evansi* in a murine model. The radiation attenuated *T. evansi* was used in immunization trial involving rats and mice. The immunized rats and mice could withstand a lethal homologous challenge, and the conferred protection was attributed to both the humoral and cellular immune responses. Based on the encouraging response achieved through irradiation attenuated parasites in the preliminary studies involving rodent model, an experimentation involving the target bovine model may be emphasized further as it has shown promise toward the development of a live attenuated vaccine against surra (Unpublished Data).

Babesiosis

Babesiosis is caused by hemotropic protozoa belonging to the genus *Babesia*, family Babesiidae and order Piroplasmida, within the phylum Apicomplexa. This protozoan parasitizes the erythrocytes of wild and domestic animals. The infection has long been recognized as an economically important disease of cattle, horses, and dogs and has gained increasing attention as an emerging zoonotic disease. Bovine babesiosis or red water fever is prevalent in cattle worldwide [45]. In India, *Babesia bigemina* is the important species infecting cattle. Clinical signs characteristic of infection in bovines are increased in body temperature, high rate of pulse, and respiration with a marked decrease in appetite and disinclination to movement. In acute infection, hemoglobinurea and hemolytic anemia are characteristic with fatal outcome in absence of chemotherapy [46].

Traditionally, the microscopic detection of *Babesia* parasites has always been considered as the gold standard for the diagnosis of acute babesiosis [47]. However, the low sensitivity of the technique is the major drawback which makes it difficult to detect low parasitemia in the chronic stage of infection as well as in the carrier animals [48,49]. Serological test-like IFAT, due to their better sensitivity, is considered as a suitable protocol for diagnosis of infection [50], but cross reactivity among species and also in genus level is really a major drawback for species-specific diagnosis. Nucleic acids-based detection methods developed in recent past with increased specificity and sensitivity. PCR-based assays have been widely used for the detection of *Babesia* parasites owing to their high specificity and sensitivity [51,52]. PCR enables detection of *Babesia* parasitemia as low as a few organisms per milliliter. Real-time PCR is useful, especially in early stage of infection when results of serological tests are negative, and the blood smear does not reveal the pathogen [53,54] or where the distinction between inter-erythrocytic forms of related organisms, viz., *Theileria* sp. and *Plasmodium* sp. required. Reverse line blot (RLB) is a more sensitive method than PCR since it is able to detect extremely low parasitemia levels and simultaneously identify

Theileria and *Babesia* species using specific oligonucleotide probes [55]. The utility of LAMP technique for diagnosis of babesiosis infection in cattle has been successfully demonstrated [56]. NASBA or transcription-mediated amplification or self-sustaining sequence replication system, which is a highly sensitive, isothermal, transcription-based amplification system specifically designed for the detection of RNA targets. NASBA employs a battery of three enzymes, i.e., RNAase H, reverse transcriptase and T7 DNA dependent RNA polymerase, and two primers leading to main amplification product of single-stranded RNA. It is recently used for diagnosis of *Babesia* and *Theileria* using RNA as an initial template [57].

The latest development in molecular biology has created exciting possibilities for improved specific diagnosis of hemoprotozoan diseases. The 18S rDNA gene (18s rDNA, SSU rDNA) encoding rRNA of the small ribosomal subunit is one of the frequently used molecular markers in diagnostic and epidemiological studies. In *Babesia*, the gene encoding 18s rRNA harbors eight variable regions numbered V_1 to V_5 and V_7 to V_9 among which the V_4 gene (300 bp) is the biggest and most changeable region. Nested PCR enables the amplification of this region characteristics for certain *Babesia* species or even strains within this species. With the aim of developing the molecular diagnostics of babesiosis, Birkenheuer *et al.*, 2003 carried out semi-nested PCR to detect and differentiate the DNA of *Babesia gibsoni*, *Babesia canis*, and *Babesia vogeli* in canine blood samples [58]. It is emphasized that in the diagnosis of babesiosis, the determination of the species, sub species, and even genotype that caused the babesiosis is very essential as virulence, prognosis, and response to treatment against *Babesia* species is different. Molecular markers such as HSP-70, β tubulin allow the precise identification of *Babesia* species with the help of PCR-RFLP technique. Recently, PCR assay targeting *B. bigemina* small subunit ribosomal RNA has been used for detection of low-level *B. bigemina* infection in yaks at the yak rearing tracts of Himalayas [59]. Microchip electrophoresis (ME) using programed field strength gradient allows the analysis of 591 and 1191 bp DNA fragments from the 18 s RNA of *B. gibsoni* and *Babesia caballi* [60]. However, none of these nucleic acid-based methods could be considered better than another. Their utility in diagnostic applications varies as per the need.

Chemotherapy

For chemotherapy of babesiosis three babesiacides, *viz.*, quinuroniumsulfate (Ludobal®, Bayer Ltd.), amicarbalideiso-thionate (Diampron®, May and Baker Ltd.), and DA (Berenil®, Hoechst Ltd.) were available in most European countries, whereas only the last one is available in India. Diaminazine works rapidly against *Babesia bovis* and *B. bigemina* at a dose rate of 3.5 mg/kg intramuscularly and well tolerated. It will protect cattle from the two diseases for 2 and 4 weeks, respectively [61]. In the 1970s, a fourth, imidocarbdipropionate was introduced (Imizol®; Schering-Plough) for chemotherapy of red water fever. Imidocarb dipropionate rapidly became the product of choice because of its prophylactic efficacy at twice the therapeutic doses. Imidocarb is used subcutaneously at 1.2 mg/kg for treatment while 3 mg/kg provides protection from *B. bovis* for 4 weeks and *B. bigemina* for at least 2 months. At high dose, imidocarb also eliminates *B. bovis* and *B. bigemina* from carrier animals [45]. Imidocarb appears to be the drug of choice for treatment of infected horses (at 2 mg/kg, 4 mg/kg for *B. caballi* and *Babesia equi*, respectively). Later quinuronium and amicarbalide were withdrawn because of safety issue and diminazene, which is still widely used in the tropics for the chemotherapy of babesiosis and trypanosomosis was withdrawn from Europe for marketing reasons [62]. In addition, supportive therapies, such as blood transfusions, anti-inflammatory drugs, tick removal, iron reparations, dextrose, vitamins (B complex), purgatives, and fluid replacements, may be necessary in severe cases of babesiosis [63].

Theileriosis

Bovine tropical theileriosis is a tick-borne infection caused by *Theileria annulata*, an intracellular protozoan parasite. It is a lymphoproliferative disease with high mortality and morbidity in cattle. *Theileria sergenti/buffeli/orientalis* cause mild or asymptomatic disease in cattle and well known as bovine benign theileriosis. Certain *Ixodid* ticks, such as *Hyalommaanatolicumanatolicum, H. m. marginatum,* and *H. a. excavatum* known to transmit *T. annulata*, are found in the Mediterranean region, especially in semi-arid areas [64]. Ticks of the genera *Amblyomma, Rhipicephalus,* and *Haemaphysalis* were suggested as a possible vector in the transmission of benign *Theileria* species [65].

Subclinical infection in cattle with *T. annulata* in endemic regions produces chronic carrier state and serves as sources of infection for ticks. Therefore, latent infections are important in the epidemiology of theileriosis [66]. The diagnosis of *Theileria* infection is based on clinical findings, and microscopic examination of Giemsa-stained thin blood and lymph node smears in acute cases. However, expertise in microscopy detection of piroplasm is required in subclinical or chronic infections because parasitemia is often extremely low and may otherwise be missed. Serological tests such as IFAT though provides adequate sensitivity and easy to perform but due to reduced specificity are not followed now a days. ELISA using recombinant proteins of *T. annulata* surface protein (TaSP) and *T. annulata* merozoite surface antigen 1 (TamS1) are being used to detect antibodies in infected animals [67]. A lateral flow device has been developed with recombinant TaSP antigen of *T. annulata* which did not show any cross reaction with hemoparasites of cattle [68]. ELISA based on 53 kDa recombinant protein from truncated EMA-2 gene of *T. equi* is able to detect *T. equi* specific antibodies as early as 9 days post-infection [69]. In recent time, PCR has been the most preferred method for detection of *Theileria* species in epidemiological studies. Several studies documented that PCR is more sensitive and specific than other conventional diagnostic techniques in determining piroplasm-carrier animals [70]. Different variants of PCR such as nested PCR [71] and real-time PCR [72], can be followed for fast and accurate diagnosis of the infection. ME is an increasingly popular technique due to its economical, time-saving nature and used successfully in the diagnosis of bovine theileriosis after amplifying the 816 bp DNA using only 200 nl of blood [73]. ME using programed field strength gradient allows amplification of 816 bp DNA fragment from the 18s RNA of *T. buffeli* [60]. RLB micro array is a recently developed technique that uses oligonucleotide probe to detect and identify *Theleria* and/*Babesia* simultaneously that by specifically amplifying the rRNA gene of V4 hypervariable region of all *Babesia* and *Theileria* species [74]. The obtained PCR products are then hybridized to nitrocellulose membrane, onto which different species-specific oligonucleotide probes are covalently linked. This assay has been extensively used in epidemiological surveys in various countries [75].

Chemotherapy

Parvaquone (2-cyclohexyl-3-hydroxy-1,4-naphthoquinone) and buparvaquone (2-(trans-4-t-butyl-cyclohexyl-methyl)-3-hydroxy-1,4-naphthoquinone) are the two important chemotherapeutic agents used for the treatment of theileriosis caused by *T. annulata* in cattle without significant side effects or relapse of disease. Buparvaquone at a dose of 2.5 mg/kg has a satisfactory therapeutic index and is more effective in the chemotherapy of *T. annulata* than parvaquone [1].

Reliable vaccines of known efficacy have been developed for *T. annulata*. Rakshavac-T - the schizont tissue culture vaccine is meant for prevention of theileriosis caused in crossbred and exotic cattle. Attenuated schizonts do not produce the clinical disease. Immunized cattle can withstand the attack of infected ticks for a period of 3-year. In areas where the vaccinated animals are constantly exposed to tick bites, the immunity is constantly boosted and hence the immunity is conferred for lifetime. Where the animals are maintained in tick free condition, revaccination in every 3 years is recommended. The prophylactic use of Rakshavac-T and chemotherapy with buparvaquone could be the most promising means of controlling theileriosis. Vaccination against *T. parva* is based on infection and treatment, in which cattle is given a subcutaneous dose of tick-derived sporozoites and a simultaneous treatment with a long-acting tetracycline formulation. Recovered animals demonstrate a robust immunity to homologous challenge, which usually lasts for the lifetime of an animal [76].

Anaplasmosis

Anaplasmosis is also known as gall sickness is an infectious non-contagious rickettsial disease caused by *Anaplasma marginale*. This is an obligate intra-erythrocyte rickettsial organism. It spreads through tick bites or by the mechanical transfer of fresh blood from infected to susceptible cattle from biting flies or by blood-contaminated fomites. The infection is also occasionally passed from an infected cow to her unborn calf through the placenta. Bovine anaplasmosis occurs in tropical and subtropical regions mainly due to *A. marginale* and *Anaplasma centrale*. Although cattle of all ages are prone to infection, adult cattle are more susceptible to infection than calves. It is worthy to note that recovered animals from primary attack remain as lifelong carriers [77]. The wild ruminants particularly cervids have been implicated as important reservoirs of infection for *A. marginale*, *Anaplasma Phagocytophilum*, and *Anaplasma ovis*. It infects the red blood cells, and the disease is characterized by fever, severe anemia, jaundice, brownish urine, loss of appetite, dullness or depression, rapid deterioration of the physical condition, muscular tremors, constipation, and pale mucous membrane and labored breathing [78].

Similar to babesiosis, diagnosis of bovine anaplasmosis can be made by microscopic detection of *Anaplasma* parasites by a well-prepared thin smear free from foreign matter, as specks of debris can confuse diagnosis. This method is suitable for clinically infected animals during the acute phase of the disease, but it is not reliable for detecting infection in pre-symptomatic or carrier animals [79]. In these cases, the diagnosis is made by serological tests. Several immunological and molecular assays have been established to detect this rickettsia in carrier animals, where parasitemia is low. Among serological tests, competitive ELISA using a recombinant antigen recombinant major surface receptor protein 5 (MSP5), and MSP5-specific monoclonal antibody has proven very sensitive and specific for detection of anaplasma-infected animals [80]. However, due to the presence of similar B epitopes in anaplasma species, the available serological tests display cross reaction among different species [81]. Nowadays, nucleic acid-based diagnostic methods with high levels of sensitivity and specificity are used. It includes arrays of tools such as RLB [82], PCR [83], PCR-ELISA [84], semi-nested PCR [85], and real-time PCR [86].

Chemotherapy

All *Anaplasma* species infections in cattle respond to tetracycline in the early stages of infection at a dose rate of 6-10 mg/kg body weight thrice in a day. Long-acting oxytetracycline sometimes preferred with a dose rate of 20 mg/kg body weight with a single dose. Chronic infection can be eliminated by administrating long-acting oxytetracycline at a dose rate of 20 mg/kg body weight with at least two injections with 7 days interval. Imidocarb is highly effective against *A. maginale* at a dose rate of 1.5 mg/kg body weight [77,87].

Presently, there are two commercially available vaccines against anaplasmosis in the United States. Anaplaz® is the first anaplasmosis vaccine manufactured for cattle in the United States made by Fort Dodge. More recently, Mallinckrodt (later Schering-Plough) marketed a vaccine called Plazvax®. Both the vaccines protect the animal against anaplasmosis by similar mechanisms. Two injections given at 4-6 weeks apart with annual boosters are recommended. This is a killed vaccine, which will prevent the death loss but not the disease [88]. In rare cases, new calves born to vaccinated dams may develop an anemia and die. In such circumstances, the early detection of the parasite becomes paramount importance.

Conclusion

Specific diagnosis of the etiological agent is most important for control of the hemoprotozoan infections [89]. Microscopy-based detection methods are still the cheapest and fastest methods for diagnosis though the techniques suffer from the limitations of sensitivity and specificity. Comparatively, newer immunological tools offer faster and higher throughput over the conventional methods [90]. Serological tests commonly used for diagnosis of hemoprotozoan diseases have become more popular because of their high sensitivity. However, the efficiency of serological tests depends on the application of specific parasite-derived diagnostic antigen molecules that are yet to be identified. Although serological tests can be used to detect circulating antibodies, cross reactivity with antibodies against other species of piroplasms have been documented by various workers [91]. Moreover, antibodies tend to disappear in long-term carriers, whereas piroplasms persist. So, animals with a negative serological test can infect ticks and be the source of infection for other animals. Another pit fall with the serological tests is that the antibodies can still be detected years after recovery even though the parasite is not present in the circulation. Most of the serological tests employ crude/native parasite antigen and/or polyclonal antiserum as test reagents which result in poor specificity and lack of uniformity. Therefore, the traditional methods have been complemented by the molecular ones.

Nucleic acid amplification-based detection methods are sensitive and reliable; they are fast and very specific. Variants of PCR such as randomly amplified polymorphic DNA (RAPD), amplified fragment length polymorphism (AFLP), amplification refractory mutation system-PCR [92], and RFLP are also useful for species-specific diagnosis, genotyping (DNA polymorphism) and hence, in epidemiological studies of parasites. RAPD able to differentiate species of *Trypanosoma* [93], *Theileria* [94], and *Babesia* [95]. Similarly, population genetics of *Trypanosoma* [96] is

investigated following AFLP. PCR-RFLP was also used to genotype trypanosome [97], *Babesia* [98], *Theileria* [99], and *A. marginale* [100,101]. Although the techniques are performed using sophisticated equipment, new methodologies are being developed to perform the tests without the need of expensive apparatus. A large reservoir of asymptomatic infections has been detected using the molecular methods [102-104]. Most of the recently developed molecular techniques are amenable to high-throughput scaling up for larger sample sizes. These methods provide novel information on prevalence and epidemiology and are suited for active detection. The tools are also useful for sensitive molecular detection of carriers, especially in endemic areas. These advanced diagnostics complemented with well-controlled and efficient chemotherapeutic usage will provide the best means of controlling the hemoprotozoan infections and emergence of drug resistance.

Authors' Contributions

BRM collected and interpreted published information as part of his post-graduate thesis work. The manuscript was jointly prepared by BRM, AKT, and BCS. AKT and BCS as principal and co-guide of BRM during his post-graduate program incorporated valuable suggestions for improvement of the manuscript. BRM, AKT, BCS, and NRS drafted and revised the manuscript. All authors read and approved the final manuscript.

Acknowledgments

The authors are highly thankful to Director ICAR-IVRI for providing the necessary facilities and support.

Competing Interests

The authors declare that they have no competing interests.

References

1. Salih, D.A., El Hussein, A.M. and Singla, L.D. (2015) Diagnostic approaches for tick borne haemoparasitic diseases in livestock. *J. Vet. Med. Anim. Health*, 7(2): 45-56.

2. Tewari, A.K., Ray, D., Mishra, A.K. and Bansal, G.C. (2001) Identification of immunodominant polypeptides common between *Babesia bigemina* and *Theileria annulata*. *Indian J. Anim. Sci.*, 71: 679-680.

3. Singh, H., Mishra, A.K., Rao, J.R. and Tewari, A.K. (2007a) A PCR assay for detection of *Babesia bigemina* infection using clotted blood in bovines. *J. Appl. Anim. Res.*, 32: 201-202.

4. Singh, H., Mishra, A.K., Rao, J.R. and Tewari, A.K. (2007b) Seroprevalence of babesiosis in cattle and buffaloes by indirect fluorescent antibody test. *J. Vet. Parasitol.*, 21(1): 1-4.

5. Singh, H., Mishra, A.K., Rao, J.R. and Tewari, A.K. (2009) Comparison of indirect fluorescent antibody test (IFAT) and slide enzyme linked immunosorbent assay (SELISA) for diagnosis of *Babesia bigemina* infection in bovines. *Trop. Anim. Health Prod.*, 41(2): 153-159.

6. Juyal, P.D., Singla, L.D. and Kaur, P. (2005) Management of surra due to *Trypanosoma evansi* in India: An overview. Infectious diseases of domestic animals and zoonosis in India. In: Tandon, V., Dhawan, B.N., editors. Proceedings

of the National Academy of Sciences of India. Vol. 75. p109-120.

7. Guan, G., Moreau, E., Liu, J., Hao, X. and Luo, J. (2010) Molecular evidence of experimental transmission to sheep by *Haemaphysalis qinghaiensis* and *Haemaphysalis longicornis*. *Parasitol. Int.*, 59: 265-267.

8. Terkawi, M.A., Thekiso, O.M., Katsande, C. and Igarashi, I. (2011) Serological Survey of *Babesia bovis* and *Babesia bigemina* in cattle of South Africa. *Vet. Parasitol.*, 182: 337-342.

9. Parida, M., Sannarangaiah, S., Dash, P.K., Rao, P.V. and Morita, K. (2008) Loop mediated isothermal amplification (LAMP): A new generation of innovative gene amplification technique; Perspectives in clinical diagnosis of infectious diseases. *Rev. Med. Virol.*, 18(6): 407-421.

10. Gasser, R.B. (2006) Molecular tools - Advances, opportunities and prospects. *Vet. Parasitol.*, 136(2): 69-89.

11. Tewari, A.K., Rao, J.R., Mishra, A.K. and Yadav, M.P. (2005) Recent trends in the diagnosis of trypanosomosis (surra) in domesticated animals. *Proc. Natl. Acad. Sci. India*, 75(B): 121-133.

12. Kurup, S.P. and Tewari, A.K. (2012) Induction of protective immune response in mice by a DNA vaccine encoding *Trypanosoma evansi* beta tubulin gene. *Vet. Parasitol.*, 187: 9-16.

13. Bossard, G., Boulange, A., Holzmuller, P., Thévenon, S., Patrel, D. and Authie, E. (2010) Serodiagnosis of bovine trypanosomosis based on HSP70/BiP inhibition ELISA. *Vet. Parasitol.*, 173(1-2): 39-47.

14. Singh, V. and Tewari, A.K. (2012) Bovine surra in India: An update. *Rumin. Sci.*, 1(1): 1-7.

15. Deborggraeve, S. and Buscher, P. (2010) Molecular diagnostics for sleeping sickness: What is the benefit for the patient? *Lancet Infect. Dis.*, 10: 433-439.

16. Mitashi, P., Hasker, E., Lejon, V., Kande, V., Muyembe, J.J., Lutumba, P. and Boelaert, M. (2012) Human African trypanosomiasis diagnosis in first-line health services of endemic countries, a systematic review. *PLoS Negl. Trop. Dis.*, 6(11): e1919.

17. Mugasa, C.M., Schoone, G.J., Ekangu, R.A., Lubega, G.W., Kager, P.A. and Schalling, H.D.F. (2008) Detection of *Trypanosoma brucei* parasites in blood samples using real-time nucleic acid sequence-based amplification. *Diagn. Microbiol. Infect. Dis.*, 61: 440-445.

18. Buscher, P., Mumba, N.D., Kabore, J., Lejon, V. and Robays, J. (2009) Improved Models of mini anion exchange centrifugation technique (mAECT) and modified single centrifugation (MSC) for sleeping sickness diagnosis and staging. *PLoS Negl. Trop. Dis.*, 3: e471.

19. Lanham, S.M. and Godfrey, D.G. (1970) Isolation of salivarian trypanosomes from man and other mammals using DEAE-cellulose. *Exp. Parasitol.*, 28: 521-534.

20. Watson, E.A. (1920) Dourine in Canada. History, Research, Suppression. Dominion of Canada, Department of Agriculture.

21. Randall, R. and Schwartz, S.C. (1936) A survey for the incidence of surra in the Philippine islands. *Vet. Bull. US Army*, 30: 99-108.

22. Luckins, A.G., Boid, R., Rae, P., Mahmoud, M.M., EI-Malik, K.H. and Gray, A.R. (1979) Sero diagnosis of infection with *Trypanosoma evansi* in camels in the Sudan. *Trop. Anim. Health Prod.*, 11: 1-12.

23. Desquesnes, M., Dargantes, A., Lai, D.H., Lun, Z.R., Holzmuller, P. and Sathaporn, J. (2013) *Trypanosoma evansi* and surra: A review and perspectives on transmission, epidemiology and control, impact, and zoonotic aspects. *Biomed. Res. Int.*, 2013: 321237.

24. Bajyana-Songa, E., Hamers-Casterman, C., Hamers, R., Pholpark, M., Pholpark, S., Leidl, K, Tangchaitrong, S., Chaichanopoonpol, I., Vitoorakool, C. and Thirapataskum, T. (1987) The use of a card agglutination test (Testryp CATT) for use in detection of *T. evansi* infection: A comparison with

25. Rayulu, V.C., Singh, A. and Chaudhri, S.S. (2007) Monoclonal antibody based immunoassays for detection of circulating antigens of *Trypanosoma evansi* in buffaloes. *Ital. J. Anim. Sci.*, 6: 907-910.

26. Shyma, K.P., Gupta, S.K., Singh, A. and Chaudhri, S.S. (2011) Latex agglutination test for detection of trypanosomosis in equines. *J. Vet. Parasitol.*, 25(2): 132-134.

27. Shyma, K.P., Gupta, S.K., Singh, A. and Chaudhri, S.S. (2012) Efficiency of monoclonal antibody based latex agglutination test in detecting *Trypanosoma evansi* under field condition for improving the productivity in buffaloes. *Buffalo Bull.*, 31: 163-172.

28. Kundu, K., Tewari, A.K., Kurup, S.P., Baidya, S., Rao, J.R. and Joshi, P. (2013) Sero-surveillance for surra in cattle using native surface glycoprotein antigen from *Trypanosoma evansi. Vet. Parasitol.*, 196: 258-264.

29. Shahardar, R.A., Rao, J.R., Mishra, A.K. and Tewari, A.K. (2007) Detection of *Trypanosoma evansi* in Indian dromedary camels by polymerase chain reaction using ribosomal DNA target. *J. Vet. Parasitol.*, 21(2): 105-108.

30. Ranjithkumar, M., Saravanan, B.C., Yadav, S.C., Kumar, R., Singh, R. and Dey, S. (2014) Neurological trypanosomiasis in quinapyramine sulfate-treated horses - A breach of the blood-brain barrier? *Trop. Anim. Health Prod.*, 46: 371-377.

31. Duffy, T., Cura, C.I., Ramirez, J.C., Abate, T., Cayo, N.M., Parrado, R., Bello, Z.D., Velazquez, E., Muñoz-Calderon, A., Juiz, N.A., Basile, J., Garcia, L., Riarte, A., Nasser, J.R., Ocampo, S.B., Yadon, Z.E., Torrico, F., de Noya, B.A., Ribeiro, I. and Schijman, A.G. (2013b) Analytical performance of a multiplex real-time PCR assay using TaqMan probes for quantification of *Trypanosoma cruzi* satellite DNA in blood samples. *PLoS Negl. Trop. Dis.*, 7(1): e2000.

32. Thuy, N.T., Goto, Y., Lun, Z.R., Kawazu, S. and Inoue, N. (2012) Tandem repeat protein as potential diagnostic antigen for *Trypanosoma evansi* infection. *Parsitol. Res.*, 110: 733-739.

33. Rudramurthy, G.R., Sengupta, P.P., Balamurugan, V., Prabhudas, K. and Rahman, H. (2013) PCR based diagnosis of trypanosomiasis exploring invariant surface glycoprotein (ISG) 75 gene. *Vet. Parasitol.*, 193: 47-58.

34. Geysen, D., Delespaux, V. and Geerts, S. (2003) PCR-RFLP using Ssu-rDNA amplification as an easy method for species-specific diagnosis of *Trypanosoma* species in cattle. *Vet. Parasitol.*, 110: 171-180.

35. Njiru, Z.K., Mikosza, A.S., Matovu, E., Enyaru, J.C., Ouma, J.O., Kibona, S.N., Thompson, R.C. and Ndung'u, J.M. (2008) African trypanosomiasis: Sensitive and rapid detection of the sub-genus *Trypanozoon* by loop-mediated isothermal amplification (LAMP) of parasite DNA. *Int. J. Parasitol.*, 38: 589-599.

36. Mugasa, C.M., Laurent, T., Schoone, G.J., Kager, P.A., Lubega, G.W. and Schalling, H.D. (2009) Nucleic acid sequence-based amplification with oligochromatography for detection of *Trypanosoma brucei* in clinical samples. *J. Clin. Microbiol.*, 47: 630-635.

37. Mugasa, C.M., Adams, E.R., Boer, K.R., Dyserinck, H.C., Buscher, P., Schalling, H.D. and Leeflang, M.M. (2012) Diagnostic accuracy of molecular amplification tests for human African trypanosomiasis–systematic review. *PLoS Negl. Trop. Dis.*, 6(1): e1438.

38. O.I.E. (2010) *Trypanosoma evansi* infections. In: Terrestrial Manual. Office International Des Epizooties, World Health Organization for Animal Health, Paris, France, Vol. 1. Ch. 2.1.17. p352-360.

39. Yadav, S.C., Kumar, R., Kumar, V., Jaideep, K.R., Gupta, A.K., Bera, B.C. and Tatu, U. (2013) Identification of immunodominant antigens of *Trypanosoma evansi* for detection of chronic trypanosomosis using experimentally infected equines. *Res. Vet. Sci.*, 95(2): 522-528.

40. Singh, V., Singh, A. and Chhabra, M.B. (1995) Polypeptide

profiles and antigenic characterization of cell membrane and flagellar preparations of different stocks of *Trypanosoma evansi*. *Vet. Parasitol.*, 56: 269-279.

41. Maharana, B.R., Rao, J.R., Tewari, A.K. and Singh, H. (2011a) Isolation and characterization of PFR1 in *Trypanosoma evansi* and its conservation among other kinetoplastid parasites. *Indian J. Anim. Res.*, 45(4): 283-288.

42. Maharana, B.R., Rao, J.R., Tewari, A.K., Singh, H. (2011b) Cloning and expression of paraflagellar rod protein gene 2 (PFR2) in *Trypanosoma evansi*. *J. Vet. Parasitol.*, 25(2):118-123.

43. Maharana, B.R., Rao, J.R., Tewari, A.K., Singh, H., Raina, O.K., Allaie, I.M. and Varghese, A. (2014a) Molecular characterization of paraflagellar rod protein gene in *Trypanosoma evansi*. *J. Appl. Anim. Res.*, 42: 1-5.

44. Maharana, B.R., Tewari, A.K. and Singh, V. (2014b) An overview on kinetoplastid paraflagellar rod. *J. Parasit. Dis.*, 39(4): 589-595.

45. EI-Ashker, M., Hotzel, H., Gwida, M., EI-Beskawy, M., Silaghi, C. and Tomaso, H. (2015) Molecular, biological identification of *Babesia*, *Theileria*, and *Anaplasma* species in cattle in Egypt using PCR assays, gene sequence analysis and a novel DNA microarray. *Vet. Parasitol.*, 207(3): 329-334.

46. Behera, S.K., Banerjee, P.S., Garg, R. and Maharana, B.R. (2012) A case of *Babesia equi*. *Indian Vet. J.*, 89(12): 87-88.

47. O.I.E. (2010) Bovine babesiosis. In: Terrestrial Manual. Vol. 1. Ch. 2.4. Office International Des Epizooties, World Health Organization for Animal Health, Paris, France. p1-15.

48. Tewari, A.K., Mishra, A.K. and Rao, J.R. (2000) Isolation and purification of cationic proteins from microaerophilus stationary phase culture supernatants of *Babesia bigemina*. *J. Appl. Anim. Res.*, 18: 41-48.

49. Almeria, S., Castella, J., Ferrer, D., Ortuno, A., Estrada-Peña, A. and Gutierrez, J.F. (2001) Bovinepiroplasms in minorca (Balearic Islands, Spain): A comparison of PCR-based and light microscopy detection. *Vet. Parasitol.*, 99: 249-259.

50. Krause, P.J., Telford, S.R. 3rd, Ryan, R., Conrad, P.A., Wilson, M., Thomford, J.W. and Spielman, A. (1994) Diagnosis of babesiosis: Evaluation of a serologic test for the detection of *Babesia microti* antibody. *J. Infect. Dis.*, 169: 923-926.

51. Mtshali, M.S. and Mtshali, P.S. (2013) Molecular diagnosis and phylogenetic analysis of *Babesia bigemina* and *Babesia bovis* hemoparasites from cattle in South Africa. *B.M.C. Vet. Res.*, 9: 154.

52. AbouLaila, M., Yokoyama, N. and Igarashi, I. (2010) Development and evaluation of two nested PCR assays for the detection of *Babesiab ovis* from cattle blood. *Vet. Parasitol.*, 172: 65-70.

53. Kim, C., Iseki, H., Herbas, M.S., Yokoyama, N., Suzuki, H., Xuan, X., Fujisaki, K., Kawazu, S. and Igarashi, I. (2007) Development of TaqMan-based real-time PCR assays for diagnostic detection of *Babesia bovis* and *Babesia bigemina*. *Am. J. Trop. Med. Hyg.*, 77(5): 837-841.

54. Teal, A.E., Habura, A., Ennis, J., Keithly, J.S. and Madison-Antenucci, S. (2012) A new real-time PCR assay for improved detection of the parasite *Babesia microti*. *J. Clin. Microbiol.*, 50(3): 903-908.

55. Gubbels, J.M., de Vos, A.P., van der Weide, M., Viseras, J., Schouls, L.M., de Vries, E. and Jongejan, F. (1999) Simultaneous detection of bovine *Theileria* and *Babesia* species by reverse line blot hybridization. *J. Clin. Microbiol.*, 37(6): 1782-1789.

56. Liu, A., Guan, G., Du, P., Gou, H., Liu, Z., Liu, J., Ma, M., Yang, J., Li, Y., Niu, Q., Ren, Q., Bai, Q., Yin, H. and Luo, J. (2012) Loop-mediated isothermal amplification (LAMP) method based on two species-specific primer sets for the rapid identification of Chinese *Babesia bovis* and *B. bigemina*. *Parasitol. Int.*, 61(4): 658-563.

57. Skotarczak, B. and Sawczuk, M. (2008) Molecular diagnostics of *Babesia* and *Theileria*. *Przegl. Epidemiol.*, 62(1): 100-108.

58. Birkenheuer, A., Levy, M. and Breitschwerdt, E. (2003) Development and evaluation of seminested PCR for detection and differentiation of *Babesia gibsoni* and *Babesia canis* DNA in canine blood samples. *J. Clin. Microbiol.*, 41: 4172-4177.

59. Saravanan, B.C., Das, S.J., Tewari, A.K., Sankar, M., Kataktalware, M.A. and Ramesha, K.P. (2013) *Babesia bigemina* infection in yak (*Poephagus grunniens L.*): Molecular detection and characterization. *Vet. Parasitol.*, 194: 58-64.

60. Kim, D.K. and Kang, S.H. (2005) On channel bare stacking in microchip capillary gel electrophoresis for high sensitive DNA fragment analysis. *J. Chromatogr. A.*, 1064: 121-27.

61. Mosqueda, J., Olveria-Ramirez, A., Canto, G.J. (2012) Current advances in detection and treatment of Babesiosis. *Curr. Med. Chem.*, 19(10): 1504-1518.

62. Vial, H.J. and Gorenflot, A. (2006) Chemotherapy against babesiosis. *Vet. Parasitol.*, 138: 147-160.

63. Zintl, A., Mulcahy, G., Skerrett, H.E., Taylor, S.M. and Gray, J.S. (2003) *Babesia divergens*, a bovine blood parasite of veterinary and zoonotic importance. *Clin. Microbiol. Rev.*, 16(4): 622-636.

64. Durrani, A.Z., Ahmad, M., Ashraf, M., Khan, M.S., Khan, J.A., Kamal, N. and Mumtaz, N. (2008) Prevalence of theileriosis in buffaloes and detection through blood smear examination and polymerase chain reaction test in district Lahore. *J. Anim. Plant Sci.*, 18(2-3): 59.

65. Kohli, S., Atheya, U.K. and Thapliyal, A. (2014) Prevalence of theileriosis in cross-bred cattle: Its detection through blood smear examination and polymerase chain reaction in Dehradun district, Uttarakhand, India, *Vet. World,* 7(3): 168-171.

66. Saravanan, B.C., Bansal, G.C., Manigandan, L., Sankar, M., Ravindran, R. and Rao, J.R. (2011) Development of a non-radioactive probe generated by RAPD-PCR for the detection of *Theileria annulata*. *Indian J. Anim. Sci.*, 81(11): 1089-1092.

67. Vanlalhmuaka, Bansal, G.C., Saravanan, B.C., Rao, J.R. and Ray, D.D. (2010) Evaluation of pre-erythrocytic stage recombinant proteins of *Theileria annulata* for early diagnosis of bovine tropical theileriosis in Indian cattle. *Indian J. Anim. Sci.*, 80(9): 822-825.

68. Abdo, J., Kristersson, T., Seitzer, U., Renneker, S., Merza, M. and Ahmed, J. (2010) Development and laboratory evaluation of a lateral flow device (LFD) for serodiagnosis of *Theileria annulata* infection. *Parasitol. Res.*, 107(5): 1241-1248.

69. Kumar, S., Kumar, R., Gupta, A.K., Yadav, S.C., Goyal, S.K., Khurana, S.K. and Singh, R.K. (2013) Development of EMA-2 recombinant antigen based enzyme-linked immunosorbent assay for seroprevalence studies of *Theileria equi* infection in Indian equine population. *Vet. Parasitol.*, 198: 10-17.

70. Vatansever, Z. and Nalbantoglu, S. (2002) Detection of cattle infected with *Theileria annulata* in fields by nested PCR, IFAT and microscopic examination of blood smears. *Turk. J. Vet. Anim. Sci.*, 26: 1465-1469.

71. Parthiban, M., Saranya, R., Magesh, M. and Raman, M. (2010) Detection of *Theileria* parasite in cattle of Tamil Nadu using nested PCR. *Tamil Nadu J. Vet. Anim. Sci.*, 6(4): 162-165.

72. Ros-García, A., Nicolás, A., García-Pérez, A.L., Juste, R.A. and Hurtado, A. (2012) Development and evaluation of a real-time PCR assay for the quantitative detection of *Theileria annulata* in cattle. *Parasit. Vectors.*, 5: 171.

73. Sangmin, J. and Keunchangcho, J.H.K. (2004) Fast diagnosis of bovine theleriosis by whole blood PCR and microchip electrophoresis. *Bull. Korean Chem. Soc.*, 25: 757.

74. Sanmartin, J.G., Nagore, D., Garciaperez, A.L., Juste, R.A.

and Hurtaldo, A. (2006) Molecular diagnosis of *Theleria* and *Babesia* species infecting cattle in Northern Spain using reverse line blot microarrays. *BMC Vet. Res.*, 2: 16-21.

75. Niu, Q., Luo, J., Guan, G., Ma, M., Liu, Z. and Liu, A. (2009) Detection and differentiation of ovine *Theleria* and *Babesia* by reverse line blotting in China. *Parasitol. Res.*, 104: 1417-1423.

76. Salih, D.A., El Hussein, A.M., Kyule, M.N., Zessin, K.H. and Ahmed, J.S. (2007) Determination of potential risk factors associated with *Theileria annulata* and *Theileria parva* infections of cattle in the Sudan. *Parasitol. Res.*, 101: 1285-1288.

77. Amorim, L.S., Wenceslau, A, Carvalho, F.S. and Albuquerque, G.R. (2013) Bovine babesiosis and anaplasmosis complex: Diagnosis and evaluation of the risk factors from Bahia, Brazil. *Braz. J. Vet. Parasitol.*, 23(3): 328-336.

78. Awad, H., Sandra, A.S. and El Hussein, A.M. (2011) Prevalence and genetic diversity of Babesia and Anaplasma species in cattle in Sudan. *Vet. Parasitol.*, 181: 146-152.

79. Aubry, P. and Geale, D.W. (2011) A review of bovine anaplasmosis. *Transbound. Emerg. Dis.*, 58(1): 1-30.

80. Reinbold, J.B., Coetzee, J.F., Sirigireddy, K.R. and Ganta, R.R. (2010) Detection of *Anaplasma marginale* and *A. phagocytophilum* in bovine peripheral blood samples by duplex real-time reverse transcriptase PCR assay. *J. Clin. Microbiol.*, 48: 2424-2432.

81. Stik, N.I., Alleman, A.R., Barbet, A.F., Sorenson, H.L., Wansley, H.L., Gaschen, F.P., Luckschander, N., Wong, S., Chu, F., Foley, J.E., Bjoersdorff, A., Stuen, S. and Knowles, D.P. (2007) Characterization of *Anaplasma phagocytophilum* major surface protein 5 and the extent of its cross-reactivity with *A. marginale*. *Clin. Vac. Immunol.*, 14: 262-268.

82. Oura, C.A.L., Bishop, R.P., Wampande, E.M., Lubega, G.W. and Tait, A. (2004) Application of a reverse line blot assay to study the haemoparasites in cattle in Uganda. *Int. J. Parasitol.*, 34(5): 603-613.

83. Torioni de Eschaide, S., Bono, M.F., Lugaresi, C., Aguirre, N., Mangold, A., Moretta, R., Farber, M. and Mondillo, C. (2005) Detection of antibodies against *Anaplasma marginale* in milk using a recombinant MSP5 indirect ELISA. *Vet. Microbiol.*, 106: 287-292.

84. Gale, K.R., Dimmock, C.M., Gartside, M. and Leatch, G. (1996) *Anaplasma marginale*: Detection of carrier cattle by PCR-ELISA. *Int. J. Parasitol.*, 26(10): 1103-1109.

85. Courtney, J.W., Kostelnik, L.M., Zeidner, N.V. and Massung, R.F. (2004) Multiplex Real-Time PCR for detection of *Anaplasma phagocytophilum* and *Borrelia burgdorferi*. *J. Clin. Microbiol.*, 42: 3164-3168.

86. Picoloto, G., Lima, R.F., Olegário, L.A., Carvalho, C.M., Lacerda, A.C., Tomás, W.M., Borges, P.A., Pellegrin, A.O. and Madruga, C.R. (2010) Real time polymerase chain reaction to diagnose *Anaplasma marginale* in cattle and deer (*Ozotoceros bezoarticus leucogaster*) of the Brazilian Pantanal. *Rev. Bras. Parasitol. Vet.*, 19(3): 186-188.

87. Ashuma, S.A., Singla, L.D., Kaur, P., Bal, M.S., Batth, B.K. and Juyal, P.D. (2013) Prevalence and haemato-biochemical profile of *Anaplasma marginale* infection in dairy animals of Punjab (India). *Asian Pac. J. Trop. Med.*, 6(2): 139-144.

88. Kocan, K.M., Fuente, J., Alberto, A. and Mele'ndez, R.D. (2003) Antigens and alternatives for control of *Anaplasma marginale* infection in cattle. *Clin. Microbiol. Rev.*, 16(4): 698-712.

89. Reetha, T.L., Thomas, K.S. and Babu, M. (2012) Occurrence of haemoprotozoan infection in bovines. *Int. J. Appl. Biores.*, 13: 1-2.

90. Nadeem, A., Aslam, A., Chaudhary, Z.I., Ashraf, K., Saeed, K., Ahmad, N., Ahmed, I. and Rehman, H.U. (2011) Indirect fluorescent antibody technique based prevalence of surra in equines. *Pak. Vet. J.*, 31(2): 169-170.

91. Papadpoulos, B., Perie, N.M. and Uilenberg, G. (1996) Piroplasms of domesticated animals in the Macedonia region of Greece. Serological cross reactions. *Vet. Parasitol.*, 63(4): 41-56.

92. Munoz, C., Talquenca, S.G. and Volpe, M.L. (2009) Tetra primer ARMS-PCR for identification of SNP in beta-tubulin of *Botrytis cinerea*, responsible of resistance to benzimidazole. *J. Microbial. Methods*, 78: 245-246.

93. Duarte, D.P., Tavares, K.C.S., Lazzarotto, C.R., Komati, L.K.O., de Araújo Ferreira, E.R., Bahia, D. and Miletti, L.C. (2014) Genetic profile of two isolates of *Trypanosoma evansi* from southern Brazil with different parasotemias. *Biotemas*, 27(3): 73-80.

94. Saravanan, B.C., Sankar, M., Bansal, G.C., Sreekumar, C., Tewari, A.K., Rao, J.R. and Ray, D. (2010) Random amplified polymorphic DNA profiles in two Indian strains of *Theileria annulata*. *J. Vet. Parasitol.*, 24(1): 39-43.

95. Ravindran, R., Mishra, A.K. and Rao, J.R. (2008) Randomly amplified polymorphic DNA-polymerase chain reaction fingerprinting of *Babesia bigemina* isolates of India. *Vet. Arch.*, 78(6): 545-551.

96. Masiga, D.K., Ndungu, K., Tweedie, A., Tait, A. and Turner, C.M. (2006) *Trypanosoma evansi*: Genetic variability detected using amplified restriction fragment length polymorphism (AFLP) and random amplified polymorphic DNA (RAPD) analysis of Kenyan isolates. *Exp. Parasitol.*, 114(3): 147-153.

97. Rozas, M., de Doncker, S., Adaui, V., Coronado, X., Barnabé, C., Tibyarenc, M., Solari, A. and Dujardin, J.C. (2007) Multilocus polymerase chain reaction restriction fragment—Length polymorphism genotyping of *Trypanosoma cruzi* (Chagas Disease): Taxonomic and clinical applications. *J. Infect. Dis.*, 195(9): 1381-1388.

98. Genis, A.D., Perez, J., Mosqueda, J.J., Alvarez, A., Camacho, M., Muñoz Mde, L., Rojas, C. and Figueroa, J.V. (2009) Using msa-2b as a molecular marker for genotyping Mexican isolates of *Babesia bovis*. *Infect. Genet. Evol.*, 9(6): 1102-1107.

99. Zaeemi, M., Haddadzadeh, H., Khazraiinia, P., Kazemi, B. and Bandehpour, M. (2011) Identification of different *Theileria* species (*Theileria lestoquardi*, *Theileria ovis*, and *Theileria annulata*) in naturally infected sheep using nested PCR-RFLP. *Parasitol. Res.*, 108(4): 837-843.

100. Noaman, V. and Shayan, P. (2010) Comparison of microscopy and PCR-RFLP for detection of *Anaplasma marginale* in carrier cattle. *Iran. J. Microbiol.*, 2(2): 89-94.

101. O.I.E. (2010) Bovine anaplasmosis. In: Terrestrial Manual. Vol. 1. Ch. 2.4.1. Office International Des Epizooties, World Health Organization for Animal Health, Paris, France. p589-600.

102. Sharma, A., Das Singla, L., Tuli, A., Kaur, P., Batth, B.K., Javed, M. and Juyal, P.D. (2013) Molecular prevalence of *Babesia bigemina* and *Trypanosoma evansi* in dairy animals from Punjab, India, by duplex PCR: A step forward to the detection and management of concurrent latent infections. *Biomed. Res. Int.*, 2013: 893862.

103. Sengupta, P.P., Balumahendiran, M., Suryanarayana, V.V.S., Raghavendra, A.G., Shome, B.R., Ganjendragad, M.R. and Prabhudas, K. (2010) PCR-based diagnosis of surra-targeting VSG gene: Experimental studies in small laboratory rodents and buffalo. *Vet. Parasitol.*, 171: 22-31.

104. Pruvot, M., Kamyingkird, K., Desquesnes, M., Sarataphan, N. and Jittapalapong, S. (2010) A comparison of six primer sets for detection of *Trypanosoma evansi* by polymerase chain reaction in rodents and Thai livestock. *Vet. Parasitol.*, 171: 185-193.

2

Comparative efficacy of anthelmintics and their effects on hemato-biochemical changes in fasciolosis of goats of South Gujarat

R. G. Shrimali, M. D. Patel and R. M. Patel

Department of Veterinary Medicine, College of Veterinary Science & Animal Husbandry, Navsari Agricultural University, Navsari - 396 450, Gujarat, India.
Corresponding author: M. D. Patel, e-mail: drmanish911@yahoo.com,
RGS: trivedironak89@yahoo.in, RMP: rmpatel05@gmail.com

Abstract

Aim: Fasciolosis is a parasitic disease caused by *Fasciola* spp. of the family *Fasciolidae (trematodes)* characterized by bottle jaw, anemia, progressive debility, and potbelly condition. There are many aspects of fasciolosis remaining unknown thus hemato-biochemical alterations in closantel, triclabendazole + ivermectin, and oxyclozanide + levamisole treated goats were studied.

Materials and Methods: A total of 40 naturally fasciolosis infected goats having egg per gram more than 100 were randomly divided into four groups. Goats of Group I-III were treated with three different anthelmintics, whereas, goats of Group-IV were kept as control or untreated. Whole blood, serum, and fecal samples were collected on 0, 7th, and 30th day of treatment.

Results: During the study, values of hemoglobin, total erythrocyte count, pack cell volume, and total protein were significantly elevated to their normal levels in anthelmintics treated groups. Whereas, values of total leukocyte count, aspartate transaminase (AST), lactate dehydrogenase (LDH), and gamma-glutamyl transferase (GGT) were significantly reduced to their normal level in anthelmintics treated groups. The efficacy of closantel (T1), triclabendazole + ivermectin (T2), and oxyclozanide + levamisole (T3) was 99.63%, 100%, and 94.74% and 100%, 100%, and 97.38% on 7th and 30th day of treatment, respectively.

Conclusions: Fasciolosis in goats can be diagnosed on the basis of fecal sample examination, but alterations in important biomarkers such as AST, GGT, and LDH are also helpful for early diagnosis. The use of newer anthelmintic either alone or in combination showed a higher therapeutic response in fasciolosis of goats.

Keywords: anthelmintics, efficacy, fasciolosis, goats, hemato-biochemical changes.

Introduction

Parasitic infections pose a serious health threat and limitation to the productivity of small ruminants due to the associated morbidity, mortality, cost of treatment, and control measures. Among various parasitic infections of small ruminants, fasciolosis is the most important pathogenic parasitic infection which is widely distributed in India causing severe infection, anemia, and hypoalbuminemia. The prevalence of fasciolosis largely depends on rainfall and production systems [1].

The pathogenic effects of these flukes on the host organism begin with the ingestion of encysted metacercaria with vegetation or freshwater. After migration of juvenile forms through the hepatic parenchyma, flukes reside and graze on the mucosa of the bile ducts, which result in the massive tissue damage.

The lesions in the liver are only partially a result of the mechanical action of liver fluke because the injury of the liver can be induced by parasites excretory products, decomposed products of parasites, bile, and hepatic tissue. Pathological changes, caused by mechanical and toxic effects of *Fasciola hepatica*, affect the complex vascular and biliary system in the liver. Properly functioning of these two systems is the most important factor for preservation of normal liver functions. In complexity of patho-physiological examination, the determination of serum transaminases, (alanine aminotransaminase [ALT] and aspartate transaminase [AST]) which are the most sensitive indicator of hepatocellular injury. Further, elevation in alkaline phosphatase (ALP), lactate dehydrogenase (LDH), gamma-glutamyl transferase (GGT), serum proteins, and bilirubin having significant importance in the degree of cholestasis and synthetic capacity of the liver [2,3].

A wide range of broad-spectrum anthelmintics are available for use in cattle, sheep, and goats including the benzimidazoles, the avermectins, tetrahydropyrimidines, and imidothiazoles, which are having varying efficacy against parasitic gastroenteritis and bronchitis. The activity of each of these drugs is variable against the different stages of the parasites' development. Some, like triclabendazole are very effective against immature flukes, whereas others, *viz.*, nitroxynil or closantel, are highly efficient against adults [4]. Fasciolosis may be controlled with the salicylanilide and related phenolic compounds. Salicylanilides are effective against a wide range of hepatic and intestinal trematodes in a variety of animals [5]. The later being the first fasciolicide with excellent activity against all stages of *Fasciola hepatica* infection. The implication of strategies for Helminth's resistance and individual immunity require periodic evaluation of these drugs. During this study, three anthelmintics claimed to be effective against fasciolosis were evaluated by studying their effects on important hemato-biochemical parameters in fasciolosis infected goats in the absence of such systemic studies on fasciolosis in goats in study areas.

Materials and Methods

Ethical approval

The prior approval from the Institutional Animal Ethics Committee was obtained for use of farmer's animals in this study.

Selection of animals

During an epidemiological survey, on gastrointestinal parasites in goats of Navsari and Valsad districts of south Gujarat (Figure-1), goats with poor body condition, history of diarrhea, anemia were suspected to be having parasitic infection and were screened for the presence of parasitic ova. Goats those having *Fasciola* spp. infection and egg per gram (EPG) for more than 100/g of fecal sample were included for evaluating anti-fasciolosis drugs. A total of 40 naturally fasciolosis infected local goats between 1.5 and 3 years of age and 20-35 kg body weight were included. They were randomly divided into four treatment groups, i.e. Group-I: Closantel,

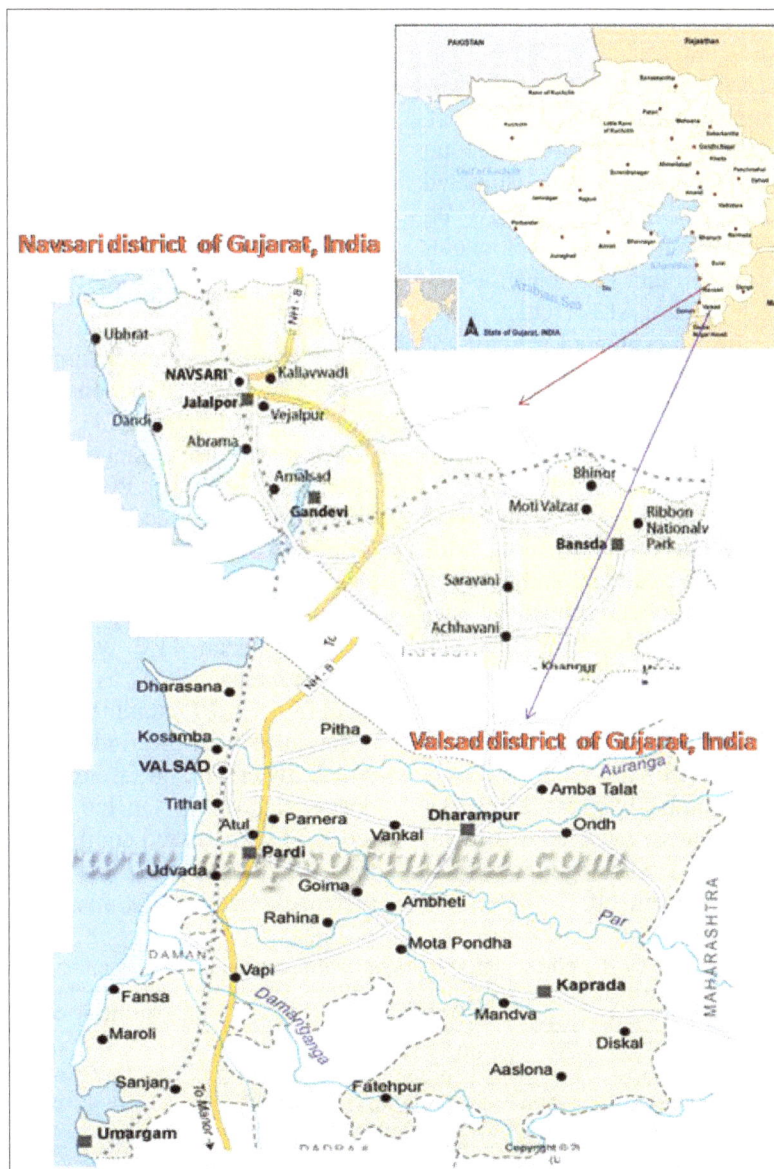

Figure-1: Area covered under the research work.

Group-II: Triclabendazole + ivermectin, Group-III: Oxyclozanide + levamisole, and Group-IV: Control or untreated. The detailed treatment protocol is given in Table-1.

Sample collection and processing

Fecal, whole blood, and serum samples from goats of all treatment groups were collected at 0, 7th, and 30th day of treatment. Fresh fecal samples were collected directly from the rectum of goats and kept immediately in plastic containers containing 10% formalin for preservation until used for examination. The qualitative examination was carried out for the presence of parasitic eggs/oocysts under ×10 magnifications under a microscope for best identification. Quantitative examinations of fecal samples of *Fasciola* spp. were carried out within 48 h of collection using a modified McMaster's technique to count EPG [6].

Blood samples for hematological and biochemical analysis were collected separately into 6 ml capacity marked vacutainers and transported to the laboratory at 4°C in pre-cooled ice-box. Serum was separated out and stored at −20°C till the further use. Hemoglobin (Hb, g%), packed cell volume (PCV, %), total erythrocyte count (TEC, × 10^6/cu.mm), and total leukocyte count (TLC, × 10^3/cu.mm) were estimated in fully automatic hematology cell counter (Exigo Vet, Sweden) on the same day. Whereas, various biochemical parameters, *viz.*, total protein (TP, g/dl), aspartate transaminase (AST, IU/L), ALT (IU/L), LDH (IU/L), and GGT (IU/L) were estimated in semi-automatic biochemistry analyzer (Microlab 300, Merck, Netherland) using commercially available diagnostic kits (Coral Clinical System, Goa) within a day or two.

Statistical analysis

Data were statistically analyzed using IBM SPSS statistical software version 20.0. Significant differences between days within treatment and between treatment at different times were determined by one-way ANOVA test for variance analysis at $p < 0.05$ [7]. The descriptive data are presented as the means ± standard error. The efficacy of anthelmintics was evaluated based a formula [8]:

% of drug efficacy = P-R/P×100

Where, R = Average number of parasite egg in a gram of fecal sample after treatment,

P = Average number of parasite egg in a gram of fecal sample before treatment.

Results and Discussion

Hematological alterations in different treatment groups

The changes in different hematological parameters at different time intervals in various treatment groups are given in Table-2. The mean Hb concentrations in treatment groups (T1, T2, T3, and T4) was comparatively lower than normal values in goats (8-12 g%). Similarly, lower Hb concentration in *Fasciola* spp. infected animals was also reported (9-12). At day 7, the mean Hb concentrations were increased significantly in anthelmintics treated groups (T1, T2, and T3) as compared to control group (T4) ($p < 0.01$). The mean Hb values were further significantly increased in T1, T2, and T3 ($p < 0.01$) on the 30th day of anthelmintic treatment. The findings of increased Hb concentrations in anthelmintic treated goats are in accordance with previous report [9] of increased Hb concentrations to normal level in anthelmintic treated animals in the treatment group at 28th day post-treatment.

Initially, the mean PCV values in all treatment groups (T1, T2, T3, and T4) were lower than normal range (22-38%). The present findings are in agreement with previous reports of lower PCV values in *Fasciola* spp. infected animals [10-13]. On 7th day, the mean PCV increased significantly in T1 and T3, whereas the increase in mean PCV value was non-significantly in the T2 group. Further, a significant increase in PCV was also observed in T1, T2, and T3 from day 7 to day 30 ($p < 0.01$). A similar trend of increase in PCV in anthelmintic treated animals at 7th and 28th day post-treatment was also observed by Khalil *et al.* [9]. In the control group (T4), the mean PCV remained lower than normal range of PCV at different time intervals. The lower PCV could be attributed to an abnormal loss of red blood cells due to feeding habits of flukes or to an excessive destruction of RBCs caused by some hemolyzing factors produced by the flukes Okoye *et al.* [13].

The mean TEC was comparatively lower in all treatments groups as compared to normal TEC level (8-18 × 10^6/cu.mm) in goats. The results are in accordance with the findings of previous reports, in which lower TEC in fasciolosis affected animals was observed [10-13]. On the 7th day of treatment, the mean TEC increased significantly in T1, T2, and T3 than the control group (T4) ($p < 0.01$). Subsequently, increasing trend in TEC in anthelmintic treated groups

Table-1: Treatment protocols to study the efficacy of various anthelmintics in fasciolosis infected goats of South Gujarat.

Groups	Treatment protocols	Dose rate	Number of animals	Mean EPG
T1	Closantel	15 mg/kg body wt. PO	10	110.90
T2	Triclabendazole+ivermectin	10.2 mg/kg body wt. PO	10	110.00
T3	Oxyclozanide+levamisole+silymarin	10 mg/kg body wt. PO	10	110.80
T4	Control group	No treatment	10	110.80

EPG=Egg per gram

(T1, T2, and T3) was also observed on 30th day of treatment. A similar trend of increasing TEC in goats treated for fasciolosis was observed by Khalil *et al.* [9], whereas in control group decreasing trend in TEC was observed from day 0 to day 30. The decrease in TEC in fasciolosis affected animal could be attributed to chronic blood loss due to the blood-sucking activity of the adult flukes and leakage of blood from the bile duct to the intestine Okoye *et al.* [13].

During the study, the mean TLC was higher in all treatment groups on day 0 as compared to normal range (4-11 × 10³/cu.mm) in goats. A similar trend of higher TLC in fasciolosis infected animals was also observed in previous reports [10,11,13]. The mean TLC was decreased significantly in T1, T2, and T3 from day 0 to day 30 (p<0.01), whereas the mean TLC values remained static without significant difference over time intervals in the control group (T4).

Biochemical alterations in different treatment groups

F. hepatica causes the release of reactive oxygen which result in damage of cell wall and hepatic tissue necrosis [11]. These changes have an influence on biochemical parameters in serum, and determination of specific liver enzymes is very valuable tool for diagnosis of hepatobiliary diseases. Physiologically, the normal levels of the enzymes in cells or serum are maintained by constant synthesis, simultaneous degradation, inactivation, and elimination of enzymes [9-11]. However, due to disruption of hepatocellular integrity, enzymes from damaged cells are released into the blood serum and their concentration increase/decrease above the physiological values. The changes in certain biochemical parameters at different

time intervals in fasciolosis infected goats under different treatment groups are given in Table-3.

During the study, initial mean AST levels in all treatment groups were comparatively higher (304.9-331.75 IU/L) as compared to normal level (66-230 IU/L) in goats. The present findings are in accordance with previous reports [9,14-16]. The mean AST level decreased significantly from day 0 to day 7 and further from day 7 to day 30 in T1, T2, and T3 (p<0.01). Similarly, decrease in mean AST in animals treated for fasciolosis was also reported by Khalil *et al.* [9]. The mean AST levels in the untreated group (T4) remained constantly higher or static with the non-significantly difference between time intervals. The enzyme AST is a sensitive indicator of parenchymal damage of the liver. The significant elevation of AST indicates chronic fasciolosis in infected goats. Higher levels of AST suggest lack of hepatocellular damage and probably indicate a chronic fasciolosis (biliary phase) and regenerative changes in the parenchyma [11]. The means ALT levels in all treatment groups was also higher than its normal range (7-24 IU/L). However, the mean ALT levels in different treatment groups (T1, T2, T3, and T4) at different time intervals (day 0-7 and day 7-30) varied from each other but difference was non-significant which indicates chronic fasciolosis [14,15].

In this study, the mean TP levels in all treatment groups were comparatively lower than normal range (6.4-7.8 g/dl). The decrease in total serum protein in fasciolosis infected animals was also reported in previous reports [14-17]. In fasciolosis, decreased TP level is suggestive of loss of plasma protein through

Table-2: Hematological changes in various treatment groups at different time intervals in fasciolosis of goats.

Parameters	Time intervals	Treatment groups				F value
		T1	T2	T3	T4	
EPG	0	110.90±0.32ʸ	110.00±0.36ʸ	110.80±0.21ᶻ	110.80±0.32ˣ	0.10
	7	0.40±0.30ˣᵃ	0.00±0.00ˣᵃ	5.80±1.36ʸᵃ	236.90±6.01ʸᵇ	1445.67**
	30	0.00±0.00ˣᵃ	0.00±0.00ˣᵃ	2.90±0.92ˣᵃ	347.80±10.14ᶻᵇ	1158.90**
F value		61162.40**	90750.00**	4044.83**	302.90**	
Hb (g %)	0	6.70±0.05ˣᶜ	6.56±0.09ˣᶜ	4.93±0.05ˣᵃ	5.79±0.18ᵃ	55.68**
	7	8.01±0.04ʸᵈ	7.73±0.03ʸᶜ	6.82±0.04ʸᵇ	5.63±0.17ᵃ	123.07**
	30	9.00±0.03ᶻᵈ	8.72±0.03ᶻᶜ	8.82±0.05ᶻᵇᶜ	5.51±0.14ᵃ	387.09**
F value		679.36**	267.28**	1393.85**	0.68	
PCV (%)	0	18.90±0.27ˣᶜ	18.32±0.40ˣᶜ	14.70±0.15ˣᵃ	16.11±0.27ᵇ	44.51**
	7	24.02±0.15ʸᵇ	18.96±2.75ˣᵃ	19.85±0.22ʸᵃ	16.27±0.44ᵃ	5.24*
	30	27.10±0.11ᶻᵇ	26.69±0.35ʸᵇ	26.86±0.28ᶻᵇ	16.05±0.33ᵃ	354.32*
F value		450.79**	8.24**	729.47**	0.102	
TEC (×10⁶/cu.mm)	0	5.72±0.05ˣᵇ	5.43±0.07ˣᵃ	5.38±0.04ˣᵃ	5.29±0.01ʸᵃ	12.42**
	7	5.96±0.03ʸᶜ	5.94±0.03ʸᶜ	5.78±0.03ʸᵇ	5.22±0.03ʸᵃ	98.04**
	30	8.56±0.10ᶻᵇ	8.70±0.05ᶻᵇ	8.72±0.04ᶻᵇ	5.07±0.04ˣᵃ	675.04**
F value		463.81**	903.43**	1919.15**	10.46**	
TLC (×10³/cu.mm)	0	12.55±0.17ᶻᵃ	12.67±0.13ᶻᵃ	13.16±0.07ᶻᵇ	12.61±0.17ᵃ	3.64*
	7	8.47±0.17ʸᵃ	8.98±0.03ʸᵇ	9.24±0.14ʸᵇ	12.79±0.15ᶜ	205.13**
	30	4.80±0.04ˣᵃ	4.67±0.05ˣᵃ	4.91±0.03ˣᵃ	12.94±0.17ᵇ	1848.05**
F value		745.13**	2083.08**	1902.36**	0.94	

Means with different superscripts a, b, c, and d along a row differ significantly at p<0.01, Means with different superscripts x, y, and z along a column differ significantly at p<0.01, **Highly significant at p<0.01, *Significant at p<0.05. EPG=Egg per gram, Hb=Hemoglobin, PCV=Packed cell volume, TEC=Total erythrocyte count, TLC=Total leukocyte count

Table-3: Biochemical changes in various treatment groups at different time intervals in fasciolosis of goats.

Parameters	Time intervals	Treatments				F value
		T1	T2	T3	T4	
AST (IU/L)	0	313.11±4.70za	304.9±5.19za	331.75±3.23zb	309.50±7.04a	5.68*
	7	295.51±1.92yab	280.90±2.78ya	280.60±11.12ya	308.84±6.24b	4.193*
	30	140.90±1.90xa	146.83±2.15xa	147.69±2.09xa	315.96±4.61b	861.86**
F value		915.09**	552.62**	195.42**	2.10	
ALT (IU/L)	0	44.99±1.31	42.71±0.34	43.31±0.23	43.62±0.70	3.85*
	7	45.13±0.69	43.01±0.36	43.66±0.22	44.69±1.34	1.50
	30	45.83±0.86	38.97±3.79	43.17±0.46	44.92±1.21	2.195
F value		0.205	1.035	0.59	1.92	
TP (g/dl)	0	4.03±0.04xc	3.79±0.03xb	3.50±0.10xa	3.61±0.06ab	11.10**
	7	4.64±0.10yc	4.21±0.02yb	4.28±0.03yb	3.65±0.09a	32.52**
	30	6.39±0.0zc	6.13±0.06zb	6.08±0.12zb	3.54±0.09a	225.77**
F value		282.56**	809.68**	189.69**	0.42	
LDH (IU/L)	0	2287.88±14.31zc	2049.67±26.33ya	2301.06±4.50zc	2146.56±39.58b	23.24**
	7	2009.24±1.55yab	1921.08±79.31ya	2068.15±12.85ybc	2154.63±40.05c	4.7*
	30	1186.29±15.59xab	1138.53±14.40xa	1213.50±17.69xb	2161.47±40.60c	401.31**
F value		2183.98**	101.42**	1972.49**	0.035	
GGT (IU/L)	0	231.08±1.91zb	219.29±1.43za	227.60±1.83zb	227.26±1.95xb	7.70**
	7	105.32±1.22ya	107.19±1.27ya	113.06±1.21yb	231.30±2.13xyc	1652.22**
	30	53.71±0.99xa	51.26±0.868xa	49.63±1.70xa	234.52±1.86zb	4115.53**
F value		4068.77**	4946.15**	3157.55**	3.34*	

Means with different superscripts a, b, c, and d along a row differ significantly at p<0.01, Means with different superscripts x, y, and z along a column differ significantly at p<0.01, **Highly significant at p<0.01, *Significant at p<0.05. AST=Aspartate transaminase, LDH=Lactate dehydrogenase, GGT=Gamma-glutamyltransferase, ALT=Alanine aminotransaminase, TP=Total protein

bile ducts into intestine as a result of increased permeability of the hyperplastic bile duct epithelium and loss of plasma proteins through the fluke's digestive tract [11,15]. The mean TP levels showed a significantly increasing trend in T1, T2, and T3 from day 0 to day 30, whereas in the control group (T4), it remained more or less static. Significantly increase in TP levels in fasciolosis infected animals after treatment was also reported by Sheikh et al. [15], whereas Khalil et al. [9] observed a non-significant increase in TP in anti-fasciolosis anthelmintics treated animals.

The mean LDH levels in treatment groups were highly elevated than normal range (78-265 IU/L) before initiation of treatment. The findings are accordance with previous reports which reported increased LDH level in animals in fasciolosis infection. Increases levels of LDH are related to the inflammatory state of liver and tissue destruction provoked by the parenchymal migration of juvenile flukes [9,11,16]. Thereafter, mean LDH levels in T1 and T3 decreased significantly from day 0 to day 7 (p<0.01), whereas the value decreased from 2049.67 to 1921.08 (IU/L) in T2 at 7th day but the difference was non-significant. Further, mean (LDH) levels in T1, T2, and T3 decreased significantly from 7th to 30th day (p<0.01). The results are in accordance with findings of the previous report of Khalil et al. [9], who had reported a significant decrease in the level of LDH in fasciolosis infected animals on the 14th and 28th day post-treatment (p<0.05). In the control group (T4), the LDH level remained at higher side throughout trail period.

The mean GGT levels were comparatively higher as compared to normal range (20-50 IU/L) in all treatment groups of goats before initiation of drug

trial. Similarly, higher GGT was observed in fasciolosis infected animals in previous reports [9,10,14-17]. Thereafter, significantly decreasing trend was observed in anthelmintic treated groups (T1, T2, and T3) on day 7 and day 30, whereas the mean GGT level in control animals increased significantly (p<0.05) from day 0 (227.26) to day 30 (234.52). The damage to the bile duct epithelium causes the release of GGT into circulation. This enzyme increases its level in serum mainly after flukes entered in the bile duct. The elevated levels of GGT were an indicator of epithelial damage in the bile duct. The marked increase in GGT level associated with cholestasis and bile duct damage [10,11].

Efficacy of anthelmintics

Based on EPG, the efficacy of closantel and triclabendazole + ivermectin was about to cent percent at 7th and 30th day of treatment (Table-4). The results are in accordance with the observations of previous reports [18-22], whereas the efficacy of oxyclozanide + levamisole was 94.74% and 97.83% at 7th and 30th day of treatment, respectively. In context to efficacy of oxyclozanide + levamisole, an earlier report of Ratnaparkhi et al. [23] reported higher efficacy (100%) in Fasciola spp. infections. However, in a recent report of Tadesse et al. [22] recorded only 28.14% efficacy of these drugs in Fasciola spp. infections of small ruminants. The reduction in efficacy of oxyclozanide + levamisole may be due to anthelmintic resistance as result of prolonged and repeated use of the same drug [24].

Conclusions

Activities and concentration of AST, ALT, GGT, and LDH in serum are reliable indicators of fasciolosis and could be used as biomarkers for early diagnosis

Table-4: Efficacy of different anthelmintics drugs in fasciolosis of goats.

Particulars	Efficacy (%)	
	On 7th day	On 30th day
T1 (closantel)	99.63	100
T2 (triclabendazole+ivermectin)	100	100
T3 (oxyclozanide+levamisole)	94.74	97.38
T4 (control)	-	

and to test the effectiveness of anthelmintic therapy. Use of newer anthelmintics showed a higher therapeutic response in fasciolosis of goats. Therefore, it can be concluded that the knowledge of epidemiology and ecology of the parasites is needed not only for planning better strategies of fasciolosis but also provide insight into the natural processes of controlling parasite population. Further, an early diagnosis and treatment with newer drugs for fasciolosis in goats could be advised to reduce economic losses. The results of this study can be useful to future research and planning out proper control of parasitic infections in goats of South Gujarat.

Authors' Contributions

RGS carried out the study and tabulated and analyzed the data. MDP analyzed data and drafted the manuscript and revision of the manuscript. RMP rendered necessary infrastructure facilities and revision of the manuscript. All authors read and approved the final manuscript.

Acknowledgments

The authors are thankful to Research Scientist, Livestock Research Station as well as Principal Investigator of AICRP on goat improvement-Surti field unit for providing infrastructure facilities available at LRS and funds for diagnostic kits.

Competing Interests

The authors declare that they have no competing interests.

References

1. Ahmadi, N.A. and Meshkehkar, M. (2010) Prevalence and long term trend of liver fluke infections in sheep, goats and cattle slaughtered in Khuzestan, Southwestern Iran. *J. Paramed. Sci.,* 1(2): 26-31.
2. Hauptman, K., Tichý, F. and Knotek, Z. (2001) Clinical diagnostics of hepatopathies in small mammals: Evaluation of importance of individual methods. *Acta Vet. Brno.,* 70: 297-311.
3. Limdi, J.K. and Hyde, G.M. (2003) Evaluation of abnormal liver function tests. *Postgrad. Med. J.,* 79: 307-312.
4. Rapic, D., Dzakula, N., Sakar, D. and Richards, R.J. (1988) Comparative efficacy of triclabendazole, nitroxynil and rafoxanide against immature and mature *Fasciola hepatica* in naturally infected cattle. *Vet. Rec.,* 122: 59-62.
5. Campbell, W.C. and Rew, R.S. (1986) Chemotherapy of Parasitic Diseases. Plenum Press, New York.
6. Anonymous. (1977) Manual of Veterinary Parasitological Laboratory Techniques. 2nd ed. Ministry of Agriculture, Fisheries, and Food. Agriculture Development Advising Services, Technical Bulletin, No. 18. p67-68.
7. Snecdacor, G.W. and Cochran, W.G. (1994) Statistical Methods. Indian Edition (Revised). Oxford and I. B. M. Publishing Company. New Delhi. p345.
8. Khayatnouri, M.H., Garedaghi, Y., Arbati, A.R. and Khalili, H. (2011) The effect of ivermectin pour-on administration against natural *Heterakis gallinarum* infestation and its prevalence in native poultry. *Am. J. Anim. Vet. Sci.,* 6(1): 55-58.
9. Khalil, F.J., Kawan, M.H. and Hayder, B.A. (2006) Clinical, hematological and biochemical pictures as a monitor of caprine fascioliasis. *I.A.S.J.,* 19(3): 15-19.
10. Matanović, K., Severin, K., Martinković, F., Šimpraga, M., Janicki, Z. and Barišić, J. (2007) Hematological and biochemical changes in organically farmed sheep naturally infected with *Fasciola hepatica. Parasitol. Res.,* 101: 1657-1661.
11. Taleb, D.F., Soliman, E.K. and El-Khalek, A. (2007) Effect of fascioliasis on hematological, serum biochemical and histopathological changes in sheep. *Egypt. J. Sheep Goat Sci.,* 2: 15-34.
12. Al-Saffar, T.M. (2008) Some haematological changes in sheep with chronic fascioliasis in Mosul. *AL-Qadisiya J. Vet. Med. Sci.,* 7(1): 1-4.
13. Okoye, I.C., Egbu, F. and Ubachukwu, M.I. (2013) Haematological changes due to bovine fascioliasis. *Afr. J. Biotechnol.,* 12(15): 1828-1235.
14. Alam, M.M., Samad, M.A., Chowdhury, N.S. and Ahmed, M.U. (1994) Haemato-biochemical changes and therapeutic management of clinical fasciolosis in a mixed flock of sheep and goats. *Bangladesh Vet. J.,* 28(1/4): 7-14.
15. Sheikh, G.N., Dar, M.S. and Das, J. (2005) Efficacy of triclabendazole on biochemical profile in ovine fascioliasis. *Indian J. Small Rumin.,* 11(2): 223-225.
16. Prakash, V. and Bano, S. (2009) Clinico-biochemical studies in goats infected with *Fasciola gigantic. Asian J. Anim. Sci.,* 4(1): 67-68.
17. Hodžić, A., Zuko, A., Avdić, R., Alić, A., Omeragić, J. and Jažić, A. (2013) Influence of fasciola hepatica on serum biochemical parameters and vascular and biliary system of sheep liver. *Iran. J. Parasitol.,* (1): 92-98.
18. Hassan, M.M., Hoque, M.A., Islam, S.K.M., Khan, S.A., Hosaain, M.B. and Banu, Q. (2012) Efficacy of anthelmintics against parasitic infections and their treatment effect on the production and blood indices in Black Bengal goats in Bangladesh. *Turk. J. Vet. Anim. Sci.,* 36(4): 400-408.
19. Singh, J., Bal, M., Aradhana, S. and Gumber, S. (2004) Efficacy of different flukicides against fascioliosis in sheep and goats. *J. Res.,* 41(2): 287-289.
20. Abouzeid, N.Z., Selim, A.M. and El-Hady, K.M. (2010) Prevalence of gastrointestinal parasites infections in sheep in the zoo garden and Sinai district and study the efficacy of anthelmintic drugs in the treatment of these parasites. *J. Am. Sci.,* 6(11): 544-551.
21. Shokier, K.M., Aboelhadid, S.M. and Waleed, M.A. (2013) Efficacy of five anthelmintics against a natural *Fasciola* species infection in cattle. *B.J.B.A.S.,* 2(1): 41-45.
22. Tadesse, D., Eshetu, L., Hadush, B., Amsalu, K. and Teklu, A. (2014) Study on the efficacy of selected antitrematodal drugs in naturally infected sheep with fasciolosis. *Acta Parasitol. Glob.,* 5(3): 210-213.
23. Ratnaparkhi, M.R., Shastri, U.V., Rajurkar, S.R. and Jamkhedkar, P.P. (1993) Efficacy of distodin® (Pfizer) against fasciolosis in cattle, buffaloes and goats under field condition. *Indian Vet. J.,* 70(2): 157-159.
24. Sharma, P., Sharma, D., Dogra, P.K. and Mandial, R.K. (2014) Comparative efficacy of fenbendazole and oxyclozanide-tetramisole combination against gastrointestinal nematodes in naturally infected Gaddi goats. *Vet. Res. Int.,* 2(1): 15-17.

3

Maggot debridement therapy as primary tool to treat chronic wound of animals

Vijayata Choudhary[1], Mukesh Choudhary[2], Sunanda Pandey[2], Vandip D. Chauhan[1] and J. J. Hasnani[1]

1. Department of Veterinary Parasitology, Veterinary College, Anand Agricultural University, Anand, Gujarat, India;
2. Department of Veterinary Pathology, Veterinary College, Anand Agricultural University, Anand, Gujarat, India.
Corresponding author: Vijayata Choudhary, e-mail: dr.viz.vet@gmail.com,
MC: mukesh.vety@gmail.com, SP: drsunandapandey@gmail.com, VDC: drvandip@gmail.com, JJH: Jhasnani@gmail.com

Abstract

Maggot debridement therapy (MDT) is a safe, effective, and controlled method of healing of chronic wounds by debridement and disinfection. In this therapy live, sterile maggots of green bottle fly, *Lucilia* (*Phaenicia*) *sericata* are used, as they prefer necrotic tissues over healthy for feeding. Since centuries, MDT is used in human beings to treat chronic wounds. Lately, MDT came out as a potent medical aid in animals. In animals, although, this therapy is still limited and clinical studies are few. However, with the increasing antibiotic resistance and chronic wound infections in veterinary medicine, maggot therapy may even become the first line of treatment for some infections. This paper will present a brief discussion of MDT and its role in veterinary medicine that may add one more treatment method to utilize in non-healing wounds of animals and overcome the use of amputation and euthanasia. The objective of this review paper is to assemble relevant literature on maggot therapy to form a theoretical foundation from which further steps toward clinical use of maggot therapy in animals for chronic wounds can be taken.

Keywords: chronic wounds, debridement, *Lucilia sericata*, maggots, maggot debridement therapy.

Introduction

Maggot debridement therapy (MDT) is a form of therapeutic wound treatment in which sterile or disinfected larvae of certain blowfly species are used to remove non-vitalized tissue, pus, slough, and metabolic wastes on the wound and promote healing [1]. MDT is also known as maggot therapy, biodebridement, larval therapy [2], biosurgery [3,4], biotherapy, and biosurgical debridement [5,6]. The larvae of the sheep blowfly, *Lucilia* (*Phaenicia*) *sericata* are the most widely used species for MDT due to its preference for feeding on necrotic tissues over healthy [6-8]. In this therapy live, sterile fly larvae commonly known as medicinal maggots are applied to the wound to effect debridement, disinfection, and ultimately wound healing [3]. The success rate of MDT was reported in literature ranges from 70% to 80% [6,9,10]. However, use of MDT in veterinary medicine has been neglected but has recently emerged as an effective treatment for chronic wounds of animals. MDT is most commonly used in horses and small animals to treat a different kind of wounds. Maggots are used less often in pets, but some small animal veterinarians are now using MDT for problematic dog and cat wounds [11,12].

History of MDT

The first observation of maggots and their beneficial effects in wounds were made in 1557 by Ambrose Paré [13,14]. In 1829, Baron D.J Larrey, a military surgeon in Napoleon's army used the fly larvae in wounds to reduce the threat of bacterial infection and stated that "maggots promoted healing without leaving any damage" [14,15]. Zacharias and Jones were the first, who clinically applied maggots to the wounds during the American Civil War [16]. In 1928, William Baer, an orthopedic surgeon, is credited with the first use of blowfly maggots to treat osteomyelitis wounds in hospital [17]. Maggots were used extensively in hospitals during the 1930s and 1940s, especially in the United States. After the invention of penicillin and better surgical techniques, the interest in MDT gradually disappeared in the early 1940s until 1980s when methicillin-resistant *Staphylococcus aureus* (MRSA) became a problem [10].

With the appearance of antibiotic resistance and increasing problems in treating chronic wounds worldwide, MDT re-emerged as a useful therapy for surgical wounds infected with antibiotic-resistant *S. aureus* [4,18,19]. Afterward in 1989, Ronald Sherman used larvae or maggots to treat decubital ulcers [10].

Current status of maggot therapy

In 2004, Food and Drug Administration (FDA) granted permission for "the production and distribution of medical maggots" to be marketed as a medical device for wound care [11,19-21]. As MDT has approved by FDA, maggots are produced aseptically and delivered by commercial companies to wound care centers and hospitals worldwide and regulates medicinal maggots as a medical device [19]. Currently, there are 12 laboratories in 20 countries dispensing maggots at low cost [22], but these larvae are sometimes sold at a very high price to veterinarians who occlude their use for economic reasons [23].

Biology of Blow Fly

The common green bottle fly, *L. sericata* (Diptera: Calliphoridae), formerly *Phaenicia sericata*, belonging to the Diptera order of insects, is a necrophagous fly which feeds on carrion, feces and garbage, and plays an important role in forensic, veterinary, and medical science [24,25]. *L. sericata* is commonly known as blow fly, sheep blow fly and green bottle fly, which is commonly found in cool-temperate habitats [26]. Adult flies of *L. sericata* are metallic green or copper green [27]. The average longevity of an adult female is about 7 days [1,28]. In forensic science, the larvae or maggots are used as a biological indicator in the determination of post-mortem interval [29]. In the field of veterinary medicine, *L. sericata* is characterized as a facultative ectoparasite responsible for primary cutaneous myiasis. Medical treatment using maggots can help to heal chronic injuries that do not respond to conventional treatments [25] and in more acute wounds, especially when surgical debridement is difficult to perform because of the location of the wound and the anatomical structures involved.

Lifecycle

Life cycle begins when adult female flies deposit clusters of eggs (about 2000-3000) on animal corpses, infected wounds of humans or animals and excrement, where they hatch in 18-24 h [1,28,30]. Eggs are usually white, elongated with one end tapered slightly, and hatch in 4-7 days [27]. Development of larvae includes three stage, i.e., 1st, 2nd and 3rd instars. The size of 1st and 3rd instar larvae (mature larvae) are 1-2 and 10 mm, respectively [29,30]. Mature larvae are smooth, yellowish-white, conical shaped, and have both anterior and posterior spiracles. After maturation of 3rd instar larvae, they leave the host or carrion and burrow into the soil or substrate surrounding it where they pupate after 7-10 days. The pupal case is hard, reddish-brown to black. After a pupal period of 6-14 days the adult fly emerges from the puparium, it reproduces and starts the cycle all over again [31]. The life cycle of *L. sericata* depends on ambient temperature, but normally completes within 4-6 weeks [32].

Production of disinfected larvae of L. (Phaenicia) sericata

The larvae of *L. sericata* are relatively small (1-2 mm) when they are applied for wound management. After feeding on necrotic tissue in the moist environment of wounds, they can grow up to 1 cm in 2-3 days [10], after that they will be changed for new ones [33]. For the production of sterile maggots in the laboratory, eggs are collected from gravid females of *L. sericata* (laboratory colony). These eggs are disinfected with a dilute phenol disinfectant (3% Lysol Brand Disinfectant, Reckitt and Coleman Inc.) or 0.525% sodium hypochlorite [12], transferred to sterile vials and left at room temperature overnight. About 500-1000 larvae hatch in each vial and are available for clinical use after quality assurance [12,34].

Maggots are microbiologically tested before use, to certify that no infection will be induced by MDT [35]. The maggots are shipped in a temperature controlled package and are approximately 1-day-old when they arrive for the treatment [36]. They should be used as soon as possible, but essential maturation can be detained by storing at refrigerator temperature (4-8°C) for 2-5 days [34-37]. In case maggots transport is expected to take 2 days then it is worth ordering more as only half of the maggots are alive and able to debride on delivery after a 2 days transport [23]. Maggots are supplied either in free range or in biobag (contained) by constructed laboratories owned by companies such as "BioMonde (formerly 'ZooBiotic') Ltd." based in Brigend, South Wales [5,38].

Mechanism of Action

Medicinal maggots (larvae) have the following beneficial effects on a wound: Tissue debridement, disinfection, stimulation of healing, biofilm inhibition, and eradication [5,28]. *L. sericata* larvae do not penetrate tissues deeply as they depend on aerobic conditions. Thus the larvae interrupt wound surfaces by crawling around using their hook-like mouthparts [39].

Maggots move over the surface of the wound secreting a powerful mixture of digestive enzymes such as carboxypeptidases A and B, leucine aminopeptidase, collagenase, and serine proteases (trypsin-like and chymotrypsin-like enzymes metalloproteinase, and aspartyl proteinase) [8]. These proteolytic enzymes, break down the dead tissue, liquidizing it and ingest the resulting liquefied material [19]. Chymotrypsin-like serine proteinase plays a significant role in the digestion of wound matrix and effective debridement through degradation of extracellular matrix components laminin, fibronectin, and collagen Types I and III [1]. Mechanical action of maggots and secretion of proteolytic enzymes helps in efficient tissue debridement. There is no danger to healthy tissue as these enzymes are neutralized when they come into contact with intact tissue. In this way, they remove cellular debris, dead contaminated tissue, microbes, and foreign material [39,40].

Secretions of maggots increase the wound pH through secretion of sodium bicarbonate, thereby inhibiting the growth of bacteria [37,39]. Maggots also ingest and digest bacteria within the devitalized tissue in the wound, which are killed in their gut [41]. It was shown that excretions/secretions contain bactericidal components with healing properties, such as allantoin, urea, phenylacetic acid, phenylacetaldehyde, and calcium carbonate, especially against MRSA (the most common organism in wounds) [8,28].

In vitro studies have shown that maggot secretions can disrupt biofilms created by *Staphylococcus epidermidis*, *S. aureus* and *Pseudomonas aeruginosa*, and maggots also decrease surface bacterial load by ingesting *Escherichia coli* [1,42]. Maggot secretions have chemotactic factors and fatty acids that affect migration of fibroblasts and induce granulation tissue formation subsequently along with tissue oxygenation [37,40].

Therefore, MDT helps to separate necrotic tissue from the underlying bed, kills microorganisms, disrupts biofilm, and hastens wound healing through a broad range of factors including leukocyte adhesion, growth factor production, collagen production, increased angiogenesis, increased macrophage responsiveness, increased fibrinolysis, and increased nitric oxide levels [43].

Techniques of Maggot Application

Maggot therapy is a controlled method in which safe and effective species and strains of maggots are selected and made germ-free by chemical disinfection. These maggots are called as medicinal maggots and apply on the wound with special dressings that prevent them from leaving the wound unescorted [5]. Maggots of *L. sericata* are used in this technique as they are non-invasive [44]. The maggots available in the United States belong to the (currently named) LB-01 strain of *Phaenicia* (*Lucilia*) *sericata* [5].

Before application, the wound is cleaned (without the use of antiseptics), with normal salt solution or sterilized water to remove the grease and dirt [45]. Maggots are applied on the wound in two-ways, i.e., free range (direct contact method) and biobag (indirect contact method) dressing [23,46,47]. In free range dressing, maggots are applied directly to the wound for 3 days, and allowed to roam freely over [47,48], the surface seeking out areas of slough or necrotic tissue due to which maggots can escape out from the wound site. In biobag dressing, the maggots are enclosed in net pouches containing pieces of hydrophilic polyurethane foam, which are placed directly upon the wound surface for 5 days, so that maggots cannot escape dressing, and the structure of the mesh enables the proteolytic secretions to reach the necrotic tissue, and maggots can still aid in debridement [46]. It also prevents the sensation of tingling due to movement of maggots on the normal skin [45]. Maggots are obligate air breathers, so the dressing must also allow fresh air to enter the area, and let the liquefied necrotic tissue to drain freely from the wound [8,36,49].

Biobag method of maggot application is less complicated as it requires less experience, saves labor, time and resources saving during dressing changes, and is less painful than free range dressing [37]. The disadvantage of the biobag method is that debridement is less effective as the maggots cannot use mouth hooks through the biobag [46]. According to Steenvoorde *et al.*, biobag have a significant negative impact on

the successful outcome of MDT [9]. In another study, Blake *et al.*, compared the two techniques and found that debridement efficiency appears to be similar [37]. Statistical analysis revealed no difference between the use of freely crawling maggots and maggots in a biobag regarding the total amount of debrided tissue after 3 or 4 days of treatment.

Maggots are applied to the wound at a dose of 5-10 maggots/cm² of wound surface area in human medicine [5,50,51]. In veterinary medicine, use of 5-10 maggots/cm² of wound surface area [12,23] and 8-12 maggots/cm² has been reported [52]. The number of maggots applied to the wound depends on the amount of necrotic tissue, wound depth, and width of wound area [23,30]. According to Blake *et al.* a standard dose of 100 maggots can debride 50 g of necrotic tissue during one treatment cycle while taking larval death in the wound into account [37]. In a study on horses, the surface area was multiplied by the depth of the wound for the deeper wound (>2 cm) [23].

During the first 2 days, there is a slight amount of odor due to the phagocytic activity of maggots, later on this odor ceases, wound become alkaline and granulation tissue starts developing across the wound. Usually, wounds have an acidic reaction which turns into alkaline, 24 h after application of maggots. Alkaline reaction is helpful in the sterilization of the wound and killing of the bacteria [45]. Maggots are left within their dressing (cage dressing) for 3-4 days, after that, maggots are satiated and can no longer remove any necrotic tissue [44,53]. At this point, maggots should be removed, the wound should be thoroughly washed out with physiological saline solution, and a new batch of maggots should be applied to the wound until the wound is completely debrided [44,45]. At the end of the second application, the wound is completely filled with granulation tissue [45]. This therapy is very effective for pressure ulcers (bed sores) [44], venous stasis ulcers, diabetic foot ulcers [44], non-healing traumatic and post-surgical wounds, burns, and gangrene in human medicine [8,54].

MDT in Animals

For centuries, MDT has been used to treat chronic infections in humans [22,23,55], but rarely has it been reported in the treatment of infections in animals [56]. Recently, MDT regressed as a powerful and effective therapy for incurable wounds of animals. This therapy is most effective for deep penetrating wounds that have hard to reach soft tissue necrosis such as infections of the palmer regions of the foot, navicular apparatus, digital cushion, and coffin joint [35]. At present, many veterinarians use MDT to treat problematic wounds due to the non-traumatic debridement and disinfection of blowfly maggots in humans [5,57].

Maggot therapy has been reported to be used successfully in a wounded bull [58], two donkeys [56,59], two ponies [23], mule and horses [53]. The first study of MDT in donkeys was carried out by Bell in 2001 [56] and in horses was done by Jurga and Morrison 2004 [60]. In horses, MDT is used in the management of supraspinous bursitis [23], septic navicular bursitis, complicated laminitis [35,61] infected abscess with pedal bone osteomyelitis and other hoof diseases [60]. Kociova *et al.* reported the use of MDT in 6 sheep with 3 cases of acute inflammation of the interdigital skin and 4 cases of purulent inflammation of the pododerm. Four sheep exhibited a marked improvement and initiation of healing already after the first application, two sheep required additional treatment during which 100-120 new larvae were applied beneath the keratin hoof capsule. The effect of a single application for 3-6 days was evaluated. Debridement was rapid and selective. The treatment was well tolerated by animals. New layers of healthy tissue were formed over the wounds [52]. Morrison *et al.* treated 41 cases of coffin bone osteomyelitis, 18 cases of chronic laminitis, 8 cases of septic navicular bursa, 4 cases of chronic distal interphalangeal joint sepsis, 3 cases of canker, 2 cases of non-healing foot ulcers (palmer region of the foot), 1 case of acute caudal coffin bone rotation and 1 case of necrosis of collateral cartilage (Quittor) in horse of both sexes with MDT [35]. Once stability is achieved, maggot therapy has been able to rid the infection. None of the cases described were euthanized for failure to treat the infection. The only side effect of maggot therapy is the occasional patient may experience irritation or itching at the wound site. The movement of the larvae within the wound may be a cause for this [40]. A total of 20 cases were treated with MDT in which 7 cases of small animals (2 dogs, 4 cats, 1 rabbit) and 13 cases of horses [12]. In this study, maggot therapy was associated with limb salvage in three of the five canines and felines that were expected to require amputation or euthanasia. One rabbit was treated with maggot therapy over the entire hock, due to a septic wound. One cycle of maggot debridement was applied, with significant debridement. No adverse events were attributed to maggot therapy for any of these cases. It should be noted, however, that two animals with serious infections succumbed to sepsis during therapy, and the septic rabbit died 4 days following maggot therapy.

Later on, Sherman *et al.*, used MDT to treat a 6-year-old horse with an extensive laceration of the left proximal hind limb, a newborn foal suffering from an obliterative vasculitis involving the hoof, a 9-year-old mare with puncture wound involving the navicular bursa, digital flexor tendon, coffin joint and digital cushion of the right hind limb, a 14-year-old Arabian stallion with a puncture wound to the lateral heel. Following maggot therapy, all infections were eradicated or controlled, and only one horse had to be euthanized. No adverse events were attributed to maggot therapy for any of these cases, other than presumed discomfort during therapy [53]. Lepage *et al.* treated 41 equids (35 horses, 4 donkeys and 2 ponies of all

ages and both sexes) by MDT with various lesions *viz.*, septic navicular bursa, fistulous withers in a donkey, keratoma, septic pedal bone osteitis, chronic proliferative wound dorsal left hind cannon bone, chronic proliferative wound proximo plantar aspect right hind tarsus, soft tissue abscess (1 buttock, 3 neck, 1 scrotum, 1 prepuce), various acute or subacute limb laceration, chronic tuber coxae fracture with fistulization and MRSA infected wounds [23]. In 38 cases a favorable outcome was reached in <1 week. In all cases, debridement, disinfection and enhanced healing were observed. In 3 cases, complete healing of the wound failed to occur. In one of these cases, healing occurred uneventfully after a bony sequestrum was removed. In 2 other horses, squamous cell carcinoma and melanoma were involved in chronic infected wounds and complete healing was not achieved because of recurrence of underlying tumors [23].

MDT were found successful in small animals and horse with complete healing in wounds that had already failed to respond to conventional medical and surgical therapy [12,34,53]. This therapy assists with wound healing by debridement of necrotic wounds [23,34,52,53], disinfection [23,53] and granulation tissue formation [23,52] occur after 3 days of application [12]. If complete debridement of the wound does not occur, the second application of maggots is required [12]. In some cases of small animals and horses, light surgical debridement was performed along with MDT to remove debris and dry necrotic tissue [23,44,53]. MDT has potent antibacterial effects as it controls difficult infections such as MRSA or other multi-antibiotic resistant bacteria [23,56]. It is an effective way to prevent the establishment of serious infections including complicated and deep lacerations, abscesses, abdominal wound dehiscence, and infections even in the presence of internal fixation [23], severe distal phalanx displacement and solar penetration [8]. It is reported that maggot therapy was associated with limb salvage in three of the five canines and felines that were expected to require amputation [12]. Other treatments, such as systemic antibiotic injections, local perfusion with antibiotics and use of disinfectants (e.g., dilute betadine or chlorine dioxide) before application of maggot therapy, have no effect on the viability of the maggots [8]. In some cases, antibiotic treatment was not used with MDT for the better assessment of the efficacy of this therapy [12]. Occasionally, general anesthesia was needed to control the animal and for the application of the dressing in a proper way [12]. Few animals died or were euthanized due to the severity of pre-existing diseases, and not due to treatment failure [12,33].

Maggot therapy is a safe and useful technique for debriding and disinfecting some severe wounds and has emerged as an alternative to amputation in dogs and cats. Progressively, small animal veterinarians are turning to MDT to treat problematic wounds [12].

Contraindications and Side Effect of MDT

Adverse reactions to MDT usually does not happen [61,62] and only side effects observed are irritation, itching and hypersensitivity [34] at the wound site. Sometimes it also causes pain, discomfort and malodor at the first change of dressing [38,44,62,63]. In the case of horses, discomfort was observed by the movement and stamping of the limb and repeated rubbing of the bandage [23,34]. No adverse effects have been identified in small animals [12].

Maggots should be avoided to treat dry wounds as they require a moist environment [22,36]. Maggot therapy should not be used in open wounds of body cavities or sinuses, fistulae, wounds in close proximity to large blood vessels [36,46], wounds close to the brain, wounds with neoplasia [23] and wounds with large necrotic areas such as a large area of osteomyelitis or a sequestrum [23,44]. Patients with rapidly advancing infection [46] and sepsis should not initially be treated with MDT [9].

During application of maggots, excessive pressure on the wound can kill maggots in that area, leading to uneven wound debridement. Maggots should be changed every 4th day [34] as they have limited "shelf-life" and need to be applied soon after delivery [64,65]. The wound should be entirely filled with the maggots so that every part is attacked by the maggots at the same time [45]. Large number of maggots for a short period should be used rather than a small number for an extended period [46].

In veterinary medicine, use of MDT was limited by the relatively high cost of treatment, time required for shipping (usually 24-48 h after ordering) and the fact that a portion of maggots failed to survive on arrival [12,23]. Another common problem was the time and effort involved in applying the dressings in such a way that they are not removed by the animal [12].

Conclusion and Future Aspects

MDT is frequently used in human medicine although this therapy is still limited in animals and clinical studies are few. However, with the increasing antibiotic resistance and chronic wound infections in veterinary medicine, maggot therapy may even become the first line of treatment for some infections. Clinical studies evaluated that MDT is more efficient and safe technique for chronic wounds as compared to conventional therapy. Maggots are supplied by licensed laboratories in sterile bottles, which make it very safe, efficient, and easy method of healing for chronic wounds and prevents secondary bacterial infections. There is an overwhelming need for improved wound care in countries which are under-provided for medical veterinary facilities. In veterinary medicine, further clinical studies are needed in several fields, including establishing a number of maggots required for safe and efficient treatment and identification of adverse effect during treatment. There is also a need

to assure the safety and efficiency of the treatment in small animals, increase awareness in owners and encourage veterinarians to take the first steps toward using MDT in dogs, cats and horses, and can help to make MDT as accessible. In addition, MDT will add one more treatment method to utilize in non-healing wounds of animals and overcome the use of amputation and euthanasia.

Authors' Contributions

This topic was studied and reviewed by VC and MC and revised by SP and VDC under the guidance of JJH. All authors read and approved the final version of the article.

Acknowledgments

The authors are thankful to all staff of Department of Veterinary Parasitology, College of Veterinary Science and Animal Husbandry, Anand Agricultural University, Anand, Gujarat, India for their help.

Competing Interests

The authors declare that they have no competing interests.

References

1. Valachova, I., Bohova, J., Kozanek, M., Takac, P. and Majtan, J. (2014) Lucilia sericata medicinal maggots: A new source of antimicrobial compounds. Microbial Pathogens and Strategies for Combating Them: Science, Technology and Education. FORMATEX, Spain. p1745-53.
2. Turkmen, A., Graham, K. and McGroutherc, D.A. (2010) Therapeutic applications of the larvae for wound debridement. J. Plast. Reconstr. Aesthet. Surg., 63(1): 184-188.
3. Cickova, H., Cambal, M., Kozanek, M. and Taka, P. (2013) Growth and survival of bagged Lucilia sericata maggots in wounds of patients undergoing maggot debridement therapy. Evid. Base. Complement Alternat. Med., 2013: 192149.
4. Sun, X., Jiang, K., Chen, J., Wu, L., Lu, H., Wang, A. and Wang, J. (2014) A systematic review of maggot debridement therapy for chronically infected wounds and ulcers. Int. J. Infect. Dis., 25: 32-37.
5. Sherman, R.A. (2009) Maggot therapy takes us back to the future of wound care: New and improved maggot therapy for the 21st century. J. Diabetes. Sci. Technol., 3(2): 336-344.
6. Gottrup, F. and Jorgensen, B. (2011) Maggot debridement: An alternative method for debridement. J. Plast. Surg., 11: 290-305.
7. Whitaker, I.S., Twine, C., Whitaker, M.J., Welck, M., Brown, C.S. and Shandall, A. (2007) Larval therapy from antiquity to the present day: Mechanisms of action, clinical applications and future potential. Postgrad. Med., 83: 409-413.
8. Dholaria, S., Dalal, P., Shah, N. and Narkhede, R. (2014) Maggots debridement therapy [MDT]. Gujarat Med. J., 69: 1.
9. Steenvoorde, P., Jacobi, C.E., Van Doorn, L. and Oskam, J. (2007) Maggot debridement therapy of infected ulcers: Patient and wound factors influencing outcome - A study on 101 patients with 117 wounds. Ann. R. Coll. Surg. Engl., 89(6): 596-602.
10. Sylvia, A. and Steenvoorde, P. (2011) Maggot debridement therapy. Proc. Neth. Entomol. Soc. Meet., 22: 61-66.
11. The Bio Therapeutics, Education & Research (BTER) Foundation. Biotherapeutics, Biotherapy, Maggot Therapy, Larval Therapy. In: Sherman, R.A., editor. Vol. 2(2). Available from: http://www.bterfoundation.org/indexfiles/

MDT. Retrieved on 23-09-2005.

12. Sherman, R.A., Stevens, H., Ng, D. and Iversen, E. (2007) Treating wounds in small animals with maggot debridement therapy: A survey of practitioners. *Vet. J.,* 173(1): 138-143.

13. Pare, A. (1557, 1952) The battell of quintin. In: Keynes G, editor. The Apologie and Treatise of Ambroise Paré. The University of Chicago Press, Chicago. p68-70.

14. Goldstein, H.I. (1931) Maggots in the treatment of wound and bone infections. *J. Bone Joint Surg. Am.,* 13(3): 477-478.

15. Erdmann, G.R. (1987) Antibacterial action of myiasis-causing flies. *Parasitol. Today,* 3(7): 214-216.

16. Chan, D.C., Fong, D.H., Leung, J.Y., Patil, N.G. and Leung, G.K. (2007) Maggot debridement therapy in chronic wound care. *Hong Kong Med. J.,* 13(5): 382-386.

17. Baer, W.S. (1931) The treatment of chronic osteomyelitis with the maggot (larva of the blow fly). *J. Bone Joint Surg. Am.,* 13: 438-475.

18. Tse, T.W. (2006) Maggot therapy in Hong Kong: A case report. *Hong Kong J. Dermatol. Venereol.* 14: 78-81.

19. Andersen, A.S., Sandvang, D., Schnorr, K.M., Kruse, B., Joergensen, S.N., Karlsmark, T. and Krogfelt, K.A. (2010) A novel approach to the antimicrobial activity of maggot debridement therapy. *J. Antimicrob. Chemother.,* 65(8): 1646-1654.

20. Geary, M.J., Smith, A. and Russell, R.C. (2009) Maggots down under. *Wound Pract. Res.,* 17(1): 36-42.

21. Cazander, G., van de Veerdonk, M.C., Vandenbroucke-Grauls, C.M., Schreurs, M.W. and Jukema, G.N. (2010) Maggot excretions inhibit biofilm formation on biomaterials. *Clin. Orthop. Relat. Res.,* 468(10): 2789-2796.

22. Michelle, L.M., Mark, T.H., Karen, M.S. and Lawrence, J.E. (2011) Maggot debridement therapy in the treatment of complex diabetic wounds. *Hawaii Med. J.,* 70(6): 121-124.

23. Lepage, O.M., Doumbia, A., Perron-Lepage, M.F. and Gangl, M. (2012) The use of maggot debridement therapy in 41 equids. *Equine Vet. J. Suppl.,* 44(43): 120-125.

24. Rueda, L.C., Ortega, L.G., Segura, N.A., Acero, V.M., Bello, F. (2010) *Lucilia sericata* strain from Colombia: Experimental colonization, life tables and evaluation of two artificial diets of the blowfly *Lucilia sericata* (Meigen) (Diptera: Calliphoridae), Bogotá, Colombia strain. *Biol. Res.,* 43(2): 197-203.

25. Anderson, M. and Kaufman, P.E. (2011) Common green bottle fly sheep blow fly *Lucilia sericata* (Meigen) (Insecta: Diptera: Calliphoridae). Department of Entomology and Nematology, University of Florida, Gainesville. Available from: http://www.edis.ifas.ufl.edu. Accessed on 02-03-2016.

26. Mun, J., Seung-Min, R., Sang-Chang, K., Jun-Ouk, H., Young-Hoon, K., Dong-Hyun, K., Soon-Myung, J., Soon-I, L., Woon-Mok, S., Hee-Jae, C. and Meesun, O. (2013) A case of oral myiasis caused by *Lucilia sericata* (Diptera: Calliphoridae) in Korea. *Korean J. Parasitol.,* 51(1): 119-123.

27. Apperson, C.S., Arends, J.J., Baker, J.R., Carter, C.C. and Payne, C.S. (2011) Blow flies. *Insect. Related Pests. Man. Anim.* Available from: http://www.ipm.ncsu.edu/ag369/notes/blow_flies.html. Accessed on 03-03-2016.

28. Du Plessis, H.J.C. and Pretorius, J.P. (2011) The utilisation of maggot debridement therapy in Pretoria, South Africa. *Wound Health. South Afr.,* 4(2): 80-83.

29. Shiravi, A.H., Mostafavi, R., Akbarzadeh, K. and Oshaghi, M.A. (2011) Temperature requirements of some common forensically important blow and flesh flies (Diptera) under laboratory conditions. *Iran. J. Arthropod-Borne Dis.,* 5(1): 54-62.

30. Abdolmaleki, A., Mirarab Razi, J., Nourzad Moghaddam, M. and Mastari Farahani. H. (2015) Maggot debridement therapy: Concepts, methods, issues and future. *Int. J. Pharmacother.,* 5(1): 27-31.

31. Youssefi, M.R., Rahimi, M.T. and Marhaba, Z. (2012) Occurrence of nasal nosocomial myiasis by *Lucilia sericata* (Diptera: Calliphoridae) in North of Iran. *Iran. J. Parasitol.,* 7(1): 104-108.

32. Yaghoobi, R., Tirgari, S. and Sina, N. (2005) Human auricular myiasis caused by *Lucilia sericata*: Clinical and parasitological considerations. *Acta Med. Iran.,* 43(2): 155-157.

33. Steenvoorde, P. (2008) Maggot debridement therapy in surgery. *Proc. Neth. Entomol. Soc. Meet.,* 22: 61-66.

34. Morrison, S. (2010) Maggot debridement therapy for laminitis. *Vet. Clin. North Am. Equine Pract.,* 26(2): 447-450.

35. Wolff, H. and Hansson, C. (2005) Rearing larvae of *Lucilia sericata* for chronic ulcer treatment - An improved method. *Acta Derm. Venereol.,* 85(2): 126-131.

36. Dar, L.M., Hussain, S.A., Abdullah, S., Rashid, A., Parihar, S. and Rather, F.A. (2013) Maggot therapy and its implications in veterinary medicine: An overview. *J. Adv. Vet. Anim. Res.,* 3(1): 47-51.

37. Blake, F.A.S., Abromeit, N., Bubenheim, M., Li, L. and Schmelzle, R. (2007) The biosurgical wound debridement: Experimental investigation of efficiency and practicability. *Wound Repair Regen.,* 15(5): 756-761.

38. Andersen, A.S., Joergensen, B., Bjarnsholt, T., Johansen, H., Karlsmark, T., Givskov, M. and Krogfelt, K.A. (2010) Quorumsensing - Regulated virulence factors in *Pseudomonas aeruginosa* are toxic to *Lucilia sericata* maggots. *Microbiol.,* 156: 400-407.

39. Patricia, A.S. (2011) Use of medicinal maggots in wound healing. The Surgical Summit Proceedings of the ACVS Veterinary Symposium, Chicago. p563-566.

40. Nigam, Y., Dudley, E. and Bexfield, A. (2010) The physiology of wound healing by the medicinal maggot, *Lucilia sericata. Adv. Insect. Physiol.,* 39: 39-81.

41. Viv, P. (2011) The use of larval therapy in modern wound care. *Wounds Int.,* 2(4): 23-27.

42. Sherman, R.A. (2014) Mechanisms of maggot-induced wound healing: What do we know, and where do we go from here? *Evid. Base. Complement Alternat. Med.,* 2014: 592419.

43. Cornell, R.S., Andrew, J., Meyr, J., Steinberg, S. and Christopher, E.A. (2010) Debridement of the non-infected wound. *J. Vasc. Surg.,* 52(12): 31-36.

44. Morrison, S. (2007) How to utilize sterile maggot debridement therapy for foot infections of the horse (Reprinted from 2005 AAEP Proceedings), 10th Geneva Congress of Equine Medicine and Surgery (Organization: Pierre A. Chuit, Founex; Dr. Stephane Montavon, Avenches), Geneva, (CH). p210-212. Available from: http://www.ivis.org. Accessed on 16-05-2016.

45. Baer, W.S. (2011) The classic, the treatment of chronic osteomyelitis with the maggot (Larva of the Blow Fly). *Clin. Orthop. Relat. Res.,* 469(4): 920-944.

46. Jones, G. and Wall, R. (2007) Maggot-therapy in veterinary medicine. *Res. Vet. Sci.,* 85(2): 394-398.

47. Brown, A. (2013) The role of debridement in the healing process. *Nurs. Times,* 109(40): 16-19.

48. (2012) Guidelines for the use of sterile maggot therapy in wound management. Derby City Primary Care Trust, 1(2): 1-14.

49. Sherman, R.A. (2014) Using maggots in wound care: Part 1. *Wound Care Advisor,* 3(4): 12-19.

50. Singh, N.M., Bhatia, S.K. and Singh, G. (2014) Maggots therapy in facilitating wound debridement: Present status. *Med. J. DY. Patil. Univ.,* 7(5): 639-642.

51. Waniczek, D., Kozowicz, A., Muc-Wierzgon, M., Kokot, T., Swietochowska, E. and Nowakowska-Zajdel, E. (2013) Adjunct methods of the standard diabetic foot ulceration therapy. *Evid. Base Complement Alternat. Med.,* 2013: Article ID:243568, 12.

52. Kociova, A., Pistl, J., Link, R., Conkova, E. and Goldova, M. (2006) Maggot debridement therapy in the treatment of foot rot and foot scald in sheep. *Acta Vet.,* 75: 277-281.

53. Sherman, R.A., Morrison, S. and Ng, D. (2007b) Maggot debridement therapy for serious horse wounds - A survey of

practitioners. *Vet. J.*, 174(1): 86-91.

54. Kuffler, D.P. (2010) Techniques for wound healing with a focus on pressure ulcers elimination. *Open Circ. Vasc. J.,* 3: 72-84.

55. Sherman, R.A. (2002a) Maggot therapy for foot and leg wounds. *Int. J. Low Extrem. Wounds*, 1(2): 135-142.

56. Bell, N.J. and Thomas, S. (2001) Use of sterile maggots to treat panniculitis in an aged donkey. *Vet. Rec.,* 149(25): 768-770.

57. Sherman, R.A. (2002b) Maggot versus conservative debridement therapy for the treatment of pressure ulcers. *Wound Repair Regen.*, 10(4): 208-214.

58. Dicke, R.J. (1953) Maggot treatment of actinomycosis. *J. Econ. Entomol.*, 46: 706-707.

59. Thiemann, A. (2003) Treatment of a deep injection abscess using sterile maggots in a donkey: A case report. World Wide Wounds. Available from: http://www.worldwide. wounds.com/2003/November/Thiemann/Donkey-Maggot-therapy.html. Retrieved on 05-04-2005.

60. Jurga, F. and Morrison, S.E. (2004) Maggot debridement therapy. Alternative therapy for hoof infection and necrosis. *Hoof Care Lameness,* 78: 28-31.

61. Bras, R.J. and Morrison, S. (2009) Retrospective case series of 20 horses (2002-2009) Sustaining puncture wounds to the navicular bursa with maggot debridement therapy as an adjunctive treatment. *Proc. Am. Ass. Equine Practnrs.,* 55: 241-250.

62. Wollina, U., Karte, K., Herold, C. and Looks, A. (2000) Biosurgery in wound healing-the renaissance of maggot therapy. *J. Eur. Acad. Dermatol. Venereol.,* 14: 285-289.

63. Daniel, J.B. (2013) Traumatic foot injuries in horses, surgical management *Compend. Contin. Educ. Vet.*, 35: 1-9.

64. Dominic, C.W.C., Daniel, H.F.F., June, Y.Y.L., Patil, N.G. and Gilberto, K.K.L. (2007) Maggot debridement therapy in chronic wound care. *Hong Kong Med. J.*, 13: 382-386.

65. Nancy, T., Abdel-Meguid, A. and El-ebiarie, A. (2010) Application of native excretory/secretory products from third larval instar of *Chrysomya megacephala* (Diptera: Calliphoridae) on an artificial wound. *J. Am. Sci.,* 6(7): 313-317.

4

Episodes of clinical mastitis and its relationship with duration of treatment and seasonality in crossbred cows maintained in organized dairy farm

Narender Kumar[1], A. Manimaran[2], A. Kumaresan[1], L. Sreela[1], Tapas Kumar Patbandha[3], Shiwani Tiwari[1] and Subhash Chandra[1]

1. Theriogenology Laboratory, Livestock Production Management Section, ICAR - National Dairy Research Institute (NDRI), Karnal - 132 001, Haryana, India; 2. Southern Regional Station, ICAR - National Dairy Research Institute, Adugodi, Hosur road, Bengaluru - 560 030, Karnataka, India; 3. Polytechnic in Animal Husbandry, College of Veterinary Science and A.H., Junagadh Agricultural University, Junagadh - 362 001, Gujarat, India.
Corresponding author: Tapas Kumar Patbandha, e-mail: patbandhavet@gmail.com,
NK: nklangyan@gmail.com, AM: maranpharma@gmail.com, AK: ogkumaresan@gmail.com; LS: sreela312@gmail.com,
ST: shiwanitiwari@gmail.com, SC: subhashchandra20july@gmail.com

Abstract

Aim: Present study aimed to evaluate the different episodes of clinical mastitis (CM) and influence of duration of treatment and seasonality on the occurrence of different episodes of CM in crossbred cows.

Materials and Methods: A total of 1194 lactation data of crossbred CM cows were collected from mastitis treatment record from 2002 to 2012. Data of CM cows were classified into types of episodes (pattern of repeated or multiple episodes occurrence) and number of episodes (magnitude of multiple cases). Types of episodes were divided as single (clinical cure by a single episode of treatment), relapse (retreatment of the same cow within 21 days), recurrence (new CM at least 21 days after treatment), and both (relapse and recurrence). The season was classified as winter (December to March), summer (April to June), rainy (July to September), and autumn (October to November). The difference between incidences of different types of CM episodes and the association between number or type of CM episodes with duration of treatment and seasons of CM occurrence were analyzed by Chi-square test.

Results: Among 1194 animals suffered with CM, 53, 16, and 18% had the single episode, relapse, and recurrence, respectively; while 13% suffered by both relapse and recurrence. We estimated the duration of treatment and found 80% of the cows treated 1-8 days, in which 65% treated for 1-4 days, while 35% cows were treated for 5-8 days. Further, 12% cows treated for 9-15 days and 7.5% cows treated >15 days. The relationship between duration of treatment and different episodes of CM revealed that 1-8 days treated cows were mostly cured by the single episode with less relapse and recurrence. In contrast, the incidences of recurrence and relapse episodes were higher in cows treated for more than 9 days. The highest incidence of relapse was noticed in winter (36%) than other seasons (10-28%), while the recurrence was less during autumn (9%) compared to other seasons (20-40%).

Conclusion: Cows those suffered by both relapse and recurrence were more susceptible to CM, and they need to be culled from farm to control the transmission of infections. Although the influence of seasonality was difficult to understand, the higher magnitude of relapse and recurrence during winter suggested the adverse effects of cold stress on treatment outcome.

Keywords: clinical mastitis, duration of treatment, episodes, recurrence, relapse, season.

Introduction

Mastitis continues to be the most frequent and costly disease of dairy animals across the globe. The recent report suggested that the incidence of mastitis has been increased from 20% to 50% in the Indian dairy animals [1]. The environmental and contagious pathogens are the major cause of clinical mastitis (CM), and outcome of clinical cases are depends on the affected cows, mastitis pathogen, treatment, and management including environment related factors [2]. Although the role of genetics background for mastitis susceptibility has been recently suggested, it is believed that mastitis is the management related disease. Hence, prevention through better management has been suggested as a better strategy for controlling the mastitis than therapeutic management. Although, CM has been traditionally considered as single episode disease per lactation, effects of repeated episodes of CM on milk yield, its quality and negative impact on reproduction were suggested by many workers [3-5]. Mastitis is one of the top most reasons for culling and chances of culling or death were increased in repeated or multiple episode cases [5]. Higher productivity of dairy animals over the period of time and its positive correlation with mastitis incidence makes that treatment of CM during lactation is an inevitable tool, and thus it is an important part of economic losses in CM affected dairy animals. However, "successful treatment" of all mastitis cases remains the challenging task for dairy farmers and veterinarians across the globe. Complex nature of disease caused very little progress in understanding the reasons for low cure rate.

The decrease in milk production was observed with repeated episodes CM caused by different organisms, whereas patterns of milk loss varied with both case number and organism [6]. Among the various factors, duration of treatment is believed to be an important determinant of treatment outcome. Although, the minimum recommended duration of treatment against CM was 3 days, the data regarding real practices in organized Indian dairy farm is not available. On other hand, this data would be helpful to calculate the economic losses due to CM treatment in the Indian context. During recent times, it is believed that the production and herd health-related data are very important to understand the efficiency of management in any farm. For instance, observed that changes in milk yield and electrical conductivity as early as 10 days before the actual appearance of clinical diagnosis of any health disorder in dairy cows [7]. Therefore, these data were exploited to use for herd health monitoring programs.

Since mastitis in dairy animals is one of the most important reasons for antibiotic usage, periodical evaluation of mastitis treatment efficacy is an important tool to assess the effectiveness of existing treatment protocol and formulation of effective future treatment strategy in dairy farms. However, mastitis treatment related data were not analyzed as much as production related data. Further, data regarding the overall prevalence of clinical or sub-CM in dairy animals, how many days the CM was treated? How many CM cows in a herd were re-treated? How many cows have multiple mastitis episodes in the single lactation, are important to assess the effectiveness of mastitis treatment protocol [8]. The understandings of various risk factors associated with treatment outcome are important to improve better treatment decision and select the CM cases that are expected to very respond to treatment [9]. However, to our knowledge, no work has been done this area under organized Indian dairy farming conditions.

It is well-known that particular percentage (about 8%) of animals in the farm was responsible for most incidences (about 40%) of CM. Therefore, identification and culling of those most susceptible animals would be very helpful to reduce the transmission of CM in a particular farm. The recent development of Marker Assisted Selections is seemed to be long-term solution for identification of most susceptible animals. On the other hand, where the management and environment are similar to all animals, repeated incidence of CM (more than one episode) in particular cows indirectly suggesting that they could be more susceptible in the farm. Therefore, we quantified the different episodes of CM in organized dairy farm and influence of duration of treatment and seasonality on the occurrence of different episodes of CM in cross-bred cows.

Materials and Methods

Ethical approval

The present retrospective study was duly approved by the Institutional Animal Ethics Committee (IAEC), ICAR - National Dairy Research Institute, Karnal, Haryana, India.

Study site

The study was conducted on crossbred cows (Karan Fries) in Livestock Research Centre, ICAR -National Dairy Research Institute, Karnal (Haryana) in the northern part of India. Livestock Research Centre is located at an altitude of 250 m above the mean sea level at 29.42°N latitude and 79.54°E longitude in Eastern Haryana, which comes under the Trans-Gangetic plain agro-climatic zone of India. Meteorological conditions include subtropical weather (hot, humid in summer and near freezing temperature in winter), average annual rainfall about 760-960 mm (received mostly during the months of July and August), and relative humidity 41-85%. The atmospheric temperature varies from near freezing (4°C) during peak winter months at night to about 40°C in summer months during the late afternoon. There are four major seasons that prevail in a year, viz., winter (December to March), summer (April to June), rainy (July to September), and autumn (October to November).

General management with reference to mastitis

The farm animals were maintained under the loose housing system with milking parlors and a well-equipped veterinary health care facility. The nutrient requirements of the animals were mostly met with ad lib green fodder, dry fodder, silage, and measured amount of concentrate. The green fodders, grown in the institute farm, were supplied according to the seasonal availability. Three times milking of animals in a day (morning 5.00-6.00 am, noon 12.00-1.00 pm, and in evening 6.00-7.00 pm) using milking machine was the routine practice in the farm. Before milking, pre-stripping and observation of lactating animals for symptoms related to CM by well-trained farm personal and milkers were also a routine procedure in the farm. All the diagnosed animals were immediately treated by a veterinarian as per standard farm practices. Treatment based on personal experience of veterinarians in farm and evaluation through clinical signs and associated physiological changes such as milk yield, feed intake, etc., are the routine follow-up procedure to assess the treatment response in the farm. Mastitis treatment registers were maintained separately in the farm, in which information of animal identification number, quarter affected, symptoms, treatment details, and date of clinical cure were mentioned.

When CM was detected, cleaning and complete removal of milk from affected quarters before administration of antibiotic through intramammary and/or systemic route were routine treatment procedures in the farm. Besides antibiotics, administration of anti-inflammatory, antihistaminic, vitamins, and other preparations as supportive therapy were also routine treatment procedure in farms.

Data collection, classification, and case definition

The data of CM related information of crossbred cows were collected from mastitis treatment record (n = 1194 lactation with CM) of the institute farm between January 2002 and December 2012. CM was defined as the occurrence of abnormal milk (flakes or chunks in normal or watery milk) with or without swelling of the affected quarter and systemic signs. Clinical cure was defined as the return of quarter and milk secretion to normal, as assessed by visual observation and palpation, at or before milking. Data of CM cows were classified into types of episodes (pattern of repeated or multiple episodes occurrence) and number of episodes (magnitude of multiple cases). Types of episodes were classified as single, relapse, and recurrence. The single episode was defined as CM was clinically cured by the single episode of treatment. Relapse was defined as a retreatment of the same cow within 21 days following an apparent clinical cure. A recurrence was defined as detection of a new CM episode in the same cow 21 days after treatment of the previous episode of CM. Percent higher episodes for multiple or repeated episodes of CM (relapse, recurrence and both) cases were calculated from the incidence of CM (number of animals suffered by CM) and number of CM episodes. Season of CM occurrence was classified as per prevalence in the study site. During classification of the duration of treatment, 1-8 days was kept as minimum due to mastitis caused by potentially invasive pathogens should be treated for 5-8 days [10]. However, the 1-8 days treated cows were divided into 1-4 days and 5-8 days as CM cases mostly treated for 3-5 days.

Statistical analysis

The frequency of CM incidence in different types of episodes, duration of treatment and seasonality of CM occurrence are represented in percentage of the total incidence. Chi-square test was used to compare the difference between incidences of different types of CM episodes through percent of higher episodes. The association between number or type of CM episodes with duration of treatment and seasons of CM occurrence were also analyzed by Chi-square test through percent calculation. All the analyzes were performed using Sigma Plot 11® software package (Systat software Inc., CA, USA).

Result and Discussion

The total number of cows suffered with CM during the study period was 1194, and the total episodes of CM were 2277 which is classified into single, relapse, recurrent, and both (relapse and recurrent) CM episodes (Table-1). Among the total animals suffered with CM, 53% of animals (n=638) suffered with single episode, whereas 46% animals (n=556) had multiple episodes (relapse, recurrence, and both relapse or recurrence). The multiple episodes affected animals had 194.78 percent higher episode than total affected animals (i.e. higher episode about 90.7%). We estimated the different types of CM episodes (Table-2) and found 53% of the cows were suffered single episode, 16% cows (n=187) suffered with relapse, and 18% cows (n=214) suffered with recurrence. About 13% of the cows (n=155) were suffered by both relapse and recurrence. Various researchers reported the recurrent episodes of CM [11,12] and suggested as a sensitive indicator of treatment efficacy [13]. The high rates of recurrence may indicate the presence of organisms resistant to the antibiotics used in treatment, and/or poor cure rates [14]. Apparao et al. [15] reported the occurrence of recurrent mastitis in quarters defined as cured as well as treatment failures. Recurrent episodes of CM in the same quarter can be caused by persistent intra mammary infection (IMI) or may be associated with recurrent IMI. Bradley and Green [16] reported recurrent episodes of mastitis by the same Escherichia coli strain and Bar et al. [17] reported 48% to 50% of the third CM episode due to the same pathogen in primiparous and multiparous cows. Very limited duration of immunological memory after each episode of CM could also be the reason for recurrent episodes as it was observed after either vaccination or a full challenge [3,18].

We estimated the duration of treatment (Table-3) for clinical cure (2277 mastitis episodes from 1194 cows) and found 80% of the cows (n=961) were treated 1-8 days against 1796 episodes, in which 65%

Table-1: Incidence of different episodes of CM in crossbred cows.

Episodes	Incidence of CM (%)	No. of CM episodes (%)	% higher episodes
Single	638 (53)	638 (28.02)	0
Multiple	556 (46)	1639 (71.98)	194.78[a]
Total	1194	2277	90.70[b]

Values with different superscript in a column varies significantly at p<0.001, CM=Clinical mastitis

Table-2: Incidence of different types of episodes of clinical mastitis in crossbred cows.

Episodes	Incidence of CM (%)	No. of CM episodes (%)	% higher episodes
Single	638 (53)	638 (28.02)	0
Relapse	187 (16)	464 (20.38)	148.12[a]
Recurrence	214 (18)	507 (22.26)	136.91[a]
Both relapse and recurrence	155 (13)	668 (29.34)	330.12[b]
Total	1194	2277	90.70

Values with different superscript in a column varies significantly at p<0.001, CM=Clinical mastitis

cows (n=620) were treated for 1-4 days against 1146 episodes, while 35% cows (n=341) were treated for 5-8 days against 652 episodes. Further, 12% cows treated for 9-15 days against 305 episodes and 7% cows treated >15 days against 176 episodes. Various researchers reported that treatment of CM for minimum 3 days and extended therapy of 5-8 days for better cure [19]. The duration of treatment in the present study (1-8 days in 80% cows) was higher than that reported in previous studies [20,21]. This difference may be attributable to the omission of severe cases of mastitis in the previous study, different drugs, cow and herd factors, as well as milker or owner awareness of prudent antibiotic usage in lactating animals.

We estimated the relationship between duration of treatment and different episodes of CM in cows (Table-4a and -b). Among the 1-8 days treated cows (n=961), we found that the majority of cows were cured by the single episode with fewer episodes of relapse (74%) and recurrence (79%). In contrast, the incidences of recurrence and relapse were higher in cows treated more than nine days duration. It suggests that longer duration of treatment were due to multiple episodes (relapse and recurrence) of CM rather than the longer duration of treatment requirement. On the other hand, these cows may also be more susceptible to mastitis than animals cured by the single episode of treatment. Among the repeatedly suffered cows (n=556), the magnitude of higher episodes was more for those cows suffered by both relapse and recurrence (330%) followed by relapse (148%) and recurrence cows (137%). Collectively, it suggests that cows suffered by both relapse and recurrence were highly susceptible to CM, and they need to be culled from farm to control the transmission of infections.

The influence of season on incidence and number of CM episodes is presented in Table-5. The highest incidence of CM was found in winter (36%) and rainy (28%) followed by in summer (25%). The less incidence of CM was noticed in autumn (10%). Similarly, the higher incidence of relapse and recurrence were noticed during winter (36% and 40%, respectively) than other seasons (11-28% and 29-29%, respectively) (Table-6). Despite the average incidence of CM, the incidence of more episodes during summer suggested that treatment efficacy was adversely affected by heat stress. However, overall higher incidence of single or repeated episodes of CM during winter suggested the influence of cold stress-associated impairment of the immunity and thus more relapse of CM.

Conclusion

Cows those suffered by both relapse and recurrence were more susceptible to CM, and they need to be culled from farm to control the transmission of infections. Although the influence of seasonality was difficult to understand, the higher magnitude of relapse and recurrence during winter suggested the adverse effects of cold stress on treatment outcome. Further, understanding of different episodes of CM with severity, causative agent, and drugs will be really helpful to improve the therapeutic strategies in future.

Authors' Contributions

AM and AK designed the study and prepared the manuscript. NK executed while SL, ST, and SC assisted the study, and NK and TKP analyzed the data. All authors read and approved the final manuscript.

Acknowledgments

Authors are thankful to Head, SRS, and Director, ICAR-NDRI for providing needful facilities. Authors are also thankful to veterinarians and staff at LRC, NDRI. The fund for the study was provided by ICAR-NDRI, Karnal.

Table-3: Relationship between duration of treatment and number of clinical mastitis episodes in crossbred cows.

Duration of treatment (days)	No. of animals treated (%)	No. of CM episodes (%)	% higher episodes
1-8	961 (80.48)	1796 (78.87)	86.02[a]
9-15	144 (12.06)	305 (13.30)	110.41[b]
>15	89 (7.45)	176 (7.72)	97.75[c]
Total	1194	2277	90.70

Values with different superscript in a column varies significantly, 1-8 days varies from 9 to 15 and >15 at p<0.01, 9-15 varies from >15 at p<0.05, CM=Clinical mastitis

Table-4a: Relationship between duration of treatment and different episodes of clinical mastitis in crossbred cows.

Duration of treatment (days)	Single (%)	Relapse (%)	Recurrence (%)
1-8	528 (82.75)[a]	140 (74.86)[a]	171 (79.90)[a]
9-15	70 (10.97)[b]	28 (14.97)[a]	26 (12.14)[b]
>16	40 (6.26)[b]	19 (10.16)[b]	17 (7.94)[c]
Total	638	187	214

Values with different superscript in a column varies significantly at p<0.05

Table-4b: Relationship between 1 and 8 days treatment and different episodes of clinical mastitis in crossbred cows.

Duration of treatment (days)	No. of animals treated (%)	No. of mastitis episodes	% higher episodes	Single	Relapse	Recurrence
1-4	620 (65)	1146	84.83	352[a]	83	104[a]
5-8	341 (35)	652	91.20	176[b]	57	67[b]
Total	961	1798	87.09	528	140	171

Values with different superscript in a column varies significantly; 1-4 varies from 5 to 8 in single at p<0.01; 1-4 varies from 5 to 8 in recurrence at p<0.05

Table-5: Influence of season on incidence and number of clinical mastitis episodes in crossbred cows.

Season	No. of animals treated (%)	No. of mastitis episodes (%)	% higher episodes
Summer	287 (24.03)	578 (25.38)	101.39[a]
Winter	422 (35.34)	828 (36.36)	96.20[b]
Rainy	353 (29.56)	640 (28.11)	81.30[b]
Autumn	132 (11.00)	231 (10.15)	75.01[b]
Total	1194	2277	90.70

Values with different superscript in a column varies significantly at p<0.05

Table-6: Influence of season on different episodes of clinical mastitis in crossbred cows.

Season	Single (%)	Relapse (%)	Recurrence (%)
Summer	142 (22.25)[a]	46 (24.59)	61 (28.50)
Winter	208 (32.60)[b]	68 (36.36)	85 (39.71)
Rainy	207 (32.44)[b]	53 (28.34)	49 (22.89)
Autumn	81 (12.69)[c]	20 (10.69)	19 (8.87)
Total	638	187	214

Values with different superscript in a column varies significantly at p<0.05

Competing Interests

The authors declare that they have no competing interests.

References

1. Sharma, N., Srivastava, A.K., Bacic, G., Jeong, D.K. and Sharma, R.K. (2012) Epidemiology. In: Bovine Mastitis. 1st ed. Satish Serial Publishing House, New Delhi, India. p231-312.
2. Oliveira, L., Hulland, C. and Ruegg, P.L. (2013) Characterization of clinical mastitis occurring in cows on 50 large dairy herds in Wisconsin. *J. Dairy Sci.,* 96(12): 7538-7549.
3. Schukken, Y.H., Hertl, J., Bar, D., Bennett, G.J., Gonzalez, R.N., Rauch, B.J., Santisteban, C., Schulte, H.F., Tauer, L., Welcome, F.L. and Grohn, Y.T. (2009) Effects of repeated gram-positive and gram-negative clinical mastitis episodes on milk yield loss in Holstein dairy cows. *J. Dairy Sci.,* 92: 3091-3105.
4. Hertl, J.A., Grohn, Y.T., Leach, J.D.G., Bar, D., Bennett, G.J., Gonzalez, R.N., Rauch, B.J., Welcome, F.L., Tauer, L.W. and Schukken, Y.H. (2010) Effects of clinical mastitis caused by gram positive and gram-negative bacteria and other organisms on the probability of conception in New York State Holstein dairy cows. *J. Dairy Sci.,* 93: 1551-1560.
5. Hertl, J.A., Schukken, Y.H., Bar, D., Bennett, G.J., Gonzalez, R.N., Rauch, B.J., Welcome, F.L., Tauer, L.W. and Grohn, Y.T. (2011) The effect of recurrent episodes of clinical mastitis caused by gram-positive and gram-negative bacteria and other organisms on mortality and culling in Holstein dairy cows. *J. Dairy Sci.,* 94: 4863-4877.
6. Hertl, J.A., Schukken, Y.H., Welcome, F.L., Tauer, L.W. and Grohn, Y.T. (2014) Pathogen-specific effects on milk yield in repeated clinical mastitis episodes in Holstein dairy cows. *J. Dairy Sci.,* 973: 1465-1480.
7. Lukas, J.M., Reneau, J.K., Wallace, R., Hawkins, D. and Munoz-Zanzi, C. (2009) A novel method of analyzing daily milk production and electrical conductivity to predict disease onset. *J. Dairy Sci.,* 92: 5964-5976.
8. Wenz, J.R. (2004) Practical Monitoring of Clinical Mastitis Treatment Programs. Proceeding 43rd Annual National Mastitis Council Meeting Charlotte (NC). Verona (WI). National Mastitis Council. p41-46.
9. Pinzon-Sanchez, C. and Ruegg, P.L. (2011) Risk factors associated with short-term post-treatment outcomes of clinical mastitis. *J. Dairy. Sci.,* 94: 3397-3410.
10. Lago, A., Godden, S.M., Bey, R., Ruegg, P.L. and Leslie, K. (2011) The selective treatment of clinical mastitis based on on-farm culture results I: Effects on antibiotic use, milk withholding time and short-term clinical and bacteriological outcomes. *J. Dairy Sci.,* 84: 4441-4456.
11. Dopfer, D., Barkema, H.W., Lam, T.J., Schukken, Y.H. and Gaastra, W. (1999) Recurrent clinical mastitis caused by *Escherichia coli* in dairy cows. *J. Dairy Sci.,* 82: 80-85.
12. Zadoks, R.N., Allore, H.G., Barkema, H.W., Sampimon, O.C., Wellenberg, G.J., Grohn, Y.T. and Schukken, Y.H. (2001) Cow and quarter-level risk factors for *Streptococcus uberis* and *Staphylococcus aureus* mastitis. *J. Dairy Sci.,* 84: 2649-2663.
13. Lago, A., Godden, S.M., Bey, R., Ruegg, P.L. and Leslie, K. (2011) The selective treatment of clinical mastitis based on on-farm culture results: II. Effects on lactation performance, including clinical mastitis recurrence, somatic cell count, milk production, and cow survival. *J. Dairy Sci.,* 94: 4457-4467.
14. Van Eenennaam, A.L., Gardner, I.A., Holmes, J., Perani, L., Anderson, R.J., Cullor, J.S. and Guterbock, W.M. (1995) Financial analysis of alternative treatments for clinical mastitis associated with environmental pathogens. *J. Dairy Sci.,* 78: 2086-2095.
15. Apparao, M.D., Ruegg, P.L., Lago, A., Godden, S., Bey, R. and Leslie, K. (2009) Relationship between in vitro susceptibility test results and treatment outcomes for gram-positive mastitis pathogens following treatment with cephapirin sodium. *J. Dairy Sci.,* 92: 2589-2597.
16. Bradley, A.J. and Green, M.J. (2001) Adaptation of *Escherichia coli* to the bovine mammary gland. *J. Clin. Microbiol.,* 39(5): 1845-1849.
17. Bar, D., Grohn, Y.T., Bennett, G., Gonzalez, R.N., Hertl, J.A., Schulte, H.F., Tauer, L.W., Welcome, F.L. and Schukken, Y.H. (2007) Effect of repeated episodes of generic clinical mastitis on milk yield in dairy cows. *J. Dairy Sci.,* 90: 4643-4653.
18. Contreras, G.A. and Rodríguez, J.M. (2011) Mastitis: Comparative etiology and epidemiology. J. *Mammary Gland Biol. Neoplasia,* 16(4): 339-356.
19. Oliver, S.P, Almeida, R.A., Gillespie, B.E., Headrick, S.J., Dowlen, H.H. and Johnson, D.L. (2004) Extended ceftiofur therapy for treatment of experimentally induced *Streptococcus uberis* mastitis in lactating dairy cattle. *J. Dairy Sci.,* 87: 3322-3329.
20. Constable, P.D. and Morin, D.E. (2003) Treatment of clinical mastitis: Using antimicrobial susceptibility profiles for treatment decisions. *Vet. Clin. North Am. Food Anim. Pract.,* 19: 139-155.
21. Hoe, F.G.H. and Ruegg, P.L. (2005) Relationship between antimicrobial susceptibility of clinical mastitis pathogens and treatment outcome in cows. *J. Am. Vet. Med. Assoc.,* 227: 1461-1468.

5

Polymorphism in *spa* gene of *Staphylococcus aureus* from bovine subclinical mastitis

Taruna Bhati[1], Prerna Nathawat[1], Sandeep Kumar Sharma[2], Rahul Yadav[1], Jyoti Bishnoi[1] and Anil Kumar Kataria[1]

1. Department of Veterinary Microbiology and Biotechnology, College of Veterinary and Animal Science, Rajasthan University of Veterinary and Animals Sciences, Bikaner, Rajasthan, India; 2. Department of Veterinary Microbiology and Biotechnology, Post Graduate Institute of Veterinary Education and Research, Rajasthan University of Veterinary and Animals Sciences, Bikaner, Rajasthan, India.
Corresponding author: Taruna Bhati, e-mail: vetcvas.bhati@gmail.com,
PN: nathawatprerna@gmail.com, SKS: drsharmask01@gmail.com, RY: drrahul16889@gmail.com,
JB: jyotibishnoi88@gmail.com, AKK: akkataria1@rediffmail.com

Abstract

Aim: The virulence-associated protein-A of *Staphylococcus aureus*, encoded by *spa* gene shows a variation in length in different strains. In this study, the *spa* gene variation in *S. aureus* strains was studied which were isolated from subclinical cases of bovine mastitis.

Materials and Methods: About 38 isolates of *S. aureus* were recovered from Holstein–Friesian (HF) crossbred (n=16) and Rathi cattle (n=22) with subclinical mastitis as per standard procedures, and these isolates were subjected to amplification of *spa* gene (X-region) by polymerase chain reaction and calculation of number of tandem repeats were done.

Results: Of the 16 isolates from H-F crossbred cattle, all with the exception of one isolate produced *spa* amplicon. Seven isolates produced amplicons of 200 bp, one produced 160 bp, and other seven produced *spa* amplicon of 150 bp with calculated number of 6, 5, and 4 repeats, respectively, whereas nine different types of amplicons were produced by 22 *S. aureus* isolates from Rathi cattle, viz., 280, 250, 240, 200, 190, 180, 170, 150, and 140 bp with 10, 8, 8, 6, 6, 6, 5, 4, and 4 repeats, respectively. One of the isolates from Rathi cattle produced two *spa* amplicons (150 and 190 bp).

Conclusion: A greater polymorphism was observed in the *S. aureus* isolates from Rathi cattle than from H-F crossbreds with subclinical mastitis.

Keywords: cattle, polymorphism, protein-A, *spa* gene, *Staphylococcus aureus,* subclinical mastitis.

Introduction

Bovine mastitis is a well-known challenge to dairy industry in India. It affects the economy of farmers and hence of the country leading to an estimated annual loss of around US \$526 million [1]. *Staphylococcus aureus* is the most important pathogen associated with various clinical forms of mastitis [2]. Among the various clinical forms of mastitis caused by *S. aureus*, subclinical cases have special importance as they go unnoticed and affect production performance of animal to a large extent [3].

The development and severity of mastitis depend on the production of virulent protein known as protein-A [4]. This protein is encoded by *spa* gene which has been shown to have a high degree of variability in size [5]. This variation in the *spa* gene comes from the differences in the repetitive variable number of 24 bp repeats in X-region of gene. The number of

these 24 bp repeats varies among different strains of *S. aureus* and hence can be used as a molecular tool in studying the genetic diversity among the Indian strains of *S. aureus* for epidemiological tracing of source of infection and comparing the differences in virulent phenotypes among various strains. Although a lot of work has been conducted in typing of *S. aureus* from human cases in India [6-8], very limited work has been done in studying the genetic diversity using *spa* gene of *S. aureus* strains originating from bovine mastitis [9].

In view of the above facts, the present investigation was designed to study the polymorphism of *spa* gene (X-region) and evaluate its applicability in differentiating the Indian *S. aureus* strains of bovine origin.

Materials and Methods

Ethical approval

This study was conducted following approval by the research committee and Institutional Animal Ethics Committee Guidelines were followed.

Isolation of *S. aureus*
Sampling

Eighty-five milk samples were collected during early morning hours in sterilized test tubes from

Holstein–Friesian (H-F) crossbred and Rathi cattle from different locations in Bikaner (Rajasthan, India). The samples were immediately taken to the laboratory for further processing on ice.

Somatic cell counting (SCC)

A 0.1 ml amount from each properly shaken milk samples was withdrawn with Pasteur Pipette and spread evenly on a glass slide to count the SCC as per the method described earlier [10].

Identification of *S. aureus*

All the milk samples which showed SCC corresponding to subclinical mastitis were processed for isolation of *S. aureus*. Phenotypic and biochemical identification of isolates were done as per the standard protocol [11]. The isolates were further genotypically confirmed by *23S rRNA* species-specific polymerase chain reaction (PCR) using forward primer-1 (5′-AC GGAGTTACAAAGGACGAC-3′) and reverse prime r-2 (5′-AGCTCAGCCTTAACGAGTAC-3′) [12].

Amplification of *spa* gene

The amplification of *spa* gene encoding protein-A was done as described by Frenay *et al.* [13] with slight modifications using 5′-CAAGCACCAAAAGAGGAA-3′ (F) and 5′-CACCAGGTTTAACGACAT-3′ (R) primers. PCR was performed in 0.2 ml thin-walled PCR tubes. The PCR mixture contained a final concentration of 10 mM Tris–HCl, pH 9.0, 50 mM KCl, 3.5 mM MgCl$_2$, 1.0 µM concentration of each primer, 0.2 mM concentrations of each 2'-deoxynucleoside 5'-triphosphate and 1.0 U of Taq DNA polymerase. The PCR was performed in Palmcycler (Corbett Research, Australia) using following cycling parameters: Initial 34 cycle of amplification (denaturation at 94°C for 60 s, primer annealing at 55°C for 60 s and primer extension at 70°C for 60 s), and final extension at 72°C for 5 min. Two µl of trekking dye was added to the PCR products and were resolved in 1.2% agarose gels prepared in 1× TBE buffer containing 0.5 µg/ml of ethidium bromide. 100 bp DNA ladder was used as molecular marker and the amplification products electrophoresed for 1 h at 100 V. The gel was then visualized under U.V. Transillumination and photographed. Calculation of a number of tandem repeats (N) in PCR amplified *spa* gene product was done using the formula given by Frenay *et al.* [13]. Mathematically, formula is given as:

$$N = \frac{\text{Size of amplified } spa \text{ gene product} - \text{Size of primers (forward + reverse)}}{24}$$

Results

Out of the 85 milk samples, 38 milk samples showed SCC in the range of 200×10^3 to 500×10^3 cells/ml corresponding to subclinical cases of mastitis as per the IDF (2005) criterion [14]. The SCC has been detected to be the most reliable test and closest to the bacteriological results for SCM in dairy

cows by Sharma *et al.* (2010) [15]. A total of 38 isolates of *S. aureus* were isolated from these samples and identified on the basis of cultural and biochemical properties. All 38 isolates produced an amplicon of 1,250 bp in species-specific PCR targeting *23S rRNA* gene. Out of 38 isolates, 16 were isolated from H-F crossbred cattle and 22 from native Rathi cattle.

In the present investigation, out of 16 isolates from H-F crossbred cattle, 15 strains produced *spa* amplicons, whereas one isolate did not produce any amplified product (Figures-1 and 2). Seven isolates produced amplicons of 200 bp, one produced 160 bp amplicon, and other seven produced amplicon of 150 bp with calculated number of 6, 5, 4 repeats, respectively (Table-1). The *spa* gene X-region amplicons produced by 22 isolates from Rathi cattle were of greater variability (Figures-2 and 3) than that in isolates from H-F crossbred cattle as nine different types of amplicons were obtained of size 280, 250, 240, 200, 190, 180, 170, 150, and 140 bp with calculated number of 10, 8, 8, 6, 6, 6, 5, 4, and 4 repeats, respectively (Table-2). The amplicon of 150 bp size was found to be produced by maximum (15 isolates) number of isolates followed by amplicons of 200 bp (11 isolates) and 280 and 240 bp (three each). One isolate from Rathi cattle produced two bands of *spa* amplicons (150 and 190 bp).

Discussion

The PCR amplification of *spa* gene (X-region) yielded amplicons similar to that recorded by Salasia *et al.* [16] who obtained nine different sized amplicons

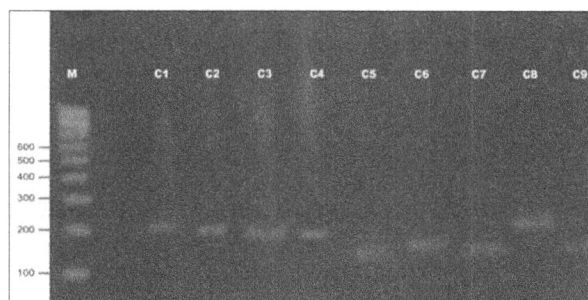

Figure-1: Polymerase chain reaction amplicons of *spa* gene (X-region) of *Staphylococcus aureus* isolates from Holstein–Friesian crossbred cattle (C1-C9) with subclinical mastitis.

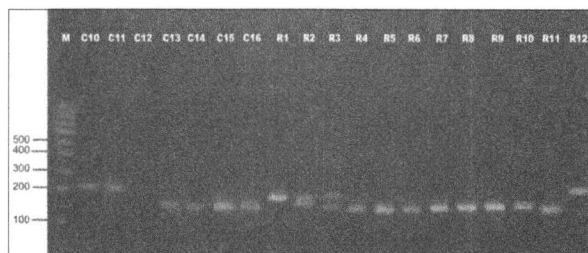

Figure-2: Polymerase chain reaction amplicons of *spa* gene (X-region) of *Staphylococcus aureus* isolates from Holstein–Friesian crossbred cattle (C10-C16) and Rathi cattle (R1-R12) with subclinical mastitis.

of 100-340 bp in *S. aureus* isolates from bovine subclinical mastitis. Bystron *et al.* [17] also recorded 10 different sizes of *spa* amplicons in the *S. aureus* isolates from unprocessed cow milk, but their amplicon size varied from 3 to 14 repeats having the highest frequency of eight to 10 repeats. In our study, however, the size varied from 4 to 10 repeats with a maximum frequency of four repeats.

The *spa* types in this study corroborated the earlier observations of Karahan *et al.* [18] who also carried out *spa* typing of *S. aureus* strains isolated from bovine subclinical mastitis and recorded nine *spa* types with amplicons ranging from 100 to 320 bp where most of the *spa* types were similar to that obtained in this study. However, contrarily, they obtained *spa* amplicons with 290 bp and 10 repeat units as predominant *spa* type, whereas in our study 150 bp *spa* amplicons with four repeats were predominant.

In our study, only seven of the isolates produced *spa* amplicons with calculated number of more than seven repeats. Freney *et al.* [19] reported that most

epidemic MRSA strains harbored more than seven repeats while non-epidemic MRSA strains contained seven or fewer repeats. They discussed that a longer X-region results in a better exposition of the Fc binding region of protein-A thereby facilitating colonization on both surfaces and contributing to the epidemic phenotypes. Considering the above fact, in the present investigation less number of isolates were detected to be pathogenic in regards to *spa* typing.

One isolate from Rathi cattle produced two bands of *spa* amplicons (150 and 190 bp) which are in conformity to the earlier observation by Rathore *et al.* [20] who recorded two *spa* bands in one isolate of *S. aureus* isolated from camel skin wounds. One of the 38 isolates did not produce *spa* amplicon. The absence of *spa*-X region gene has also been reported by Kalorey *et al.* [21] in subclinical mastitis, Momtaz *et al.* [22] from bovine clinical and subclinical mastitis, Salem-Bekhit *et al.* [23] in bovine mastitis isolates, and Shakeri *et al.* [24] in healthy carriers and human patients.

Conclusion

This study revealed polymorphism in *spa* X-region gene amplicons of *S. aureus* obtained from subclinical mastitis cases. A greater polymorphism was observed in the isolates from native breed. Based on the number of repeats, it was deduced that in this study though both pathogenic and non-pathogenic strains were recovered from sub-clinical mastitis cases but nonpathogenic strains were more in number.

Authors' Contributions

AKK was the major guide of my MVSc research work and he planned and designed the study. This work is a part of my MVSc thesis. RY and PN helped in conducting the Laboratory work. Lab analysis was carried out by SKS and JB. The manuscript was revised and edited under the guidance of AKK. All authors participated in writing and revision process and approved of the final manuscript.

Acknowledgments

The first author wishes to acknowledge the institutional fellowship provided by the Rajasthan University of Veterinary and Animal Sciences (RAJUVAS) Bikaner for MVSc thesis work. The

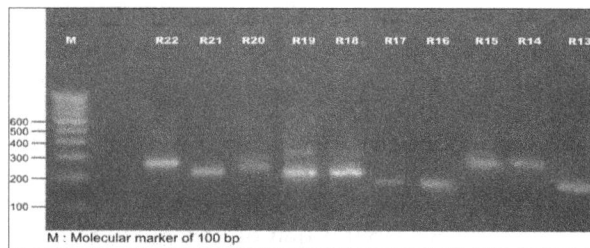

Figure-3: Polymerase chain reaction amplicons of *spa* gene (X-region) of *Staphylococcus aureus* isolates from Rathi cattle (R13-R22) with subclinical mastitis.

Table-1: *spa* gene (X-region) polymorphism in *S. aureus* isolates from H-F crossbred cattle with subclinical mastitis.

Serial number	Isolate numbers	Total isolates	*spa* gene amplicon (bp)	Total number of repeats
1	C1, C2, C3, C4, C8, C10, C11	7	200	6
2	C6	1	160	5
3	C5, C7, C9, C13, C14, C15, C16	7	150	4

S. aureus=*Staphylococcus aureus*, H-F=Holstein–Friesian

Table-2: *spa* gene (X-region) polymorphism in *S. aureus* isolates from Rathi cattle with subclinical mastitis.

Serial number	Isolate numbers	Total isolates	*spa* gene amplicon (bp)	Total number of repeats
1	R14, R15, R22	3	280	10
2	R20	1	250	8
3	R18, R19, R21	3	240	8
4	R12, R13, R16, R17	4	200	6
5	R3	1	190,150	6,4
6	R1	1	180	6
7	R2	1	170	5
8	R4, R5, R6, R7, R8, R9, R10	7	150	4
9	R11	1	140	4

S. aureus=*Staphylococcus aureus*

authors are highly thankful to the Department of Veterinary Microbiology and Biotechnology, College of Veterinary and Animal Sciences, RAJUVAS, for providing necessary facilities to carry out the research work.

Competing Interests

The authors declare that they have no competing interests.

References

1. Dua, K. (2010) Incidence, etiology and estimated economic losses due to mastitis in Punjab and India - An update. *Indian Dairyman*, 53: 41-48.

2. Aires-de-Sousa, M., Parente, C.E.S., Vieira-da-Motta, O., Bonna, I.C., Silva, D.A. and De Lencastre, H. (2007) Characterization of *Staphylococcus aureus* isolates from buffalo, bovine, ovine, and caprine milk samples collected in Rio de Janeiro State, Brazil. *Appl. Environ. Microb.* 73: 3845-3849.

3. Suleiman, A.B., Kwaga, J.K.P., Umoh, V.J., Okolocha, E.C., Muhammed, M., Lammler, C., Shaibu, S.J., Akinden, O. and Weiss, R. (2012) Macro-restriction analysis of *Staphlyococcus aureus* isolated from subclinical bovine mastitis in Nigeria. *Afr. J. Microbiol. Res.* 6(33): 6270-6274.

4. Mitra, S.D., Velu, D., Bhuvana, M., Krithiga, N., Banerjee, A., Shome, R., Rahman, H., Ghosh, S.K. and Shome, B.R. (2013) *Staphylococcus aureus* spa type t267, clonal ancestor of bovine subclinical mastitis in India. *J. Appl. Microbiol.*, 14(6): 1604-1615.

5. Brandt, K.M., Mellmann, A., Ballhausen, B., Jenke, C., van der Wolf, P.J., Broens, E.M., Becker, K. and Kock, R. (2013) Evaluation of multiple-locus variable number of tandem repeats analysis for typing livestock-associated methicillin-resistant *Staphylococcus aureus*. *PLoS One*, 8(1): 54425.

6. Nadig, S., Velusamy, N., Lalitha, P., Kar, S., Sharma, S. and Arakere, G. (2012) *Staphylococcus aureus* eye infections in two Indian hospitals: Emergence of ST772 as a major clone. *Clin. Ophthalmol.*, 6: 165-73.

7. Mehndiratta, P.L., Bhalla, P., Ahmed, A. and Sharma, Y.D. (2009) Molecular typing of methicillin-resistant *Staphylococcus aureus* strains by PCR-RFLP of *spa* gene: A reference laboratory perspective. *Indian J. Med. Microbiol.*, 27(2): 116-122.

8. Dhawan, B., Rao, C., Udo, E.E., Gadepalli, R., Vishnubhatla, S. and Kapil, A. (2014) Dissemination of methicillin-resistant *Staphylococcus aureus* SCCmec type IV and SCC mec type V epidemic clones in a tertiary hospital: Challenge to infection control. *Epidemiol. Infect.*, 2: 1-11.

9. Khichar, V., Kataria, A.K. and Sharma, R. (2014) Characterization of *Staphylococcus aureus* of cattle mastitis origin for two virulence – Associated genes (*coa* and *spa*). *Comp. Clin. Pathol.*, 23(3): 603-611.

10. Prescott, S.C. and Breed, R.S. (1910) The determination of the number of body cells in milk by a direct method. *J. Infect. Dis. 7:* 632.

11. Quinn, P.J., Carter, M.E., Markey, B.K. and Carter, G.R. (1994) Clinical Veterinary Microbiology. Wolfe Publishing, Mosby-Year Book Europe Ltd., England.

12. Straub, J.A., Hertel, C. and Hammes, W.P. (1999) A 23S rRNA target polymerase chain reaction based system for detection of *Staphylococcus aureus* in meat starter cultures and dairy products. *J. Food Protect.*, 62(10): 1150-1156.

13. Frenay, H.M.E., Bunschoten, A.E., Schouls, L.M., Van Leeuwen, W.J., Vandenbroucke-Grauls, C.M., Verhoef, J. and Mooi, F.R. (1996) Molecular typing of methicillin-resistant *Staphylococcus aureus* on the basis of protein A gene polymorphism. *Eur. J. Clin. Microbiol.*, 15(1): 60-64.

14. International Dairy Federation, (IDF). (2005) Diagnostic potential of California Mastitis Test to Detect Subclinical Mastitis 26. IDF, Maastricht, Netherlands. p15-19.

15. Sharma, N., Pandey, V. and Sudhan, N.A. (2010) Comparison of some indirect screening tests for detection of sub-clinical mastitis in dairy cows. *Bulg. J. Vet. Med.*, 13: 98-103.

16. Salasia, S.I., Khusnan, Z., Lammler, C. and Zschock, M. (2004) Comparative studies on phenol - and genotypic properties of *Staphylococcus aureus* isolated from bovine sub-clinical mastitis in central Java in Indonesia and Hesse in Germany. *J. Vet. Sci.*, 5(2): 103-109.

17. Bystron, J., Bania, J., Lis, E., Molenda, J. and Bednarski, M. (2009) Characterisation of *Staphylococcus aureus* strains isolated from Cow's milk *B. Vet. I. Pulawy*, 53: 59-63.

18. Karahan, M., Aciki, M.N. and Cetinkaya, B. (2011) Investigation of virulence genes by PCR in *Stapylococcus aureus* isolates originated from subclinical bovine mastitis in Turkey. *Pak. Vet. J.*, 31(3): 249-253.

19. Frenay, H.M.E., Theelen, J.P.G., Schouls, L.M., Vandenbroucke-Grauls, C.M.J.E., Verhoef, J., Van Leeuwen, W.J. and Mooi, F.R. (1994) Discrimination of epidemic and non-epidemic methicillin-resistant *Staphylococcus aureus* strains on the basis of protein A gene polymorphism. *J. Clin. Microbiol.*, 32: 846-847.

20. Rathore, P., Kataria, A.K., Khichar, V. and Sharma, R. (2012) Polymorphism in *coa* and *spa* virulence genes in *Staphylococcus aureus* of camel skin origin. *J. Camel. Pract. Res.*, 19(2): 129-134.

21. Kalorey, D.R., Shanmugam, Y., Kurkure, N.V., Chousalkar, K. and Barbuddhe, S.B. (2007) PCR-based detection of genes encoding virulence determinants in *Staphylococcus aureus* from bovine subclinical mastitis cases. *J. Vet. Sci.*, 8(2): 151-154.

22. Momtaz, H., Rahimi, E. and Tajbakhsh, E. (2010) Detection of some virulence factors in *Staphylococcus aureus* isolated from clinical and subclinical bovine mastitis in Iran. *Afr. J. Biotechnol.*, 9(25): 3753-3758.

23. Salem-Bekhit, M.M., Muharram, M.M., Alhosiny, I.M. and Hashim, M.E.S. (2010) Molecular detection of genes encoding virulence determinants in *Staphylococcus aureus* strains isolated from bovine mastitis. *J. Appl. Sci. Res.*, 6(2): 121-128.

24. Shakeri, F., Shojai, A., Golalipour, M., Alang, S.R., Vaez, H. and Ghaemi, E.A. (2010) *Spa* diversity among MRSA and MSSA strains of *Staphylococcus aureus* in North of Iran. *Int. J. Microbiol.*, 2010: Article ID: 351397, 5.

6

Effect of egg yolk powder on freezability of Murrah buffalo (*Bubalus bubalis*) semen

N. Kumar[1], S. A. Lone[1], J. K. Prasad[2], M. H. Jan[3] and S. K. Ghosh[2]

1. Division of Animal Reproduction, Gynecology & Obstetrics, NDRI, Karnal, Haryana, India; 2. Germ Plasm Centre, Division of Animal Reproduction, Indian Veterinary Research Institute, Izatnagar, Bareilly, Uttar Pradesh, India; 3. Central Institute for Research on Buffalo, Hisar, Haryana, India.
Corresponding author: N. Kumar, e-mail: drnishantvet@yahoo.com,
SAL: drloneshabir@gmail.com, JKP: jkprasad2001@yahoo.com, MHJ: mhjanivri@gmail.com,
SKG: skghoshivri@yahoo.com

Abstract

Aim: The aim of this study was to investigate the effect of commercial egg yolk powder as an alternative to fresh egg yolk on freezability of Murrah buffalo semen.

Materials and Methods: Semen samples (12) from 3 Murrah buffaloes (4 from each bull) with mass motility ($\geq$3+) and total motility (70% and above) were utilized in this study. Immediately after collection, each sample was divided into four groups. Groups I was diluted up to 60×10^6 sperm/ml with tris extender containing 10% fresh egg yolk and Groups II, III, and IV were diluted up to 60×10^6 sperm/ml with tris extender containing 2%, 4%, and 6% egg yolk powder, respectively. Semen samples were processed and cryopreserved followed by examination of frozen semen samples after 24 h. Semen samples from each group were evaluated for total motility, viability, acrosomal integrity, abnormality, and hypo-osmotic swelling test (HOST) response after dilution, pre-freeze, and post-thaw stage.

Results: Pre-freeze total motility was significantly (p<0.05) higher in Groups III and IV as compared to Groups I and II, and post-thaw total motility was significantly (p<0.01) higher in Group III as compared to other three groups. Viability was significantly (p<0.05) higher in Groups II, III, and IV than Group I at the pre-freeze stage. Significantly (p<0.01) higher viability and acrosomal integrity were recorded in Group III as compared to other three groups at the post-thaw stage. Abnormality was significantly (p<0.05) higher in Group IV than other three groups. HOST response was significantly (p<0.05) higher in Groups II and III than Groups I and IV at the pre-freeze and post-thaw stages.

Conclusion: Addition of egg yolk powder at 4% level yielded significantly better results in terms of post-thaw semen quality as compared to the fresh egg yolk and other concentrations of egg yolk powder (2% and 6%).

Keywords: buffalo semen, egg yolk powder, freezability.

Introduction

The beneficial effect of egg yolk on spermatozoa during liquid storage and cryopreservation was first time reported by Phillips and Lardy in 1940 [1]. Egg yolk protects spermatozoa against cold shock, reduces loss of acrosomal enzymes, and helps in preserving semen quality [2]. The protective effects of egg yolk are due to low-density lipoprotein fraction present in it. Egg yolk has been included in dilutor at concentrations ranging from 1.5% to 50% [2]. Harvesting egg yolk is a cumbersome process because it involves proper disease screening, disinfection, skilful breaking of the outer shell, and inner membrane to separate the yolk from albumin and chalazae [3].

Due to the animal origin of egg yolk, it represents a potential risk of microbial contamination in the diluent. Although egg yolk benefits spermatozoa during cryopreservation, it can represent a potential risk to cells as they may contain specific microbial agents or other contaminants that may compromise sperm quality [4]. Terrestrial Animal Health Code (OIE) recommended that products used to treat spermatozoa should originate from sources of animal origin, which are free from any health risks [5]. This can be accomplished using egg yolk powder, instead of fresh egg yolk, as it is pasteurized. The use of egg yolk powder is documented for the cryopreservation of ovine [6], Zebu bull [7], and buffalo [8] and it is reported that semen treated with egg yolk powder had higher post-thaw motility as compared to fresh egg yolk treated semen.

In buffalo semen, egg yolk powder was used at the rate of 5%, 10%, and 20%, and it was shown that at higher concentration of egg yolk powder (20%), the post-thaw quality of semen deteriorated [8]. It is, therefore, hypothesized that the use of egg yolk powder in the dilutor for the cryopreservation of buffalo bull semen at lesser concentration as reported earlier will not compromise the post-thaw attributes, and the same will reduce the cost of cryopreservation. Hence, the present study was designed to investigate the effect of egg yolk powder on quality and freezability of buffalo semen.

Materials and Methods

Ethical approval

No ethical approval was necessary to pursue this research work.

Experimental animals

Three healthy breeding buffalo bulls of approximately 4-6 years of age maintained at GermPlasm Center of Animal Reproduction Division, IVRI, Izatnagar, were utilized for the study. These bulls were kept under identical feeding and managemental conditions during the entire course of theinvestigation.

Collection of semen and its processing

Four different dilutors containing 2%, 4%, and 6% w/v egg yolk powder (Sigma, USA) and 10% v/v fresh egg yolk, respectively, were prepared and kept at 37°C. A total of 12 ejaculates (4 from each bull) were collected from three Murrah breeding bulls with artificial vagina. Ejaculates with mass motility ≥3+ and total motility 70% and above were utilized for the present study. Semen ejaculates that qualified for cryopreservation were split into four groups. Group I was diluted with tris-egg yolk-glycerol dilutor (containing 10% fresh egg yolk) up to 60×10^6 spermatozoa/ml. Groups II, III, and IV were diluted with tris dilutor containing 2%, 4%, and 6% egg yolk powder, respectively. After dilution, the percentage of various seminal attributes (total motility, viability, acrosomal integrity, abnormality, and hypo-osmotic swelling response) was recorded in each group.

Semen freezing and its evaluation

French mini straws (0.25 ml) were filled with the diluted semen samples, sealed with polyvinyl alcohol powder and kept for 4 h at 5°C for equilibration. After equilibration, straws were kept in automatic programmable biological cell freezer (IMV Technology, France) until the temperature of straws reached −140°C. Then, straws were plunged into liquid nitrogen (−196°C) for storage and stored for 24 h before thawing at 37°C for 30 s. From each group, semen samples were evaluated for various seminal attributes (total motility, viability, acrosomal integrity, abnormality, and hypo-osmotic swelling response) at pre-freeze and post-thaw stage.

Semen evaluation

Seminal attributes

A drop of the diluted semen was kept on a clean, grease free, pre-warmed glass slide; cover slip was placed, and total motility was assessed under high power magnification (400×magnification) of a phase contrast microscope. Percentage of live and abnormal spermatozoa was determined by a differential staining technique using Eosin-Nigrosin stain [9]. Acrosomal intactness was determined by Giemsa stain as per method described by Watson [10]. Hypo-osmotic swelling test (HOST) was carried out according to the method described by Jeyendran *et al.* [11].

Statistical analysis

Data were statistically analyzed by one-way ANOVA and results were expressed as mean±standard error. Means were compared using Tukey's multiple comparisons test. The statistical package of GraphPad Prism, San Diego, USA was used for analyzing the data.

Results and Discussion

Total motility

The mean values of total motility are presented in Table-1. The total motility of a semen sample gives a good indication of fertility of the bull and ability of spermatozoa to withstand the stress of the cryopreservation process. After dilution, the percentage of total motility was 74.67±1.09, 74.50±0.92, 74.58±1.03,

Table-1: Effect of egg yolk powder on seminal attributes and sperm function of buffalo semen at post-dilution, pre-freeze, and post-thaw stage.

Seminal attributes	Stage	Group I	Group II	Group III	Group IV
Total motility	PD	74.67±1.09	74.50±0.92	74.58±1.03	75.17±1.15
	PF	67.42±1.19^B	67.78±0.99^B	69.50±1.14^A	68.92±1.16^A
	PT	48.17±0.71^b	49.85±0.78^b	54.58±0.65^a	48.75±0.83^b
Viability	PD	76.25±1.07	76.25±1.28	77.17±1.22	76.83±1.17
	PF	69.67±1.19^B	70.75±1.19^A	71.08±1.31^A	70.17±1.22^A
	PT	54.78±1.44^b	55.34±0.75^b	61.33±0.71^a	54.25±1.00^b
Acrosomal integrity	PD	78.58±1.01	78.50±1.13	78.83±1.15	78.42±1.15
	PF	72.50±1.00	72.75±1.21	72.67±1.10	72.83±1.01
	PT	57.69±0.88^b	57.50±0.71^b	65.67±0.54^a	58.50±0.71^b
Abnormality	PD	10.33±0.47	10.33±0.45	9.83±0.41	10.67±0.41
	PF	11.00±0.46	10.75±0.41	10.58±0.38	11.17±0.46
	PT	11.25±0.45^B	11.25±0.48^B	10.78±0.40^B	12.50±0.50^A
HOS (%)	PD	68.75±0.87	69.83±0.74	69.33±0.78	69.75±0.81
	PF	61.08±0.81^B	63.17±0.81^A	62.67±0.69^A	60.92±0.82^B
	PT	41.76±0.69^B	44.17±0.79^A	45.50±0.94^A	40.83±0.72^B

PD=Post-dilution, PF=Pre-freeze, PT=Post-thaw. Groups I, II, III, and IV contain 10% fresh egg yolk, 2%, 4%, and 6% egg yolk powder, respectively. Mean showing different superscripts in upper case letters (A and B) and lower case letters (a and b) in row differ significantly at 5% ($p<0.05$) and 1% ($p<0.01$), respectively

and 75.17±1.15 in Groups I, II, III, and IV, respectively. No significant difference in motility percentage at post-dilution was recorded among any groups. After dilution, the percentage of motile spermatozoa was higher than the values reported by Mittal *et al.* [12]. At pre-freeze stage, the percentage of motile spermatozoa was significantly (p<0.05) higher in Groups III and IV as compared to Groups I and II. At pre-freeze stage, the percentage of motile spermatozoa was higher than the values reported by Rao *et al.* [13]. At post-thaw stage, percentage of individual motility was significantly (p<0.01) higher in Group III as compared to other three groups. The percentage reduction in total motility was 35.48, 33.08, 26.18, and 35.14 in Groups I, II, III, and IV, respectively.

Viability

Viability of spermatozoa in a semen sample is significantly and positively correlated with initial motility, post-thaw motility, and fertility of spermatozoa. Post-dilution viability was 76.25±1.07, 76.25±1.28, 77.17±1.22, and 76.83±1.17 in Groups I, II, III, and IV, respectively. The percentage of live spermatozoa was higher than the values reported by Bhakat *et al.* [14]. No significant differences in viability percentage were recorded among any groups post-dilution. At pre-freeze stage, percent viability was significantly (p<0.05) higher in Groups II, III, and IV as compared to Group I. At post-thaw stage, percent viability was significantly (p<0.01) higher in Group III as compared to Groups I, II, and IV. The percentage reduction in viability was 28.15, 27.42, 20.52, and 29.61 in Groups I, II, III, and IV, respectively.

Acrosomal integrity

Acrosomal integrity of mammalian spermatozoa is prerequisite for capacitation, normal acrosome reaction, and successful fertilization *in vivo*. The percentage of intact acrosomes after dilution in Groups I, II, III, and IV was 78.58±1.01, 78.50±1.13, 78.83±1.15, and 78.42±1.15, respectively. The percentage of spermatozoa with intact acrosome was higher than the values reported by Meena *et al.* [15] and Patel and Siddiquee [16]. After dilution and pre-freeze stage, no significant difference in the percentage of acrosomal integrity was recorded among any groups. However, at post-thaw stage, the percentage of spermatozoa with intact acrosome was significantly (p<0.01) higher in Group III as compared to other three groups. Values of acrosomal integrity in all groups were lower which can normally occur in buffalo semen and also observed by Singh *et al.* [8]. Percentage decline in acrosomal integrity was 26.58, 26.75, 16.69, and 25.40 in Groups I, II, III, and IV, respectively.

Abnormality

After dilution, the percentage of abnormal spermatozoa in Groups I, II, III, and IV was 10.33±0.47, 10.33±0.45, 9.83±0.41, and 10.67±0.41, respectively. The percentage of abnormal spermatozoa was in agreement to the reports of Bhakat *et al.* [14]. No significant difference in the percentage of abnormal spermatozoa was recorded after dilution and at the pre-freeze stage. However, at post-thaw stage, the percentage of abnormal spermatozoa were significantly (p<0.05) higher in Group IV as compared to other three groups.

HOST response

The percentage of HOST positive spermatozoa after dilution in Groups I, II, III, and IV were 68.75±0.87, 69.83±0.74, 69.33±0.78, and 69.75±0.81, respectively. The HOST (%) in our study was comparable to values of Meena *et al.* [15] but higher than the values reported by Bhakat *et al.* [14]. No significant difference in HOST response was recorded after dilution among any groups. However, at pre-freeze and post-thaw stage, the percentage of HOST positive spermatozoa were significantly (p<0.05) higher in Groups II and III as compared to Groups I and IV. The percentage reduction in HOST response was 39.25, 36.76, 34.37, and 41.46 in Groups I, II, III, and IV, respectively.

Conclusion

Addition of egg yolk powder at 4% level in the extender yielded significantly better results in terms post-thaw semen quality as compared to the fresh egg yolk and other levels of egg yolk powder (2% and 6%). Egg yolk powder at a level of 4% can be effectively used as an alternative to fresh egg yolk for cryopreservation of Murrah buffalo semen.

Author's Contributions

NK and SAL planned and carried out research work. JKP and SKG provided lab facility and necessary help during research work. MHJ helped in the statistical analysis of Data. All authors read and approved the final manuscript.

Acknowledgments

The authors are thankful to Director, Indian Veterinary Research Institute, Izatnagar- 243122, Bareilly, for providing facilities and fund during this research work.

Competing Interests

The authors declare that they have no competing interests.

References

1. Phillips, P.H. and Lardy, H.A. (1940) A yolk-buffer pabulum for preservation of bull sperm. *J. Dairy Sci.,* 2: 399-404.
2. Salamon, S. and Maxwell, W.M.C. (1995) Frozen storage of ram semen I. Processing, freezing, thawing and fertility after cervical insemination (review). *Anim. Reprod. Sci.,* 37: 185-249.
3. Andrabi, S.M.H., Ansari, M.S., Ullah, N., Anwar, M., Mehmood, A. and Akhter, S. (2008) Duck egg yolk in extender improves the freezability of buffalo bull spermatozoa. *Anim. Reprod. Sci.,*104: 427-433.
4. Gil, J., Lundeheim, N., Soderquist, L. and Rodrı´guez-Martı´nez, H. (2003) Influence of extender, temperature, and addition of glycerol on post-thaw sperm parameters in ram semen. *Theriogenology,* 59: 1241-1255.

5. OIE. (2003) Terrestrial Animal Health Code. Appendix 3.2.1, Article 3.2.2.4. Available from: http://www.oie.int/eng/normes/Mcode/A_summry.htm. Accessed on 21-07-2014.

6. Marco-Jiménez, F., Puchades, S., Mocé, E., Viudes-de-Cartro, M.P., Vicente, J.S. and Rodriguez, M. (2004) Use of powdered egg yolk vs fresh egg yolk for the cryopreservation of ovine semen. *Reprod. Domest. Anim.,* 39: 438-441.

7. Ansari, M.S., Rakha, B.A., Andrabi, S.M.H. and Akhter, S. (2010) Usefulness of powdered and fresh egg yolk for cryopreservation of Zebu bull spermatozoa. *Reprod. Biol.,* 10(3): 235-240.

8. Singh, M., Barik, N.C., Ghosh, S.K., Prasad, J.K., Rajoriya, J.S., Soni, Y.K., Kumar, A., Chaudhary, J.K. and Srivastava, N. (2015) Egg yolk powder an alternative to fresh egg yolk for buffalo semen cryopreservation. *Indian J. Anim. Sci.,* 85(1): 40-42.

9. Campbell, R.G., Hancock, J.L. and Rothschild, L. (1953) Counting live and dead bull spermatozoa. *J. Exp. Biol.,* 30: 44-45.

10. Watson, P.F. (1975) Use of Giemsa stain to detect changes in the acrosome of frozen ram spermatozoa. *Vet. Rec.,* 97: 12-15.

11. Jeyendran, R.S., Vander Ven, H.H., Parez-pelaez, M.,

Crabo, B.G. and Zaneweld, L.J.D. (1984) Development of an assay to assess the functional integrity of the human membrane and its relationship to other semen characteristics. *J. Reprod. Infertil.,* 70: 219-228.

12. Mittal, P.K., Anand, M., Madan, A.K., Yadav, S. and Kumar, J (2014) Antioxidative capacity of vitamin E, vitamin C and their combination in cryopreserved Bhadavari bull semen. *Vet. World,* 7(12): 1127-1131.

13. Rao, T.K.S., Kumar, N., Patel, N.B., Chauhan, I. and Chaurasia, S. (2013) Sperm selection techniques and antioxidant fortification in low grade semen of bulls: Review. *Vet. World,* 6(8): 579-585.

14. Bhakat, M., Mohanty, T.K., Singh, S., Gupta, A.K., Chakravarty, A.K. and Singh, P. (2015) Influence of semen collector on semen characteristics of Murrah buffalo and crossbred bulls. *Adv. Anim. Vet. Sci.,* 3: 253-258.

15. Meena, G.S., Raina, V.S., Gupta, A.K., Mohanty, T.K., Bhakat, M., Abdullah, M. and Bishist, R. (2015) Effect of preputial washing on bacterial load and preservability of semen in Murrah buffalo bulls. *Vet. World,* 8(6): 798-803.

16. Patel, B.R. and Siddiquee, G.M. (2013) Physical and morphological characteristics of Kankrej bull semen. *Vet. World,* 6(7): 405-408.

7

Comparative study on immunoglobulin Y transfer from breeding hens to egg yolk and progeny chicks in different breeds of poultry

Ritu Agrawal, S. D. Hirpurkar, C. Sannat and Amit Kumar Gupta

Department of Veterinary Microbiology, College of Veterinary Science & Animal Husbandry,
Anjora, Durg, Chhattisgarh, India.
Corresponding author: C. Sannat, e-mail: csannat@rediffmail.com,
RA: ritu2808@rediffmail.com; SDH: smpuhir@yahoo.com; AKG: dramitkumaragrahari2009@gmail.com

Abstract

Aim: This study was undertaken to compare the immunoglobulin Y (IgY) level and its efficacy in laying hens of four different breeds of poultry (*viz.*,Vanraja, Gramapriya, BlackRock, and KalingaBrown) and its relative transfer in egg yolk and chick.

Materials and Methods: This study was conducted in 48 apparently healthy laying hens vaccinated with *Salmonella* inactivated polyvalent vaccine, eggs and progeny chicks; 12 each from four different breeds of poultry,*viz.*,Vanraja, Gramapriya, BlackRock, and KalingaBrown. The methodology included measurement of egg and yolk weight, total protein and IgY in egg yolk, total serum protein and IgY in breeding hens, and progeny chicks and extent of IgY transfer from hens to yolk then to chicks. Further, *Salmonella*-specific antibodies in breeding hens, egg yolk and progeny chicks were assessed using O and H antigen by tube agglutination test.

Results: The egg weight differed nonsignificantly (p>0.05) among breeds, however, breed wise significant variation (p<0.01) was reported in yolk weight. The weight of egg yolk significantly affects the total protein and IgY concentration although these levels per unit of volume did not differ. Total protein was significantly higher (p<0.01) in KalingaBrown and Gramapriya as compared to Vanraja and BlackRock. Non-significant (p>0.05) difference among breed was found in total protein of egg yolk and chick. The IgY concentration in hens, egg yolk and chick was found to be in the range of 5.35±0.63-5.83±0.65, 2.3±0.1-2.6±0.2, and 1.3±0.11-1.7±0.16 mg/ml, respectively which is uniform and independent of total protein concentration at all the three levels. Significant breed variations were not observed in maternal IgY transfer from breeding hens to chicks and were 25.62±1.42-36.06±4.34% of total IgY in parent flock. Moderate to higher rate of seroprevalence with peak titers of 1:640 against *Salmonella*-specific antibodies was observed in only 41.6% of breeding hens.

Conclusion: No significant difference in the rate of transfer of IgY was observed in four breeds studied (*viz.*,Vanraja, Gramapriya, BlackRock, and KalingaBrown) and moderate seropositivity was detected for *Salmonella*-specific antibodies in progeny chicks.

Keywords: breeding hens, chicks, maternal immunoglobulin Y, *Salmonella* antibody, yolk.

Introduction

Chicken of all age groups are susceptible to many pathogens if innate immune response by maternal antibody transfer and/or active immune response by foreign materials (vaccine) are not evoked at its full potential [1]. In general, advanced poultry production practice promises full protection by immunization which is cleverly designed by a combination of breeder hen vaccination and active immunization of chicks at appropriate age during early life. Efficacy of breeder hen vaccination is adjudged by quantum of maternal antibodies received by progeny chicks from dam and thereby newly hatched chicks are protected

from diseases even if they lack fully developed immune system. The importance of vertical transmission of immunity to provide specific pathogen protection during the early post-hatching period has long been recognized. Immunoglobulin (Ig)-secreting B cells of chick origin have been detected in circulation after 6 days post-hatch [2], meaning that during the first days of the post-hatching period, humoral immunity is totally dependent on the maternal transfer of Igs. In the domestic chicken, 3 classes of Igs have been identified as the homologs of mammalian IgM, IgA, and IgG. Avian IgY is the evolutionary ancestor of mammalian IgG and is the main defense mechanism against systemic infections [3]. Contrary to mammals, who after birth may obtain maternal antibodies in the colostrums, all of the maternal Igs needed to protect the newly hatched chick must be incorporated into the egg before it is laid.

The transfer of IgY from the hen to the chicks is completed in two steps, first transfer of circulating IgY from the hen's bloodstream into the ovarian follicle (i.e., the egg yolk) and then to the embryo[4]. The natural transfer of antibodies that occurs from hen to chick via the egg yolk can be exploited to produce antibodies specific to a given pathogen, simply by immunizing the laying hens with an antigen from this targeted pathogen [5]. However, despite seropositivity and the presence of maternal antibodies, some of the poultry farms face the problem of disease outbreak, particularly when the pathogen has potential of vertical transmission. Salmonellosis is one such problem which intensifies many folds due to emerging antibiotic resistant *Salmonella* spp. and increasing zoonotic threat to human population [6]. Thus, overall transfer of maternal antibody and its efficacy depends mainly on individual titers of specific antibody coupled with rate at which prevalence of the pathogen is recorded.

The present study was therefore planned with a view compare the IgY level in laying hens of four different breeds of poultry (*viz.* Vanraja, Gramapriya, BlackRock, and KalingaBrown) and its relative transfer in egg yolk and chick. Finally, the efficacy of IgY transferred was judged by evaluating the presence of specific (*Salmonella*) antibodies.

Materials and Methods

Ethical approval

This study was approved by Institutional Animal Ethics Committee of Veterinary College, Anjora, Durg.

Birds under study

Apparently healthy laying hens (40-60 weeks of age) from four different breeds of poultry, *viz.*, Vanraja, Gramapriya, BlackRock, and KalingaBrown were selected on a random basis and reared under optimum feeding (as per BIS) and management condition at Government Poultry Farm, Durg. No additional supplements like IgY and other growth promoters were added in the feed. These hens were vaccinated with *Salmonella* polyvalent vaccine inactivated (Venky's). Sufficient numbers of egg were collected, and hatching of eggs was carefully undertaken. Apparently healthy day old chicks from all the four different breeds of poultry were separated immediately after hatching and then used for study within 2-3 h. 12 numbers of samples were studied for each breed of poultry.

Measurement of weight of egg and egg yolk

About 48 eggs were collected from four different breeds (12 numbers from each breed) of poultry. First, each egg was weighed and then broken so that the yolk could be separated from the egg albumin. The yolk was then separated by rolling over filter paper to remove the albumin adhered to it. Weight of each yolk so collected was recorded in gram.

Determination of total protein and IgY in egg yolk

Total protein in egg yolk was measured by colorimetric method using Biuret reagent [7] and the results were expressed as mg/ml. The total IgY concentration in egg yolk was assessed after 7 days of serum collection from breeding hens. Polyethylene glycol (PEG)-precipitationtechnique was performed for purification of IgY as per procedure described by Polson *et al*. [8] with slight modifications. The concentration of IgY extract was measured by single radial immunodiffussion (SRID) [9]. Two-fold serial dilution (1:2 to 1:32 dilution equivalent to 11.97, 5.9, 3, 1.5, and 0.74 mg/ml of standard antigen concentration, respectively) of purified chicken IgY at 23.8 mg/ml (BangaloreGenei) was used as standards to generate standard curves by plotting the zone annulus area (the area of zone minus the area of well) of the precipitation rings after 18 h diffusionin a moist chamber at room temperature.

Determination of total protein and IgY concentration in breeding hens and their progeny chicks

Serum samples were collected from breeding hens and chicks under study and stored at $-20°C$ in deep freeze. The total IgY concentration in chicks was recorded on the day of hatch. The concentration of total serum protein was measured by colorimetric method using Biuret reagent [7], and the results were expressed as g/dl. IgY concentration in serum was estimated using SRID.

Extent of IgY transfer in four different breeds

Percent transfer of maternal antibody was calculated as below:

$$\text{IgY transfer from breeding hen to egg yolk} = \frac{\text{IgY level in egg yolk}}{\text{IgY level in breeding hens}} \times 100$$

$$\text{IgY transfer from breeding hen to chick} = \frac{\text{IgY level in chick}}{\text{IgY level in breeding hens}} \times 100$$

Assessment of *Salmonella*-specific antibodies in breeding hens, egg yolk, and progeny chicks

The *Salmonella* antigens, *viz.*, Somatic (O) and Flagellar (H) from stock culture were prepared using standard protocol as mentioned in OIE terrestrial manual [10] with slight modifications. Standard titration was carried out with known serum to ensure presence of antigen and stored in a refrigerator at 4°C until required. The presence of *Salmonella*-specific antibodies was detected in serum samples from breeding hens and chicks and PEG extract for egg yolk using tube agglutination test. The highest dilution of the serum sample that gives a visible agglutination was recorded as the titer of the serum using antigen suspensions.

Results

Weight of egg and yolk

Although, nonsignificant (p>0.05) variation was reported in the egg weight among four breeds

(Table-1), but comparatively higher egg weight was observed in KalingaBrown (56.67±1.42 g) as compared to Vanraja (55±1.51 g). However, the weight of the yolk differs significantly (p<0.01) among the breeds studied. Significantly higher yolk weight was found in BlackRock (18.76±0.40g) as compared to Gramapriya (15.82±0.27 g) and KalingaBrown (17.06±0.38 g).

Total protein

Total protein (Table-2) in breeding hens was found to be significantly higher (p<0.01) in KalingaBrown and Gramapriya (5.69±0.41 and 5.18±0.31 g/dl, respectively) as compared to Vanraja and BlackRock (3.54±0.30 and 3.76±0.30, respectively). Nonsignificant (p>0.05) difference in total protein was recorded in egg yolk (164±1.82-175±6.03 mg/ml) and chick (2.03±0.10-2.38±0.16 g/dl).

IgY concentration

Nonsignificant (p>0.05) differences in IgY concentration were recorded among different breeds of poultry. The IgY concentration ranged from 5.35±0.63-5.83±0.65, 2.3±0.1-2.6±0.2, and 1.3±0.11-1.7±0.16 mg/ml in hens, egg yolk, and chicks, respectively (Table-3).

Extent of IgY transfer in four different breeds

The extent of IgY transfer were nonsignificant (p>0.05) among different breeds (Table-4). The transfer of IgY from breeding hens to egg yolk, egg yolk to chick and breeding hens to chick were in range of 46.39±1.42-54.92±5.3%, 54.39±1.93-66.52±1.99%, and 25.62±1.42-36.06±4.34%, respectively.

Salmonella-specific passive transfer of IgY

In this study, 79.16% of the serum samples from breeding hens were found to be seropositive for O antigen while 18.75% for H antigen (Table-5). In fact, only 2-10% of total specific antibody in hens is transferred to chicks. Titer of Specific antibodies against *Salmonella* in breeding hens among different breeds is shown in Table-6. More than 1:640 antibody titer for O antigen was recorded in 41.6% (20) samples, however, only 8% antibody titer was observed for H antigen.

Data recording and statistical analysis

Data were analyzed by applying general linear model for factorial experiments using SPSS computer

Table-1: Egg weight and yolk weight of four different breeds of poultry.

Particular	Breeds				Level of significance
	Vanraja	Gramapriya	BlackRock	KalingaBrown	
Egg weight (g±SEM)	55±1.51	55.33±1.66	55.83±1.21	56.67±1.42	NS
Yolk weight (g±SEM)	18.04±0.37[ab]	15.82±0.27[c]	18.76±0.40[a]	17.06±0.38[b]	**

[abc]Means having different superscripts in a row differs significantly. **p<0.01, NS=Not significant, SEM=Standard error of mean

Table-2: Total protein levels in breeding hens, egg yolk and chicks in four different breeds of poultry.

Source of samples	Breeds				Level of significance
	Vanraja	Gramapriya	BlackRock	KalingaBrown	
Breeding hens (g/dl±SEM)	3.54±0.30[b]	5.18±0.31[a]	3.76±0.30[b]	5.69±0.41[a]	**
Egg yolk (mg/ml±SEM)	168±7.94	164±1.82	175±6.03	171.62±5.81	NS
Chick (g/dl±SEM)	2.27±0.11	2.30±0.07	2.38±0.16	2.03±0.10	NS

[ab]Means having different superscripts in a row differs significantly. NS=Not significant; **Highly significant (p<0.01), SEM=Standard error of mean

Table-3: IgY levels in breeding hens, egg yolk and chicks in four different breeds of poultry.

Source of samples	Breeds				Level of significance
	Vanraja	Gramapriya	BlackRock	KalingaBrown	
Breeding hens (mg/ml±SEM)	5.83±0.65	5.35±0.63	5.42±0.70	5.59±0.69	NS
Egg yolk (mg/ml±SEM)	2.4±0.1	2.3±0.1	2.6±0.2	2.5±0.3	NS
Chick (mg/ml±SEM)	1.5±0.16	1.3±0.11	1.7±0.16	1.5±0.08	NS

NS=Not significant, SEM=Standard error of mean, IgY=Immunoglobulin Y

Table-4: Percentage transfer of IgY from breeding hens to egg yolk and chicks in four different breeds of poultry.

Sources of samples	Breed wise transfer (%±SEM)				Level of significance
	Vanraja	Gramapriya	BlackRock	KalingaBrown	
Breeding hens to egg yolk	46.39±1.42	51.10±3.39	54.92±5.3	54.86±6.1	NS
Egg yolk to chicks	60.46±3.70	54.39±1.93	66.52±1.99	58.09±2.21	NS
Breeding hens to chicks	26.84±1.82	25.62±1.42	36.06±4.34	30.34±2.45	NS

NS=Not significant, SEM=Standard error of mean, IgY=Immunoglobulin Y

Table-5: Seroprevalence of specific antibodies against *Salmonella* in breeding hens.

Breed	Total number of samples	Number of samples positive		Percentage positive	
		O antigen	H antigen	O antigen	H antigen
Vanraja	12	10	4	83.3	33.3
Gramapriya	12	11	3	91.7	25.0
BlackRock	12	9	2	75	16.6
KalingaBrown	12	8	UD	66.6	-
Total	48	38	9	79.16	18.75

UD=Undetectable

Table-6: Titer of specific antibodies against *Salmonella* in breeding hens in different breeds.

Antibody titre	Number of samples positive (%)							
	Vanraja		Gramapriya		BlackRock		KalingaBrown	
	O antigen	H antigen	O antigen	H antigen	O antigen	H antigen	O antigen	H antigen
640	5 (41.6)	-	7 (58.3)	-	7 (58.3)	1 (8)	1 (8)	-
320	3 (25)	4 (33.3)	2 (16.6)	3 (25)	2 (16.6)	1 (8)	4 (33.3)	-
160	2 (16.6)	-	2 (16.6)	3 (25)	-	3 (25)	3 (25)	-
80	1 (8)	3 (25)	1 (8)	3 (25)	2 (16.6)	2 (16.6)	-	2 (16.6)
<80	1 (8)	5 (41.6)	-	3 (25)	1 (8)	5 (41.6)	4 (33.3)	10 (83.33)

Total number of samples from each breeds - 12

software package (Version 16.0.0.247©2007). Duncan's multiple range tests were done to make specific treatment comparisons for values that were found significant by ANOVA.

Discussion

The difference in the total protein concentration in different breeds of breeding hen may be due to difference in the genetic makeup as the total serum protein is influenced by breed, age, physiological state, environment and antigen exposure and the levels can be extremely variable [11]. Values of serum protein concentration in breeding hens are well supported by El-Sheikh *et al.* [12]. On contrary, slightly lower values were reported by Malakian *et al.* [13]. The findings of total serum protein in chicks (2.03±0.10-2.38±0.16) are also in accordance with those reported by Bowes *et al.* [14]. Low serum protein in chicks as compared to hens in this study are in accordance with findings of Kaneko [15], who observed that concentration of protein is significantly lower in young animals than in adults. Some relevant reports revealed that the total proteins are the yolk precursors, which are synthesized in the liver and transported via the plasma to the ovary where they were incorporated in the oocyte [16]. In contrast to present observation, Li *et al.* [17] reported higher values of protein in egg yolk.

The IgY concentration in hens and chicks during present work are in congruence with the findings of Hamal *et al.*[18]. In agreement with present observation, Carlander *et al.* [19] also reported different levels of IgY/mL of egg yolk among strains, however, higher values (9.3-11.3 mg/g) were recorded by Ulmer-Franco *et al.*, [20]. Immunization of hens yielded higher IgY level in yolk [21]. Likewise present finding, Sun *et al.*, [22] reported significant correlation among IgY levels in hen serum, yolk, and offspring

serum in White Leghorn, Silkie, and Dongxiang blue-shelled chickens. Varied concentration of IgY might be attributed to different techniques used for extraction, purification, and concentration of IgY by different authors, as purity of the extract by PEG precipitation technique may be around 80% only [23]. However, age and feeding condition might had no or very little effect on IgY concentration as birds were of uniform age groups and optimum and uniform feeding conditions were applied during present investigation.

As regards the total protein and IgY concentration per ml egg yolk, there was no significant difference. As the total weight of yolk is less as observed in Gramapriya (15.82±0.27 g), there was proportionate decrease in the concentration of total protein and total IgY. Hence, the total protein and IgY concentration per egg yolk were found to be significantly different in four breeds studied.

Yolk weight observed are in accordance with the findings of Niranjan *et al.* [24] who also reported a significant difference in yolk weight of Vanraja and Gramapriya breeds. This is also in conformity with reports of Haunshi *et al.* [25]. Similar to present finding, Li *et al.* [17] observed that weight of yolk have direct effect on total protein and IgY levels. The high levels of IgY might be because of the prior immunization of hens with bovine serum albumin. Differences reported in this study might be due to the difference in the method used, as the PEG extraction method yield high levels of IgY from egg yolk [26]. The IgY concentration by PEG extraction method yielded almost twice than that of other methods.

Very young chicks are susceptible to many pathogens during the first few weeks of age because their immune system is not fully developed; hence, maternal antibodies are the primary means of antigen-specific protection. There are many reports in the literature regarding the transfer of pathogen-specific antibodies from hens to their chicks via the egg, and their role in the protection of newly hatched chicks from the pathogens [18,27]. It was also observed that the amount of IgY deposited in the egg and thereby transferred to the offspring were directly related to the circulating levels of IgY in the dam. During present work, the percentage transfer expressed as the percentage of the dam's plasma IgY levels circulating in the blood of day-old chicks (approximately 25-36%) did not differ significantly in the four breeds of chickens. This observation suggests that the amount of maternal antibody present in chick was ultimately decided by the levels in the dam and not the breed. However, this is not in conformity with findings of some earlier workers [28] who have detailed variation in 4 native and crossbred chicken lines with respect to the amounts of inherited maternally derived antibodies in both yolk and day-old chicks.

The present observations on percentage transfer of IgY from hens serum to chick fall in range between 25% and 36%. The differences were, however, not significant when compared among the four breeds which collaborate with findings of Hamal et al. [18]. Antibody levels in the egg yolk are directly proportional to the antibody levels in the dam's serum [29]. Thus, understanding on the relationship between maternal antibody transfer and endogenous antibody production in layer chicks, one may find its direct application in formulating strategies for protecting chicks, especially during the first few weeks of age when their own immune systems are not yet fully functional. It is reported that only minor quantities of IgA and IgM are transferred to the egg yolk from the plasma cells of the oviduct [30] and 10-15% of immunized hens might be low responders to certain antigens which correspond less IgY in egg yolk [31].

By immunizing the laying hens with an antigen from targeted pathogen induces efficient protection in chicks [5] but it is short-term and is limited to infections present in the hen's environment at the time of lay [32]. Usually, titer of 100 or more for O antigen is considered significant, and a titer in excess of 200 for H antigen is considered significant for salmonellosis. Seropositivity for *Salmonella* in this study collaborates with the finding of Betancor et al. [33] who found 24.4% of the birds sera to be positive for *Salmonella* group O: 9. It may be attributed to change in geographical conditions because a particular serotype was prevalent in a particular area. The specific antibody could not be detected in egg yolk and chicks by tube agglutination test. In fact, only 2-10% of total specific antibody in hens is transferred to chicks. Moderate to low antibody titer in hens render their chicks with undetectable levels of *Salmonella* antibodies by STAT.

The results revealed as much as cent percent immunity at flock level, out of which, only 41.6% show titer of 1:640 which can be correlated with the reports of Kumar et al. [34] in which the antibody titer was found to be highest (1:1280) which decreased gradually, but the bird remain seropositive until end of observation, i.e. 6th week. The results are slightly lower than the findings of Ahmed et al.[35] who reported seroprevalence of 49.5% in live birds and the rate decreased with advancement of age. It is opined that due to resultant low titer in hen, antibodies in chicks could not reach to level to be detected by STAT. Likewise,Hermans et al.[36] observedtiters of 1:16 000 for *Campylobacter jejuni*-specific IgY in egg yolk of hens immunized with a *C. jejuni* whole-cell lysate. This indicates that transfer of IgY to egg yolk is biologically relevant in the overall transfer of Igs into eggs after immunization of hens.

Multiple research studies using hyperimmunization of hens to produce avian [37] and interspecies-specific egg Ig [38] have been carried out.However, faster absorption of yolk sac IgY in chicks from breeding hens, might led the chicks more susceptible to localized pathogen invasion of the yolk sac during the early post-hatching period. In the post-hatching period, protein integrity within the yolk sac is critical for normal absorption of the yolk sac content and for IgY transfer to the circulation of the chick[39]. Hence, factors affecting transfer of IgY to the chick may threaten the chick's immune status and increase disease susceptibility during the early post-hatching period.

Conclusion

This study reports comparative IgY transfer from parent flock to yolk and then to chicks in four breeds of poultry, *viz*.,Vanraja, Gramapriya, BlackRock, and KalingaBrown. Extent of IgY transfer among four breeds at three different stages wasnonsignificant, as it may depend on individual dam serum IgY concentration. Moderate to high percent seropositivity was detected for *Salmonella*-specific IgY in hens immunized with polyvalent *Salmonella* vaccine.This work has initiated investigations to assess the cutoff IgY concentration received by progeny from hen that impart specific immunity to infection in the early period of life in the immunocompetent chicks.

Authors' Contributions

SDH designed the experiment and RA performed the experiment under supervision of SDH. CS and AKG helped in sample collection and analysis. Manuscript preparation was reviewed and edited by all authors. All authors read and approved the final manuscript.

Acknowledgments

The authors are pleased to Dean, College of Veterinary Science and Animal Husbandry, Anjora, Durg, Chhattisgarh, India, for providing the necessary facilities and funding to carry out this work. The study is a part of the post-graduate research work and submitted by the first author to Indira Gandhi KrishiVishwavidyalaya, Raipur.

Competing Interests

The authors declare that they have no competing interest.

References

1. Bar-Shira, E. and Friedman, A. (2006) Development and adaptations of innate immunity in the gastrointestinal tract of the newly hatched chick. *Dev. Comp.Immunol.*, 30(10):930-941.

2. Lawrence, E.C., Arnaud-Battandier, F., Grayson, J., Koski, I.R., Dooley, N.J., Muchmore, A.V. and Blaese, R.M. (1981) Ontogeny of humoral immune function in normal chickens: A comparison of immunoglobulin-secreting cells in bone marrow, spleen, lungs, and intestine. *Clin. Exp. Immunol.*, 43:450-457.

3. Warr, G.W., Magor, K.E. and Higgins, D.A. (1995) IgY: Clues to the origins of modern antibodies. *Immunol. Today*, 16:392-398.

4. Orlans, E. (1967) Fowl antibody VIII. A comparison of natural, primary, and secondary erythrocytes in hen sera; their transmission to yolk and chick. *Immunol.*,12:27-37.

5. Kovacs-Nolan, J. and Mine, Y. (2012) Egg yolk antibodies for passive immunity. *Annu. Rev. Food Sci. Technol.*, 3: 163-182.

6. Yan, S., Pendrak, M. and Abela-Ridder, B. (2003) An overview of *Salmonella* typing public health perspectives. *Clin. Appl. Immunol. Rev.*, 4: 189-204.

7. Reinhold, J.G. (1953) In: Reiner, M., editor. Standard Methods of Clinical Biochemistry. Vol. 1.Academic Press, New York & London. p88.

8. Polson, A., Von Wechmar, M.B. and Van Regenmortel, M.V.H. (1980) Isolation of viral IgY antibodies from yolks of immunized hens. *Immunol.Commun.*, 9: 475-493.

9. Mancini, G., Carbonara, A.O. and Heremans, J.F. (1965) Immunochemical quantitation of antigens by single radial immunodiffusion. *Immunochem.*, 2: 235-254.

10. OIE. (2010) Salmonellosis. Terrestrial Manual. p9-10. http://www.oie.int/fileadmin/Home/eng/Health_standards/tahm/2.09.09_SALMONELLOSIS.pdf. Accessed on 04-12-2015.

11. Bell, D.J. (1971) Plasma enzymes. In: Bell, D.J. and Freeman, B.M., editors. Physiology and Biochemistry of the Domestic Fowl. Academic Press Inc., London. p964-965.

12. EL-Sheikh, A.M.H., Abdalla, E.A. and Hanafy, M.M. (2009) Study on productive performance, haematological and immunological parameter in a local strain of chicken as affected by Mannanoligosaccharide under hot climate conditions. *Egypt. Poult. Sci.*, 29(I): 287-305.

13. Malakian, M., Hassanabadi, A. and Heidariniya, A. (2011) Effects of Safflower seed on performance, carcass traits and blood parameters of Broilers. *Res. J. Poult. Sci.*, 4(2): 18-21.

14. Bowes, V.A., Julian, R.J. and Stirtzinger, T. (1989) Comparison of serum biochemical profiles of male broilers with female broilers and White leghorn chickens. *Can. J. Vet. Res.*, 53: 7-11.

15. Kaneko, J.J. (1997) In: Serum proteins and the dysproteinemias. Clinical Biochemistry of Domestic Animals. 5th ed. Academic Press, San Diego, London, Boston, New York, Sydney, Tokyo, Toronto. p117-138.

16. Ritchie, B.W., Harrison, J.G. and Harrison, R.L. (1994) Avian Medicine. Winger's Publishing, Inc., Florida.

17. Li, X., Nakano, T., Sunwoo, H.H., Paik, B.H., Chae, H.S. and Sim, J.S. (1998) Effects of egg and yolk weights on yolk antibody (IgY) production in laying chickens. *Poult. Sci.*, 77:266-270.

18. Hamal, K.R., Burgess, S.C., Pevzner, I.Y. and Erf, G.F. (2006) Maternal antibody transfer from dams to their egg yolks, egg whites, and chicks in meat lines of chickens. *Poult. Sci.*, 85: 1364-1372.

19. Carlander, D., Wilhelmson, M. and Larsson, A. (2003) Immunoglobulin Y level in egg yolk from three chicken genotypes. *Food Agric.Immunol.*, 15(1): 35-40.

20. Ulmer-Franco, A.M., Cherian, G., Quezada, N., Fasenko, G.M. and McMullen, L.M. (2012) Hatching egg and newly hatched chick yolk sac total IgY content at 3 broiler breeder flock ages. *Poult. Sci.*, 91(3):758-764.

21. Meenatchisundaram, S. and Michael, A. (2010) Comparison of four different purification methods for isolation of anti *Echiscarinatus* antivenom antibodies from immunized chicken egg yolk. *Iran.J.Biotechnol.*, 8: 50-55.

22. Sun, H., Chen, S., Xia, C., Guiyun, X. and Lujiang, Q. (2013) Effect of transportation duration of 1-day-old chicks on post-placement production performances and pododermatitis of broilers up to slaughter age. *Poult. Sci.*, 92(12): 3300-3309.

23. Pauly, D., Chacana, P.A., Calzado, E.G., Brembs, B. and Schade, R. (2011) IgY technology: Extraction of chicken antibodies from egg yolk by polyethylene glycol (PEG) precipitation. *J. Vis. Exp.*, 51:3084.

24. Niranjan, M., Sharma, R.P., Rajkumar, U., Chatterjee, R.N., Reddy, B.L.N. and Battacharya, T.K. (2008) Egg quality traits in chicken varieties developed for backyard poultry farming in India. *Livest. Res.Rural Dev.*, 20(12): 103-105.

25. Haunshi, S., Doley, S. and Kadirvel, G. (2010) Comparative studies on egg, meat and semen qualities of native and improved chicken varieties developed for backyard poultry production. *Trop. Anim. Health Prod.*, 42(5): 1013-1019.

26. Amir, M.P., Rasaee, M.J., Qujeq, D., Asadikaram, G.H.R. and Moqhadam, M.F. (2000) A simple and economical procedure for the purification of immunoglobulin Y from egg yolk by T-Gel chromatography. *Iran. J. Allergy Asthma Immunol.*, 1(2): 53-57.

27. Liou, J.F., Chang, C.W., Tailiu, J.J., Yu, C.K., Lei, H.Y., Chen, L.R. and Tai, C. (2010)Passive protection effect of chicken egg yolk immunoglobulins on enterovirus 71 infected mice. *Vaccine*, 28: 8189-8196.

28. Abdel-Moneim, A.S. and Abdel-Gawad, M.M.A. (2006) Genetic variations in maternal transfer and immune responsiveness to infectious bursal disease virus. *Vet. Microbiol.*,114: 16-24.

29. Loeken, M.R. and Roth, R.E. (1983) Analysis of maternal IgG subpopulations which are transported into the chicken oocyte. *Immunol.*, 49: 21-28.

30. Rose, M.E., Orlans, E. and Buttress, N. (1974) Immunoglobulin classes in the hen's egg: their segregation in yolk and white. *Eur. J. Immunol.*, 4: 521-523.

31. Schade, R., Calzado, E.G., Sarmiento, R., Chacana, P.A., Porankiewicz-Asplund, J. and Terzolo, H.R. (2005) Chicken egg yolk antibodies (IgY-technology): A review of progress in production and use in research and human and veterinary medicine. *Altern. Lab. Anim.*, 33:129-154.

32. Smith, A.L. and Beal, R. (2008) The avian enteric immune system in health and disease. In: Davison, F., Kaspers, B., Schat, K.A., editors. Avian *Immunolo*gy. Elsevier Ltd., New York. p243-271.

33. Betancor, L., Pereira, M., Martinez, A., Giossa, G., Fookes, M., Flores, M., Barrios, P., Repiso, V., Vignoli, R., Cordeiro, N., Algorta, G., Thomson, N., Maskell, D., Schelotto, F. and Chabalgoity, J.A. (2010) Prevalence of *Salmonella enterica* in poultry and eggs in Uruguay during an epidemic due to *Salmonella enterica* Serovarenteritidis. *J. Clin.Microbiol.*, 48(7): 2413-2423.

34. Kumar, S., Sadana, J.R., Chaturvedi, G.C. and Michra, S.K. (2001) Studies on humoral and cellular immune response in Japanese quail (Coturnixcoturnix japonica) experimentally infected with *S. typhimurium*. *Indian J.Poult. Sci.*, 36(2): 197-200.

35. Ahmed, A.K.M., Islam, M.T., Haider, M.G. and Hossain, M.M. (2008) Seroprevalence and pathology of naturally infected salmonellosis in poultry with isolation and identification of causal agents. J. Bangladesh Agrilc. Univ., 6(2): 327-334.

36. Hermans, D., Van Steendam, K., Verbrugghe, E., Verlinden, M., Martel, A., Seliwiorstow, T., Heyndrickx, M., Haesebrouck, F., De Zutter, L., Deforce, D. and Pasmans, F. (2014) Passive immunization to reduce *Campylobacter jejuni* colonization and transmission in broiler chickens.*Vet. Res.*,45:27.

37. Gómez-Verduzco, G., Tellez, G., Quintana, A.L., Isibasi, A. and Ortiz-Navarrete, V. (2010) Humoral immune response in breeding hens and protective immunity provided by administration of purified *Salmonella Gallinarum* porins. *Poult. Sci.*, 89:495-500.

38. Machado Leal Ribeiro, A., Rudnik, L., Wageck Canal, C., RibeiroKratz, L. and Farias, C. (2005) Supply of hipperimmunized hen yolks against swine *Escherichia coli* to control newborn piglets diarrhea. *R. Bras. Zootec.,* 34:1234-1239.

39. Ulmer-Franco, A.M. (2012)Transfer of chicken immunoglobulin Y (IgY) from the hen to the chick. *Avian Biol. Res.,* 5(2): 81-87.

8

Reproductive disorders in dairy cattle under semi-intensive system of rearing in North-Eastern India

M. H. Khan[1], K. Manoj[2] and S. Pramod[3]

1. ICAR-National Research Centre on Mithun, Jharnapani, Medziphema - 797 106, Nagaland, India; 2. ICAR Research Complex for NEH Region, Umiam - 793 103, Meghalaya, India; 3. Central Institute for Research on Cattle, Meerut - 255 001, Uttar Pradesh, India.
Corresponding author: M. H. Khan, e-mail: haidermeraj@rediffmail.com,
KM: mkumar_iari@yahoo.co.in, SP: singhpramod@gmail.com

Abstract

Aim: This study was conducted to determine the incidence of major reproductive problems of dairy cattle reared under a semi-intensive system by small and marginal farmers in Meghalaya province of North-Eastern India.

Materials and Methods: In a 3 years study, a total of 576 crossbred dairy cattle (212 Holstein Friesian cross and 364 Jersey cross) from all districts (n=11) of Meghalaya were assessed with the survey, clinical examination, and personal observations.

Results: Out of the total animal assessed, 33.85% (n=195) were found to be affected with one or more of the clinical reproductive problems. Repeat breeding (RB), anestrus, retention of fetal membrane, and abortion were found to be the major clinical reproductive problems. Out of the total animal affected with reproductive disorders, the incidence of anestrus, RB, retention of fetal membrane, and abortion was found to be 31.79% (n=62), 24.61% (n=48), 14.35% (n=28), and 11.25% (n=22), respectively. In addition, dystocia (5.12%), prolapse (1.53%), endometritis (4.61%), and pyometra (6.66%) were minor clinical reproductive problems. There was a significant difference in the incidence of reproductive disorders with respect to breed, age, and parity.

Conclusion: It was revealed from this study that RB, anestrus, retention of fetal membrane, and dystocia are the major clinical reproductive problems in Meghalaya. Results indicated unsatisfactory feeding, housing, and health management practices are the main cause of low fertility of dairy cows. Lack of scientific knowledge, low access to breeding, and health services further contributed to low productivity and fertility.

Keywords: anestrus, dairy, infertility, Meghalaya, reproductive disorders.

Introduction

Meghalaya, the North-Eastern province of India, is located between 20°1' and 26°5' North latitudes and 85°49' and 92°52' East latitudes. The altitude varies from 30 to 2000 m MSL. The state has rich natural resources, and the climate ranges from tropical and subtropical to temperate. The state has almost 69.7% forest coverage and receives heavier rainfall (average rainfall 2000 mm) [1]. The annual maximum temperature ranges from 10°C to 20°C during winter and 25-35°C during summer season over different places [1].

The animal husbandry is the main component of agriculture development in India and particularly in North-Eastern part of the country owing to the hilly terrain and undulating topography where agriculture is largely rain fed. Dairy production in this part of the country has not been viewed seriously because of less intake of milk and milk products by the native tribal people [2]. Most of the dairy farming is being done by the outside settlers mainly from neighboring states or Nepal. In Meghalaya, the crossbred cattle population is only 26458 in number which is 0.67% of India's crossbred cattle population [3]. Over the last 5 years showed 3.94% increase in crossbred cattle population which is lower than the national average (7.58%) [3]. The farmers generally practice mixed crop-livestock production system with crop mostly being the primary production, and the animals are generally reared under semi-intensive system [4]. The smallholder's dairy sector in this part of the country is facing with several challenges. These include limited breeding stock, high cost of feed, non-availability of green fodder round the year, poor management, inadequate health extension services which ultimately resulted in low productivity, and poor fertility or infertility of dairy cows. Reproductive disorder among farm animals is the great economic problem. It is particularly widespread among dairy cattle [5]. Economy of the dairy farming largely depends on pregnancy rate after insemination. The 12-month calving interval is advantageous for high milk yield per cow with the good economic return. It is accepted that bovine genital infections, either specific or non-specific accounts for a large number of pregnancy failure in cows [6]. These reproductive health problems are the bottleneck in the production process and productivity in the livestock sector.

Therefore, it is justifiable to generate scientific information and database on the production system, and the major reproductive problems of dairy cows in the study area with the objective to determine the prevalence of major infertility problems of dairy cattle. It is anticipated that the information generated could be used as a basis for interventions to improve dairy cattle productivity among smallholder farmers in Meghalaya.

Materials and Methods

Ethical approval

The present study was conducted in accordance with the guidelines set by Animals Ethics Committee of the Institute.

Study area and animals

This study was conducted at Indian Council of Agricultural Research Complex for North-Eastern Hill Region, Barapani, Meghalaya, India. The study was conducted for 3 years from 2010 to 2013 to determine the prevalence of reproductive diseases in randomly selected 576 crossbred dairy cattle covering all districts of Meghalaya, India. All the animals selected for the study were reared in semi-intensive type of management where animals were stall-fed with little open area for grazing. Almost same cattle rearing pattern in terms of feeding, housing, and health care management was seen across the study area. Feed comprised broken rice, wheat/rice bran, maize, and vegetables mixed and boiled. Feed was provided twice daily. Apart from this, paddy straw and some green fodder grass were also given.

Data collection on reproductive disorders

Crossbred dairy cows (n=576) were subjected to gynecological examinations to find out the prevalence of reproductive disorders. The detailed history of the cow, including the date of previous artificial insemination (AI) or natural mating, was obtained from the cattle owner through structured questionnaire format. Diagnosis of reproductive diseases was made on the basis of history, clinical signs, and response of the treatment. The cows having apparently normal genitalia but failed to conceive through natural mating with fertile bull or using AI with quality semen consecutively for three times were considered as repeat breeders. The cows with the history of prolonged absence of estrus were examined twice at 11 days apart and those showing the smooth ovaries on both the examinations were confirmed as anestrus [7].

Biochemical analysis of blood serum

Out of 576 cows, blood sample of 240 dairy cattle was collected for estimation of total protein, albumin, and cholesterol concentration in blood serum. The animals were categorized into three group, viz.,

normal breeding (without any apparent reproductive disorder), repeat breeding (RB), and anestrus comprising of 80 animals in each group. 10 ml of blood samples were collected from jugular vein without adding anticoagulant. Serum was separated by centrifugation and transferred into a sterilized plastic vial and labeled. The serum samples were used immediately for glucose estimation using standard kit. The samples, which were not able to be analyzed on the same day of collection, were stored at −20°C until analyzed. The total protein, albumin and cholesterol concentration were estimated using the standard kit (Qualigens Diagnostic, Glaxo, Mumbai, Maharashtra, India) following the procedure given by the manufacturer.

Data processing and analysis

The collected data were sorted manually, and questionnaires were coded before processing. The data were also checked thoroughly for consistency and to make sure that there was no missing value. Animals were classified into two genotypes, viz., Holstein Friesian (HF) crossbred (HF×Indian local cattle; n=212) and Jersey crossbred (Jersey×Indian local cattle; n=364). The data were further categorized into the basis of age group and parity. There were four age groups, viz., <3 years (n=132), 3-5 years (n=170), 5-7 years (n=189), and >7 years (n=85). Similarly parity wise, four groups, viz., heifers (n=147), 1st-3rd parity (n=234), 4-6th parity (n=145), and >6th parity (50) were classified. The prevalence and relative frequencies of reproductive health problems were determined as the proportion of affected animals out of the total animals examined and the total number of particular disorder out of the total affected animals, respectively. The baseline survey data were entered and analyzed in SPSS 15.0 program. Descriptive statistics was done to explore the prevalence of reproductive diseases and Duncan t-test was used to determine the level of significance among clinical cases of cow. Blood biochemical profile data were subjected to one-way analysis of variance.

Results

Incidence of reproductive disorders

All the animals selected for the study were maintained under the semi-intensive system of management. As the animals were provided shelter, concentrate feed and water by the owner but allowed to graze in open for green fodder. The result showed that out of total 576 dairy cows examined, 33.85% (n=195) were found to be affected either with one or more reproductive health problems. Reproductive disorders reported in this study were anestrus (31.79%), RB (24.61%), retention of fetal membrane (14.35%), abortions (11.25%), dystocia (5.12%), prolapse (1.53%), endometritis (4.61%), and pyometra (6.66 %) irrespective of breed, age, and parity of the cow (Table-1). Anestrus syndrome was the most common cause of infertility of cow. In this study, RB was found to be the second highest common reproductive disease which was 26.66%.

The major reproductive problems were anestrus, RB, retention of fetal membrane, and abortions which contributed >80% of the total affected animals. However, dystocia, vaginal prolapse, endometritis, and pyometra also found to affect the fertility of dairy cattle.

Effect of breed on reproductive disorders

Out of total 576 animals examined in this study, HF cross showed a higher incidence of reproductive disorders (43.39% versus 28.29%) than Jersey crosses (Table-2). Breed had a significant effect on anestrus, abortion, dystocia, and endometritis. No significant difference was observed in cases of RB, retained fetal membrane (RFM), prolapse, and pyometra. The incidence of anestrus, abortions, dystocia, and endometritis was significantly higher in HF crossbred cattle than in Jersey cross which was found to be 11.32% versus 6.59%, 5.66% versus 2.74%, 6.13% versus 1.92%, and 2.83% versus 0.82%, respectively (Table-3).

Effect of age

Age group had significant (p<0.05) effect on RB and anestrus. Lower incidence of reproductive

disorders was reported in <3 years age group and no cases of prolapse, endometritis, and pyometra were recorded during the study period. On the contrary, significantly higher anoestrus cases were recorded in 5-7 and >7 years age group followed by 3-5 years age group and in heifers. RB was highest in >7 years age group and minimum in <3 years age group. No significant difference was recorded in RFM, abortion and dystocia, proplapse, endometritis, and pyometra between the age groups (Table-4).

Effect of parity

Parity had a significant effect on the occurrence of various reproductive disorders under smallholder's dairy cattle production system in Meghalaya. Maximum incidence of reproductive disorders was reported between 1st and 3rd parity followed by 4-5th parity. Cases of RB, anestrus, RFM, and abortion were highest in 1st to 3rd parity followed by 4-5th parity group, and minimum was reported in heifers. All cases of prolapse were reported only in 1st-3rd parity. Similarly, cases of endometritis were not reported in heifers and animals >6 parity. The prevalence of abortion was highest (5.12) in 2nd calving and the lowest (1.36%) in heifer, 1st calving, 6th calving, and >7th calving. The prevalence of stillbirth was highest (0.7%) in 1st calving and no stillbirth in heifers, 5th calving, 6th calving, and >7th calving. Similarly, retained placenta (4.5%), metritis (1.1%), pyometra (1.1%), uterine prolapsed (0.5%), and RB (5.2%) were higher in 2nd parity. Vaginal prolapsed (0.7%) and mastitis (2.8%) were highest in 3rd parity (Table-5).

Blood biochemical profile

The blood serum glucose level in normal breeding, RB, and anestrus animals were 55.45±1.34, 48.36±0.75, and 46.54±0.99 mg/dl, respectively. The

Table-1: The relative frequency of various reproductive disorders in Meghalaya.

Reproductive disorders (n=195)	Frequency	Percent of total affected animals
Anestrus	62	31.79
RB	48	24.61
RFM	28	14.35
Abortion	22	11.25
Dystocia	10	5.12
Prolapse	03	1.53
Endometritis	09	4.61
Pyometra	13	6.66
Total	195	100

RFM=Retained fetal membrane, RB=Repeat breeding

Table-2: Reproductive disorders in HF and Jersey crossbred cows.

Breed	Total number of cows examined	Number of cows affected	Number of non-affected cows	Percent affected (%)
HF cross	212	92	120	43.39
Jersey cross	364	103	261	28.29
Total	576	195	381	33.85

HF=Holstein Friesian

Table-3: Effect of breed on the prevalence of reproductive diseases of dairy cows.

Reproductive disorders	Breed N (%)		Total (n=576) N (%)	Level of significance
	HF cross (n=212)	Jersey cross (n=364)		
Anestrus	24 (11.32)	24 (6.59)	48 (8.33)	*
RB	25 (11.79)	37 (10.16)	62 (10.76)	NS
RFM	14 (6.60)	14 (3.84)	28 (4.86)	NS
Abortion	12 (5.66)	10 (2.74)	22 (3.81)	*
Dystocia	13 (6.13)	07 (1.92)	10 (1.73)	*
Prolapse	02 (0.09)	01 (0.27)	03 (0.52)	NS
Endometritis	06 (2.83)	03 (0.82)	09 (1.56)	*
Pyometra	07 (3.30)	07 (1.92)	13 (2.25)	NS
Total	92 (43.39)	103 (28.29)	195 (33.85)	

*Significant (p<0.05), n=Number of observations, N=Number of animals affected, NS=Non significant (p<0.05).
RFM=Retained fetal membrane, RB=Repeat breeding

Table-4: Effect of age group on the prevalence of reproductive diseases of dairy cows.

Reproductive disorders	Age group N (%)				Overall (n=576) N (%)	Level of significance
	<3 years (n=132)	3-5 years (n=170)	5-7 years (n=189)	>7 years (n=85)		
Anestrus	05 (3.48)	13 (7.64)	25 (13.22)	5 (5.88)	48 (8.33)	*
RB	05 (3.78)	20 (11.36)	22 (11.64)	15 (17.64)	62 (10.76)	*
RFM	06 (4.54)	10 (5.88)	07 (3.70)	05 (5.88)	28 (4.86)	NS
Abortion	03 (2.27)	07 (4.11)	06 (3.17)	06 (7.05)	22 (3.81)	NS
Dystocia	06 (4.54)	02 (1.17)	02 (1.05)	-	10 (1.73)	NS
Prolapse	-	-	02 (1.05)	01 (1.17)	03 (0.52)	NS
Endometritis	-	03 (1.76)	04 (2.11)	02 (2.35)	09 (1.56)	NS
Pyometra	-	05 (2.94)	04 (2.11)	04 (4.70)	13 (2.25)	NS
Total	25 (18.93)	60 (35.29)	72 (38.09)	38 (44.70)	195 (33.85)	

*Significant ($p<0.05$), n=Number of observations, N=Number of animals affected, NS=Non significant ($p<0.05$), RFM=Retained fetal membrane, RB=Repeat breeding

Table-5: Effect of parity on the incidence of reproductive diseases of dairy cows.

Reproductive disorders	Parity N (%)				Overall (n=576) N (%)	Level of Significance
	Heifer (n=147)	1st to 3rd (n=234)	4-5th (n=145)	>6th (n=50)		
Anestrus	5 (3.4)	26 (11.11)	14 (9.65)	3 (6.0)	48 (8.33)	*
Repeat Breeding	5 (3.4)	46 (19.65)	9 (6.20)	2 (4.0)	62 (10.76)	*
RFM	4 (2.72)	14 (5.98)	6 (4.13)	4 (8.0)	28 (4.86)	*
Abortion	2 (1.36)	12 (5.12)	6 (4.13)	2 (4.0)	22 (3.81)	NS
Dystocia	5 (3.4)	3 (1.28)	2 (1.37)	-	10 (1.73)	NS
Prolapse	-	3 (1.28)	-	-	3 (0.52)	NS
Endometritis	-	6 (2.56)	3 (2.06)	-	9 (1.56)	NS
Pyometra	2 (1.36)	7 (2.99)	3 (2.06)	1 (2.0)	13 (2.25)	NS
Total	23 (15.64)	117 (50.0)	43 (29.65)	12 (24.0)	195 (33.85)	

*Significant ($p<0.05$), n=Number of observations, N=Number of animals affected, NS=Non significant ($p<0.05$), RFM=Retained fetal membrane.

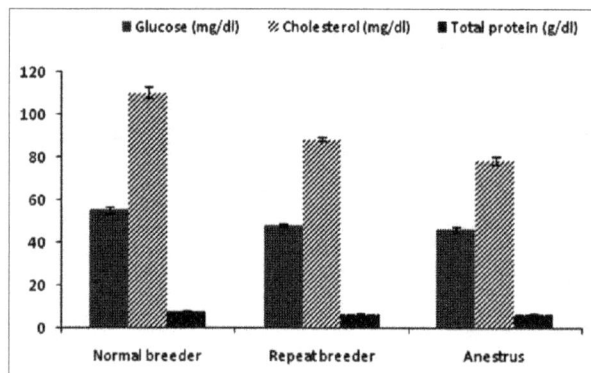

Figure-1: Blood biochemical profile of normal breeding, repeat breeding, and anestrus cows.

serum total cholesterol level of normal breeding, RB, and anestrus cows were 110.54±2.54, 88.65±0.96, and 78.64±1.79 mg/dl, respectively. Total serum protein level of normal breeding, RB, and anestrus cows were 7.54±0.68, 6.43±0.62, and 6.58±0.51 g/dl, respectively (Figure-1).

Discussion

Although livestock is an important source of income for smallholders and the landless in North-East India, still it is largely deficit in egg, pork, milk, and mutton production. Products such as milk and eggs are steady source of cash income, and live animals are important natural assets for the poor, which can be easily liquidated for cash during emergency. Smallholders and landless together control 75% of the country's livestock resources and are capable of producing at a lower cost because of availability of sufficient labor with them. Evidence shows that smallholders obtain nearly half of their income from livestock [8].

This study documented the common reproductive disorders encountered under smallholder's dairy production system in North-Eastern part of India. Livestock in India and particularly in the North-Eastern region are raised as a part of mixed farming systems which is considered environmentally most benign and sustainable because of complementarities between crop and livestock production. Animals derive most of their feed-fodder requirement from agricultural residues and by-products, and in turn provide draught power and dung manure for cropping activities.

This study revealed 37.85% of reproductive incidence out of total animal examined which is in close approximation with earlier findings of Hadush et al. [9], who reported 44.3% of the cows with major pre-partum and post-partum reproductive problems in Ethiopia. Similarly in other findings of Tesfaye and Shamble [10], it was reported that out of total 231 dairy cows included in the study, 40.25% were found to be affected at least by one reproductive health problems. Anestrus (31.79%) and RB (24.61%) were two major reproductive problems encountered in more than 50% of the cows during their lifetime which are slightly higher than reported earlier [9], where the incidence of anestrus and RB as 12.9% and 11.4%, respectively. Similarly, very high incidence of anestrus (20.4%) and RB (12.8%) reported common reproductive diseases in crossbred dairy cattle in Bangladesh [11]. On the contrary, 65% of anestrus and 35% RB cases in crossbred cattle were reported in Kerala [12]. Similarly, higher prevalence of anestrus and RB (49.9% and 15.1%, respectively) in cows was reported by Serur et al. [13]. Major reason for anestrus in dairy cattle is due to poor quality ration provided by the farmers, lack of round the year green fodder availability, higher incidence of parasitic diseases, lack of scientific knowledge, and poor managemental practices. Higher incidence of the reproductive problem in HF cross than the Jersey cross is due to less adoptability of HF cross cattle under subtropical hill ecosystem, high milk production, and low plane of nutrition. The common cause of RB was a cystic ovarian disorder, anovulation, delayed ovulation, early embryonic mortality, improper timing of AI, lack of knowledge of proper heat detection, using old and infected bull, lack of veterinary extension services, poor quality semen, and inexperienced inseminator. Error in estrus detection and improper timings of AI was also reported by earlier workers as the common cause of RB in cows [14]. Metritis (clinical and sub-clinical), milk fever, dystocia, and retained placenta had a significant association with RB [15].

Our results are in agreement with previous findings of Tesfaye and Shamble [10], who reported the major productive health problems in the dairy cows as clinical mastitis (19.3%), abortion (9.05%), dystocia (7.75%), retained placenta (7.32%), and RB (3.87%). This variation in prevalence might be due to the differences in management and breed of the animals as well as environmental factors. The higher incidence of reproductive problems was in HF cross than in Jersey cross cattle which may be due to the fact that HF cross is less adapted to tropical conditions of high temperature and humidity, disease and low feed quality than Jersey crossbred making them more susceptible. Beside this, HF cross requires more elaborated management, feeding, and better health care than the indigenous zebu to get better reproductive performance.

Genotype had a significant effect (p<0.05) on abortion, RB, dystocia, retention of placenta, endometritis, anestrus, and milk fever. In this study, two different genetic groups, viz., HF and Jersey crossbred cattle were selected, and significantly higher incidence of reproductive disorders was recorded in HF cross than in Jersey. The major reason for this is the climatic conditions of Meghalaya. The climate of Meghalaya varies with the altitude. Temperature in the study area ranges between 20 and 32°C. Due to high humidity and increased temperature, HF cross is more susceptible to heat stress which may result in high incidence of reproductive disorders. Further, this climate is more conducive for the propagation of external as well as internal parasites which can easily infect the cattle through grazing. Since deworming practice is usually not being followed by the majority of farmers, the chronic parasitic infection causes loss of production and anestrus.

All the reproductive diseases were lowest in <3 years age group cows. Since the age of first calving is more than 3 years in both genetic groups. Therefore, very less incidence of reproductive disorders was found in <3 years age group. Higher incidence of reproductive diseases in 5-7 years and >7 years age group high milk production and negative energy balance. Higher incidence of RB cases in >8 years age group might be due to endocrine disturbances. Higher incidence of abortion, metritis, cystic ovaries, vaginal prolapse, uterine prolapse, RFM, dystocia, anestrus, and RB in >8 years old cows and lower in <4 and 4-6 years old cows were also reported in Bangladesh [16]. However, no significant difference was recorded in retention of placenta, abortion, dystocia, prolapse, endometritis, and pyometra between the age groups. Other factors which significantly contribute are poor body condition score, body weight, mangemental factors, environmental factors and inadequate veterinary and extension services, etc. On the contrary, it was reported that the occurrence of overall reproductive problems was not significantly affected within the different age groups. However, the problems were seen to rise with age [10].

Parity of female is one of the most important factors associated with reproductive disorders. The parity 1st-3rd is the most productive phase of female cattle followed by parity 4th-5th. This parity falls in the age group between 3 and 8 years. Milk production is maximum up to 3rd parity after that it starts declining. Due to high milk production, animals becomes in negative energy balance. As the poor farmers could not afford the high cost of concentrate feed, the productive animals fail either to return to cyclicity resulting prolonged calving to conception interval leading to anestrus or it may result into endocrine disturbances leading failure of ovulation, failure of fertilization, early embryonic mortality resulting in RB. The usual practice in this part of the country is to cull the animal after 6th parity due to less milk production. The culled animals are being slaughtered and used as beef. Therefore, very less incidence of reproductive disorders after 6th parity was reported. It is reported that the prevalence of RB was although found to vary from 1st to 5th parity, the difference was non-significant. However, significantly lowest prevalence was recorded at 6th parity (6.25%) when compared to other parities [17].

It was also reported that the number of parity has significant (p<0.05) influence for the occurrence of reproductive problems where animals with higher parities were seen to show reproductive problems more frequently than those with low number of parities [10]. This study showed most of the reproductive disorders in 2nd parity which is similar to the findings of earlier workers [18].

The blood serum glucose level in this study agrees with the previous findings [19]. There was a significant decrease in blood glucose level of RB and anestrus cows compared to normal breeding cows. Lower blood glucose level in RB and anestrus animals might influence the pituitary function thereby interfering the fertility [20]. The serum total cholesterol level (mg/dl) of normal breeding animals were significantly higher (p<0.05) than in RB and anestrus cattle. Lower cholesterol level in RB cows was also documented in an earlier report [21]. The serum protein level (g/dl) of normal breeding cows was comparatively higher than those of RB and anestrus cows. However, no statistical significance was observed. This is in agreement with the previous work [18]. Lower serum protein level in RB and anestrus group may lead to deficiency of certain amino acids which are essential for gonadotropin synthesis [22].

Conclusion

This study revealed a high prevalence of reproductive health problems in the study area. Anestrus, RB, retention of fetal membrane, and dystocia were the major reproductive diseases in crossbred dairy cattle reared under resource poor, smallholders dairy production system in northeastern part of India. Breed, parity and age group are possible risk factors identified for the occurrence of reproductive health problems. Management and fertility of dairy cows among smallholder farms is faced with both challenges and opportunities to improve productivity that are related to feeding, housing, health, and breeding system. Both the challenges and opportunities are influenced by the extent to which farmers have accesses to important services such as extension, health, breeding, and finance. Improvement in service delivery and further capacity building of both farmers and extension staff is required in order to improve dairy management skill and subsequent productivity. Further, detailed research in specific aspects of feeding, housing, health care, and breeding systems would help to identify specific interventions that could be used to improve dairy cattle productivity.

Authors' Contributions

MHK: Involved in designing of research, data collection, statistical analysis, and drafted and revised the manuscript. KM: Involved in the collection of data and statistical analysis. SP: Involved in data collection. All authors read and approved the final manuscript.

Acknowledgments

The authors are thankful to the Director, ICAR Research Complex for NEH region, Umiam, Meghalaya, for providing financial support and facilities to carry out this work. Technical support, provided by the Department of Veterinary and Animal Husbandry, Government of Meghalaya, is highly acknowledged.

Competing Interests

The authors declare that they have no competing interests.

References

1. Anonymous. (2012) Vision Document 2050. ICAR Research Complex for NEH Region, Umiam, Meghalaya, India. p8.

2. Deka, R. (2012) International Scenario of Livestock in Respect to North Eastern Region of India. Paper Presented at North East Food Tech Summit, Guwahati, India on 21st March; 2012.

3. Livestock Census. (2012) Ministry of Agriculture, Department of Animal Husbandry, Dairying and Fisheries, Krishi Bhavan, New Delhi.

4. Anjani, K., Steven, S., Elumalai, K. and Dhiraj, K.S. (2007) Livestock sector in north-eastern region of India: An appraisal of performance. *Agric. Econ. Res. Rev.,* 20: 255-272.

5. Arther, G.H., Noaks, D.E., Pearson, H. and Parkinson, T.J. (1988) Veterinary Reproduction and Obstetrics. 7th ed. W. B. Saunders Company Ltd., London, Philadelphia, Taranto, Sydney, Tokoyo.

6. Sirohi, N.S., Monga, D.P. and Knar, S.K. (1989) Microbiological studies on some reproductive disorders of cattle. *Indian J. Anim. Sci.,* 59(5): 537-541.

7. Kumaresan, A., Prabhakaran, P.P., Bujarbaruah, K.M., Pathak, K.A., Chhetri, B. and Ahmad, S.K. (2009) Reproductive performance of crossbred dairy cows reared under traditional low input production system in the eastern Himalayas. *Trop. Anim. Health Prod.,* 41: 71-78.

8. Birthal, P.S., Deoghare, P.R. and Riyazuddin, S.K. (2003) Development of Small Ruminant Sector in India. Project Report. National Centre for Agricultural Economics and Policy Research, New Delhi, India.

9. Hadush, A., Abdella, A. and Regassa, F. (2013) Major prepartum and postpartum reproductive problems of dairy cattle in Central Ethiopia. *J. Vet. Med. Anim. Health,* 5(4): 118-123.

10. Tesfaye, D. and Shamble, A. (2013) Reproductive health problems of cows under different management systems in Kombolcha, Noetheast Ehiopia. *Adv. Biomed. Res.,* 7: 104-108.

11. Sardar, M.J.U., Moni, M.I.Z. and Aktar, S. (2010) Prevalence of reproductive disorders of cross bred cows in the Rajshahi district of Bangladesh. *SARC J. Agric.,* 8(2): 65-75.

12. Kutty, C.I. and Ramachandran, K. (2001) Bovine infertility - A field oriented categorization based on investigation among crossbred cattle in a district of Kerala. *Indian J. Anim. Sci.,* 73: 155-157.

13. Serur, B.H., Farrag, A.A. and Gomaa, A. (1982) Incidence of certain infertility problems among cows and buffaloes in Upper Egypt. *Assoc. Vet. Med. J.,* 10: 209-214.

14. O'Farrel, K.J., Langley, O.H., Hartigan, P.J. and Sreenan, J.M. (1983) Fertilization and embryonic survival rates in dairy cows culled as repeat breeders. *Vet. Rec.,* 112: 95.

15. Khair, A., Alam, A.A., Rahman, M.A., Islam, M.I., Azam, A. and Chowdhury, E.H. (2013) Incidence of reproductive and production diseases of cross bred dairy cattle. *Bangladesh J. Vet. Med.,* 11(1): 31-36.

16. Salasel, B., Mokhtari, A. and Taktaz, T. (2010) Prevalence, risk factors for and impact of subclinical endometritis

in repeat breeder dairy cows. *Theriogenology,* 74(7): 1271-1278.

17. Sardar, M.J.U. (2008) Occurrence of reproductive disorders in crossbred cows of Northern Bangladesh. 15th International Congress on Biotechnology in Animal Reproduction.

18. Bhat, F.A., Bhattacharyya, H.K. and Khan, M.Z. (2012) Studies on prevalence of repeat breeding in crossbred cattle of Kashmir valley. *Indian J. Anim. Res.,* 46: 306.

19. Bicalho, R.C., Galvao, K.N., Cheong, S.H., Gilbert, R.O., Warnick, L.D. and Guard, C.L. (2007) Effect of still birth on dam survival and reproduction performance in Holstein dairy cows. *J. Dairy Sci.,* 90(6): 2797-2803.

20. Chandrahar, D.P., Tiwari, M.K. and Dutta, G.K. (2003) Serum biochemical profile of repeat breeder cows. *Indian J. Anim. Reprod.,* 24: 125-127.

21. Arthur, G.H., Noakes, D. and Pearson, H. (1996) Veterinary Reproduction and Obstetrics: (Theriogenology). 6th ed. Tindall, UK. p83-85.

22. Khan, S., Thangavel, A. and Selvasubramaniyan, S. (2010) Blood biochemical profile in repeat breeding cows. *Tamil Nadu J. Vet. Anim. Sci.,* 6: 75-80.

9

Potential of acute phase proteins as predictor of postpartum uterine infections during transition period and its regulatory mechanism in dairy cattle

A. Manimaran[1], A. Kumaresan[2], S. Jeyakumar[1], T. K. Mohanty[2], V. Sejian[1], Narender Kumar[1], L. Sreela[3], M. Arul Prakash[3], P. Mooventhan[3], A. Anantharaj[1] and D. N. Das[1]

1. Southern Regional Station, ICAR - National Dairy Research Institute, Adugodi, Bengaluru - 560 030, Karnataka, India;
2. Theriogenology Laboratory, ICAR - National Dairy Research Institute, Karnal-132 001, Haryana, Uttar Pradesh, India;
3. ICAR - National Dairy Research Institute, Karnal - 132 001, Haryana, India.
Corresponding author: S. Jeyakumar, e-mail: jeyakumarsakthivel@gmail.com,
AM: maranpharma@gmail.com, AK: ogkumaresan@gmail.com, TKM: mohanty.tushar@gmail.com,
VS: drsejian@gmail.com, NK: nklangyan@gmail.com, LS: sreela312@gmail.com, MAP: drarullpm@gmail.com,
PM: agriventhan@yahoo.co.in, AA: cellsig2ananth@gmail.com, DND: dndasndri@gmail.com

Abstract

Among the various systemic reactions against infection or injury, the acute phase response is the cascade of reaction and mostly coordinated by cytokines-mediated acute phase proteins (APPs) production. Since APPs are sensitive innate immune molecules, they are useful for early detection of inflammation in bovines and believed to be better discriminators than routine hematological parameters. Therefore, the possibility of using APPs as a diagnostic and prognostic marker of inflammation in major bovine health disorders including postpartum uterine infection has been explored by many workers. In this review, we discussed specifically importance of postpartum uterine infection, the role of energy balance in uterine infections and potential of APPs as a predictor of postpartum uterine infections during the transition period and its regulatory mechanism in dairy cattle.

Keywords: cute phase proteins, bovine uterine infections, pro-inflammatory cytokines, negative energy balance, transition period.

Introduction

The incidence of uterine infections in cows has been reported between 10% and 50% with 10-20% of metritis, 15% of clinical endometritis, and 15% of subclinical endometritis [1-3]. Sheldon and Dobson [2] reported that up to 40% of the animals have a uterine infection during initial 2 weeks postpartum, in which 10-15% show persisted infection for at least another 3 weeks while 30-35% of cows have subclinical endometritis between 4 and 9 weeks postpartum [4]. The high prevalence of postpartum uterine infections in buffalo cows (38.54%) and in crossbred cows (up to 29.7%) was also reported in India [5,6]. Uterine infections cause inflammation, histological alteration, delayed uterine involution, reduced pituitary LH secretion, and disruption of ovarian follicular growth and its function in dairy cattle [7]. Dubuc *et al.* [8] found 3.7 kg loss of milk production per day in multiparous cows due to metritis. When considering reproductive parameters alone, reproductive inefficiency beyond 100 days postpartum results in an estimated loss of $2.5 to $3 per cow per day, while overall loss due to reproductive inefficiency has been estimated to be $5.4 per cow per day [9]. With approximately 100 dairy cows with 10% incidence of uterine infections, the cost of uterine infections/cow/month would be about $750-$1620.

Although more than 95% of the animals get exposed to bacterial contaminations during calving, only a few of them develop uterine disease, and it could be the associated outcome of pathogens, animal, and the environment. However, in a particular environment with equal chances of exposure to pathogens, the more susceptibility of some animals in the herd suggested the greater importance of animal factor over the environment or pathogen-related factors. In fact, an impairment of immune functions during the peri-partum period has an important role in determining whether an animal develops postpartum uterine disease or not. However, the exact mechanism that initiates and sustains the uterine inflammation is not clear at present. Among the various factors, the energy status of the peri-partum animals is one of the most important determinants for the development of uterine disease. Endocrine and metabolic changes around parturition are believed to depress the uterine defense mechanism, which favors the development of uterine disease in dairy cattle [10,11]. The first response of the innate immune system against uterine infection is the invasion of neutrophils into the uterus. However, the invasion of neutrophils is determined by pro-inflammatory cytokines and other factors. Recently, Galvao et al. [12] observed that lower expression of pro-inflammatory cytokines in the endometrium immediately after calving impaired the chemotaxis and activation of neutrophils which leads to the development of endometritis in cows. Further, the functional capacity of neutrophils is determined by many factors, and negative energy balance (NEB) is believed to be an important determinant [13].

Prevention and early treatment of postpartum uterine infections are more economical than treatment at a later stage when diseases get established. Thus, early diagnosis or predictions of uterine infections are important for effective postpartum management. Since the postpartum complications are of multi-factorial nature; it has been difficult to find out the biomarker for early prediction of uterine infections. Recently, many workers [7,14-16] have explored the possibility of bovine major acute phase proteins (APPs) such as haptoglobins (Hp) and serum amyloid A (SAA) as biomarkers to predict the postpartum uterine infections and found different results. Huzzey et al. [17] suggested that acute phase response (APR) precedes clinical metritis, and thus Hp screening may assist for early detection of metritis. They [18] also found that Hp concentration tended to be greater during pre-partum cows that developed more than one disorder or that died by 30 days in milk. Dubuc et al. [19] reported that Hp concentrations higher than 0.8 g/l during 1st week after parturition are a risk factor for endometritis and purulent vaginal discharge. Although several review regarding the role of APPs in dairy animals are available [20,21], we are specifically discussing here the potential of APPs as the predictor of postpartum uterine infections during the transition period and its regulatory mechanism in dairy cattle.

Uterine Immunology during Transition Period

Although, our understanding of the role of the uterine immune system is still limited, it is believed that uterine defense mechanisms play a major role during the postpartum period. Cellular defense against bacterial contaminants is mainly provided by uterine leukocytes, in which neutrophils are the major and primary defense molecule involved in bacterial clearance after uterine infection [22]. Neutrophils are short-lived (1-3 days) cells, and they have the ability to migrate and engulf the foreign invaders. They execute their functions through oxygen-dependent free radical-mediated killing (respiratory burst) or through enzymatic killing of the pathogens. It is believed that adequate recruitment of functionally active neutrophils in the uterus is foremost important for clearing the bacteria [22]. In general, pathogen recognition receptors on the endometrial cells and macrophages mainly toll-like receptors, recognize the pathogen through pathogen-associated molecular patterns and

secrete or release the mediators such as pro-inflammatory cytokines (interleukin [IL]-1β, IL-6, tumor necrosis factor-α [TNF-α], etc.) and chemokines (IL-8) [23], then IL-6, TNF-α, and IL-8 stimulate the production of antimicrobial peptides by endometrial cells or accelerate the polymorphonuclear (PMN) cells infiltration into endometrium for elimination of pathogens [24]. The function of TNF-α is to stimulate the IL-8 expression and cell adhesion molecules on vascular endothelium while IL-8 is a potent chemoattractant. However, the kinetics of neutrophils with reference to the magnitude of movement and time of appearance in the uterus depends on chemoattractant produced by inflammation or bacterial stimulation, energy state, hormonal influence, and other factors. For instance, Zerbe et al. [25] reported that infusion of human recombinant IL-8 into bovine uterus cause attraction of PMN, while anti-IL-8 antibody prevented the PMN-dependent PMN infiltration and subsequent tissue damage. Although, this observation confirmed the IL-8 role in normal animals, its role under the influence of uterine infections remains to be confirmed. They also suggested the influence of bacteria and its components on neutrophils entry into uterus [26]. Although, the cytokines are believed to play an important role in neutrophil migration and clearance of pathogens, higher or excessive expressions of pro-inflammatory cytokines are often associated with greater inflammation during the 1st or 2nd week postpartum [27,28], while their lower expression in the endometrium immediately after calving impaired the chemotaxis and activation of neutrophils which leads to development of endometritis in cows [12]. Collectively, it suggests that adequate stimulation of pro-inflammatory cytokines is critical for the healthy uterus and any changes in these cytokines synthesis will adversely affect the uterine immunity.

Several authors suggested that changes in cytokines levels during the peri-partum period could be useful for predicting postpartum complications. Ishikawa et al. [29] investigated the correlation between the IL-6 concentration and the occurrence of postpartum diseases and found that cows suffered with endometritis had a higher level of pre-partum IL-6 than control. They suggested that alteration in the IL-6 concentration during pregnancy was one the useful tool for predicting postpartum diseases in dairy cattle. Kim et al. [11] reported that dairy cows suffered with endometritis during the 3rd and 4th week postpartum period had a higher concentration of TNF-α than normal cows. Islama et al. [30] observed the significantly higher concentration of IL-10 in clinical metritis than normal cows at 15 days before calving, at calving and 15 days postpartum. However, the significant difference was found only at 30 d postpartum for clinical endometritis cows. Kasimanickam et al. [31] found that cows with metritis or clinical endometritis had higher serum concentrations of IL-1β, TNF-α, and IL-6 compared to normal cows and suggested that loss of body conditions mediated increases in cytokines and thereby prolonged the uterine inflammation in dairy cows.

Energy Balance and Postpartum Uterine Infections

Among the various factors, the energy status of the postpartum animals is one of the most important determinants for the development of uterine disease. Hammon et al. [13] reported that cows in greater NEB have more pronounced impairment of immune functions and susceptibility to develop metritis or endometritis. Among the various mediators, inflammatory cytokines are believed to be as central integrators of metabolic changes and immune function [32], particularly during the transition period. For instances, slower increase of negative APPs such as albumin and higher concentration of NEFA, BHBA in transition cows after administration of interferon alpha [33], increased risk of ketosis in cows administered TNF-α during late pregnancy [34], and possible role of IL-6 in ketosis [35] are suggestive for the role of cytokines in metabolic disorders. Collectively, it suggests that cytokines have an important role during the transition period. NEB-mediated alterations of gene expression and metabolites (NEFA or BHBA) also have an important role in uterine immunity. Beam and Butler [36] observed that cows with severe NEB had increased uterine pro-inflammatory cytokine gene expression at 2 weeks postpartum compared to moderate NEB cows. Further, it was supported by the findings of Wathes et al. [37] that NEB caused more expression of uterine inflammation-associated genes (IL-1 and IL-8 receptors). The higher concentrations of NEFA and BHBA during pre-partum have been associated with postpartum metritis and endometritis in cows, and it could be mediated through impairment of neutrophils function [13,38]. Decreased concentrations of glycogen in neutrophils and blood calcium were also suggested for reduction of neutrophil function and thus favor postpartum uterine infection [38]. Recently, Giuliodori et al. [39] found that higher pre-partum NEFA and postpartum BHBA levels increased the risk for endometritis, whereas high pre-partum BUN reduced it.

Although the major consequence of uterine infection is conception failure and subsequent culling [40], the possible mechanism for such outcome remains unclear. Therefore, proper investigation of the mechanism would be very useful for the development of diagnostic or prognostic markers for postpartum health assessment. Rossi et al. [41] reported that NEB can affect cow reproductive performances through metabolic hormonal modifications. They suggested that profound changes in the liver lead to a reduction in the concentration of growth hormone receptor (GHR), insulin-like growth factor (IGF)-I level, IGF binding proteins (IGFBPs), and the acid-labile subunit while IGFBP-2 was increased. Collectively, it causes the impairment of reproductive functions (Figure-1).

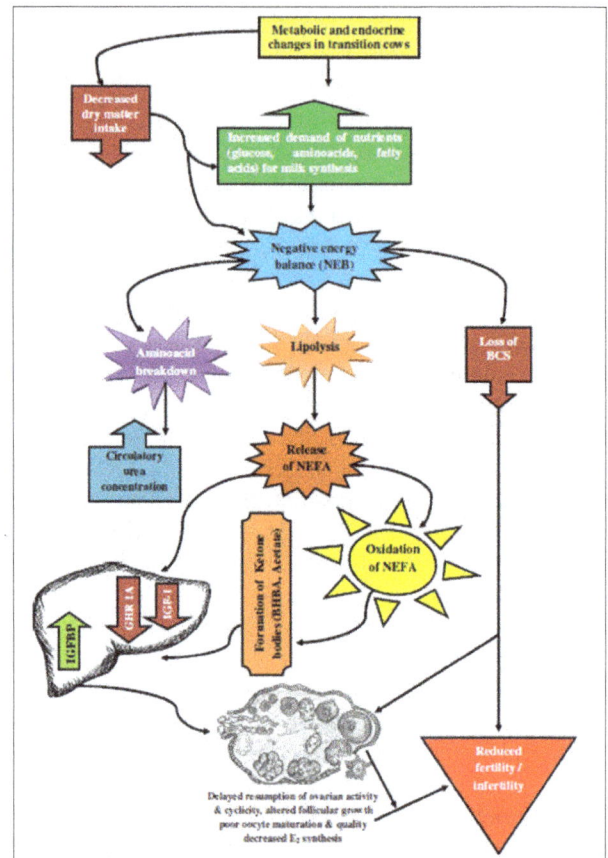

Figure-1: Effects of negative energy balance on reproductive function. Up arrow indicate increase while down arrows indicate a decrease.

Biomarkers in Uterine Infections

Identification of biomarkers against various diseases becomes a major thrust area of research in this "omic" era due to the discovery of new molecules and technologies. Identification of biomarkers would be useful to assess the pathophysiological status of the animal and thus early diagnosis, treatment, and prevention of economically important diseases including postpartum uterine infections. Though some traditional markers (such as NEFA, BHBA, and feeding behavior) are available to predict the postpartum uterine infections, they were not successful due to its variability between the conditions. Silva et al. [42] explored the possible role of COX-2 and PGE$_2$ as biomarkers (at transcription and protein level) and found that they were not useful markers. Recently, Dubuc et al. [19] suggested that higher pre-partum NEFA concentration, dystokia, and RFM as important risk factors for metritis while, ketosis as a risk factor for subclinical endometritis and dystokia, twinning, and metritis for clinical endometritis. Interestingly, they found that increased Hp concentration during the 1st week of postpartum as a common risk factor for all these conditions [19]. It suggested that despite variation in clinical manifestations of postpartum uterine infections, Hp could serve as a better indicator for the postpartum performance of dairy animals.

Cairoli *et al.* [43] found that the concentrations of Hp and α₁-acid glycoprotein (AGP) were fluctuated at the time of calving and in cows affected with postpartum endometritis.

Role of APPs in Bovine Reproduction

Following infection, injury or even with changes in normal physiological homeostasis, a number of systemic responses take place, and APR is one of them. APR is a cascade of systemic reactions (Figure-2) against inflammation, mostly coordinated by cytokines, which are produced from macrophages or any other inflammatory cells. Production of pro-inflammatory cytokines (mainly IL-1β, TNF-α, and IL-6) at the site of injury, subsequently stimulates the production of APPs from a local site or at the liver. APPs are classified into three categories based on the: (1) magnitude of elevation in blood (positive if they increase or negative if they decrease), (2) time of APPs released into blood in response to APR (first phase proteins are elevated immediately and second phase proteins are increased after 1-3 days), and (3) cytokines which are responsible for its stimulation (IL-1- and IL-6-dependent response). Collectively, it suggests that the kinetics of APPs would differ based on APR, severity of infection and time course of infections. About 40 APPs have been identified in humans. Out of which, nine APPs are well-studied in cattle. Among these nine proteins, Hp and SAA are considered as major, while AGP is moderate and fibrinogen (Fb) is minor [20,44]. Further, the major APPs (Hp and SAA) can also act as moderate APPs in bovines. Several researchers observed that Hp concentrations are often undetectable in healthy cattle [45] but increase about 50±100 times during an APR, making it the most prominent APP in cattle [46]. On the other hand, SAA is a low constitutive APP in cattle increasing around 2±5 times or 10-fold during an APR [46,47]. Nevertheless, SAA seems to react faster than Hp against APR [48], and thus SAA is considered as good marker for acute clinical conditions [49] while Hp as a better marker for chronic conditions [50].

The role of APPs following infection has been extensively evaluated in human practice to monitor pathogenesis of disease and efficacy of treatment. In veterinary practice, the application of APPs for the determination of health status in domestic and pet animals was reviewed by various authors [20,21,45,51]. In large ruminants, the role of APPs in mastitis was extensively studied [52-55]. Krakowski and Zdzisińska [56] reported that major bovine APPs plays an important role in the reproductive processes through intensification of the phagocytosis against the pathogens introduced into the uterus and by the reconstruction of the endometrium. Indeed, the role of APPs in prediction, diagnosis, and treatment evaluation of postpartum uterine infections was also reported by several researchers [18,57-59]. Mordark [60], found a higher concentration of Hp in cows with retained placenta, which is believed to be an immune-mediated disorder. Williams *et al.* [61] observed that cows with high uterine pathogen growth density had higher peripheral concentrations of AGP, SAA, and Hp compared to low uterine pathogen growth density cows during 7 and 14 days postpartum period. A positive correlation between APPs level and severity of disease and the extent of the tissue damage was also reported by Baumann and Gauldie [62]. Further, they suggested the differential kinetics of the APR between APPs,

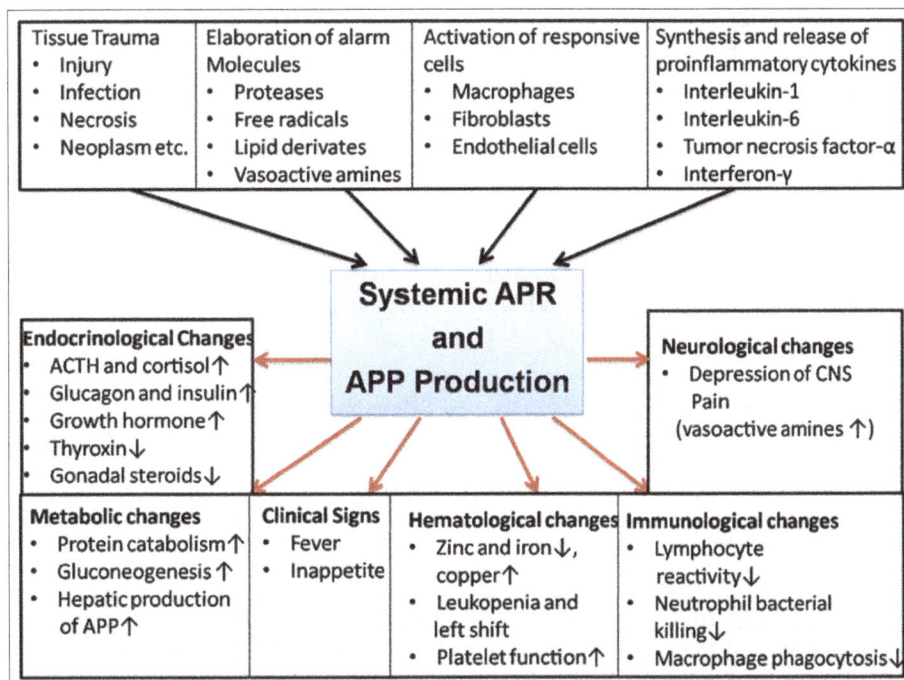

Figure-2: Acute phase responses. ↑increase, ↓decrease.

where AGP had more persistent effect than Hp or SAA. In contrast, Pyorala [51] revealed that the AGP levels did not correlate with the severity of disease compared to Hp, and thus the capacity of AGP in differentiating uterine infections was poor.

Measurements of serum Hp and SAA have been widely used to diagnose the uterine infection in postpartum cows. Hirvonen et al. [58] studied the diagnostic and prognostic efficacy of Hp and AGP in acute metritis cows during postpartum period and found increased plasma Hp concentration in metritic cows and predicted the poor condition and low fertile cows. Regassa and Noakes [63] reported that presence of intrauterine infections did not affect the uterine involution in mule ewes. However, the Hp level was significantly higher in the uterine infected ewes than the healthy ewes. Sheldon et al. [64] found that uterine involution was associated with a decrease in the concentrations of APPs (AGP, Hp, and CP). However, the bacterial contamination increased the APPs irrespective of uterine involution status. It suggested that APPs could be useful to differentiate between postpartum infections with normal physiological events. Horadagoda et al. [50] reported that assays of APP, particularly Hp and SAA, might differentiate the chronic from the acute inflammation in cattle in a better way than the hematological tests. In contrast, Humblet et al. [14] suggested that Hp and SAA were good markers for identification of healthy animals, but their ability to identify the diseased animals was low as most of the postpartum diseases were chronic in nature. Further, they reported that physiological status of a cow, particularly at parturition, can have an influence on serum Hp concentration. Heidarpour et al. [65], found that cows suffered with clinical and subclinical endometritis had significantly higher concentration of Hp. Schneider et al. [66] found that cows diagnosed with uterine infection had a higher concentration of Hp during 7 days postpartum. Besides, Kováč et al. [67] studied the relationship between APPs (Hp and SAA) and energy metabolites (NEFA and BHBA) in dairy cows and found significant correlations between Hp with NEFA as well as BHBA and SAA with only NEFA. Various workers reported a positive correlation between hormonal status (estrogens, progesterone, and cortisol) and Hp level during the last trimester of pregnancy and after calving [68,69].

Smith et al. [57] evaluated the therapeutic efficacy of different antimicrobial regimens through serum Hp concentrations in cows suffered with toxic puerperal metritis and found that the 5-day treatments reduced the serum Hp concentration (19 mg/dl vs. 7.35 mg/dl). Heidarpour et al. [65] reported that Hp level was reduced after treatment in cows suffered with clinical endometritis and cows had a lower concentration of Hp (before treatment), shown a better response to further treatment. In contrast, Jeremejeva et al. [60] evaluated the effect of two treatment strategies (ceftiofur + NSIAD and ceftiofur + PGF2α) in acute puerperal metritis and clinical metritis cows through APPs (SAA and Hp) and found no significant difference. Mordak [70] found that the cows with highest Hp concentration were expelled placenta after 4 days (2.22 g/l) and cows with the lowest concentration of Hp had been easily removed the placenta (0.9 g/l).

Besides, the diagnostic and prognostic applications of APPs few studies were attempted to see the dynamics of APPs with postpartum performance to consider the potential role of APPs as a predictor for uterine infections and subsequent conception. Chan et al. [71] reported that cows suffered by postpartum reproductive disorders had a significantly greater concentration of Hp than the healthy animals with no significant influence of season or pregnancy. It suggests that Hp is not influenced by environment or physiological status and thus a useful indicator for cows with postpartum reproductive disorders. Huzzey et al. [17] reported that mild and severe metritis cows had higher Hp concentrations than healthy cows in early postpartum period (between 0 and 12) and cows with ≥ 1 g/L Hp concentrations on day 3 postpartum were 6.7 times more susceptible for severe or mild metritis with 50% sensitivity and 87% specificity. They suggested that APR precedes clinical metritis, and thus Hp screening may assist for early detection of metritis and opportunities for early treatment or prevention. Chan et al. [16] found that serum Hp concentrations in cows suffered with acute puerperal metritis were significantly higher than clinically healthy animals from 1 week pre-partum to 6-month postpartum period. In addition, among the successfully pregnant animals, the number of days open was significantly higher in cows had a higher concentration of Hp than cows with a lower concentration of Hp; suggest that Hp may also be a useful predictor of postpartum reproductive performance. Sabedra et al. [72] reported that elevated serum Hp concentrations were associated with disease status (healthy vs. infected), severity (healthy, moderate, severe, or died), number, and type of disease (one or more diseases such as metritis, ketosis and mastitis), birth complications, and clinical onset of disease in early lactation. Further, they suggested that serum Hp concentrations may assist in early detection and treatment of diseases in early lactation. Burke et al. [73] reported that among successfully pregnant animals, the number of days open was significantly higher in cows with a high concentration of Hp suggesting its prediction ability of postpartum performance even in the absence of uterine infections.

Recently Huzzy et al. [74] evaluated the association between peri-partum (3 weeks before calving to 10 days after calving) markers of stress (cortisol), inflammation (Hp), and energy balance (NEFA and BHBA) and milk yield and reproductive performance in HF cows and found negative association of Hp and other markers with milk yield and reproductive performance. It suggested that understanding of Hp dynamics during peri-partum would be useful for assessing the opportunities for improved milk yield and reproduction. Krause et al. [75] evaluated the association between resumption of postpartum ovarian activity, uterine health (PMN cells and P₄ levels), severity of the NEB (through NEFA, glucose and insulin levels), and the synthesis of inflammatory mediators (albumin and Hp levels and paraoxonase activity) during the transition period and found that cows resumed ovarian activity early in the postpartum period had higher albumin concentrations during peri-partum period. However, they found no association between APPs levels with subclinical endometritis incidence and markers of energy indicators or milk yield with postpartum cyclicity. It suggested that influences of energy on APPs dynamics need to be further evaluated. Nightingale et al. [76] investigated the relationship between the intensity of the APR (through classification of cows with low, medium and high concentrations of Hp) and the metabolic status and leukocyte responses of early postpartum cows and found that postpartum reproductive performance was impaired in cows with a greater APR (days open in these groups were 123, 139, and 183 days, respectively). They suggested that a stronger APR during the early postpartum period is characterized by an activated innate immune system, and a suppressed mitogen-induced interferon-γ secretion resulted in impaired reproductive efficiency.

APPs and Cytokines Expression in Uterine Tissues

APPs are primarily synthesized by the liver against APR. However, there is increasing evidence for the extra-hepatic expression of APPs for the local needs. For instance, the APP synthesis in the mammary gland is a well-known phenomenon during mastitis or physiological changes such as involution. Chapwanya et al. [28] reported that expression of SAA3 mRNA was increased in early postpartum (2 weeks) compared to late postpartum (9 weeks) cows and SAA reflected the severity of inflammation. They also revealed that the SAA expression was higher than Hp mRNA expression. Gabler et al. [77] revealed time-related expression of inflammatory cytokines and APPs, with significant peak expression on the day 17 postpartum period as a possible mucosal immune response in the uterus. In addition, they found that IL-1β, IL-8, and Hp mRNA expression were correlated significantly with the proportion of PMN. Collectively, it suggests that the dynamics of these APPs differs between normal and inflamed uterus and it needs further investigation. Further, the moderate level of expression of AGP in the healthy uterus has been reported by some researchers [78,79], but there is no information on AGP expression in the infected uterus.

Fischer et al. [24] found that the expression of IL-1β, IL-8, and TNF- α mRNA was significantly higher in cows with subclinical or clinical endometritis compared with healthy cows while there was no indication or correlation with uterine health for IL-6 and Hp transcripts. They suggested that IL-1β, IL-8, and TNF-α might represent potential marker genes for the detection of cows with subclinical endometritis and for monitoring new therapeutic approaches. Ghasemi et al. [80] found 20, 30, and more than 50-fold higher mRNA expression of TNF-α, IL-6, and IL-8 level, respectively, in subclinical endometritis than healthy cows. They suggested that IL-8 gene expression might be useful to predict endometrial inflammation. Galvão et al. [81] found that Escherichia coli-stimulated monocytes from cows with metritis had lower expression of TNF-α, IL-1β, and IL-6 than healthy counterpart while there were no significant differences in IL-8 or IL-10 expression in these cows. Collectively, it suggested that pro-inflammatory cytokines expressions are differentially altered during postpartum uterine infections.

Loyi et al. [82] found several fold higher expression of cytokines (IL-1β, IL-6, IL-8, and TNF-α) in endometritic samples while significant up-regulation of CD14, IL-6, IL-8, and TNF-α mRNA in subclinical endometritic buffaloes samples collected from the abattoir. Chapwanya et al. [83] found that expression of IL-1β, TNF-α, and SAA3 genes were increased by 121-, 357-, and 721-fold, respectively, during 6 h post E. coli stimulation. However, IL-1β, IL-6, IL-8, and TNF-α gene expression was decreased, whereas SAA3 expression was further increased to 3452-fold after 24 h of E. coli stimulation compared to 6 h. They suggested that better understanding of localized endometrial expression of SAA3 was needed to use SAA as a sensitive diagnostic marker for E. coli infection in cattle.

Transcriptional Regulation of APP Production

Although, APR and subsequent changes in serum concentrations of APPs are known for almost a century, the biological importance of the different APPs and molecular mechanisms controlling their expression is just beginning to emerge. The expressions of APPs in hepatocytes are mostly controlled at the transcriptional level by different transcriptional factors such as signal transducer and activator of transcription (STAT) family [84] and NF-kB [85]. However, the transcription factors involved in the regulation of each APPs and in species are differed. For instance, the transcriptional regulation of SAA gene is mainly controlled by NF-kB [86], while of fibrinogens, α₂-macroglobulin, or α₁-antichymotrypsin strongly depends on STAT3. Regarding individual APP regulation, NF-kB plays an essential role for the transcriptional up-regulation of the SAA [87,88] or AGP expression [89]. Several reports further indicated that the expression of SAA is cooperatively regulated by NF-kB and

STAT3 [90,91]. Therefore, understanding the role of APPs in innate immunity, detailed knowledge of its regulations and functions of different proteins, and their mutual interrelationship are required [92].

Conclusion

Early predictions of economically important diseases including postpartum uterine infections are very important for optimizing productive and reproductive performance in dairy animals. On other hand, estimation of major APPs such as Hp and SAA are seems to be very useful during the transition period for prediction of animals at risk, evaluation of treatment outcome and prognosis of the disease. Although the available results suggested that APPs could differentiate the healthy and inflamed uterus in advance, studies on the cellular and molecular mechanism of APPs regulation during transition or early postpartum period are required. Such studies in naturally infected (with appropriate diagnosis) animals could further strengthen the existing evidence as transition period has differential immune, hormonal, and energy status. Further, it is believed that the Indian cattle are less susceptible or more resistant to diseases due to the strong innate immune system in these animals. Therefore, the correlation between APPs level and postpartum performance during early lactation are needed to be studied in indigenous animals for better understanding.

Authors' Contributions

AM, AK, SJ, TKM, VS, and DND conceptualized the concept of this review paper. AM and SJ prepared the final figures and manuscript. NK, SL, MAP, PM, and AA assisted in collecting and compiling the resource material and in manuscript preparation. All authors read and approved the final manuscript.

Acknowledgments

The authors are thankful to Head, SRS, and Director, ICAR - NDRI for providing needful facilities. The fund for the study was provided by ICAR - NDRI, Karnal.

Competing Interests

The authors declare that they have no competing interests.

References

1. Lewis, G.S. (1997) Symposium: Health problems of the postpartum cow. *J. Dairy Sci.*, 80: 984-994.
2. Sheldon, I.M. and Dobson, H. (2004) Postpartum uterine health in cattle. *Anim. Reprod. Sci.*, 82-83: 295-306.
3. LeBlanc, S.J., Osawa, T. and Dubuc, J. (2011) Reproductive tract defense and disease in postpartum dairy cows. *Theriogenology*, 76(9): 1610-1618.
4. LeBlanc, S.J. (2008) Production diseases of the transition cow. Postpartum uterine diseases and dairy herd reproductive performance: A review. *Vet. J.*, 176(1): 102-114.
5. Rantibioticn, S.R.P. and Bawa, S.J.S. (1977) Incidence of pre and postpartum reproductive disorders in buffaloes. *Haryana Vet.*, 16: 99-101.
6. Pal, S. (2003) Investigation on health disorder in dairy cattle and buffaloes during pre and postpartum period. M.V.Sc. Thesis Submitted to NDRI, Karnal.
7. Williams, E.J., Fischer, D.P., Pfeiffer, D.U., England, G.C.W., Noakes, D.E., Dobson, H. and Sheldon, I.M. (2005) Clinical evaluation of postpartum vaginal mucus reflects uterine bacterial infection and the immune response in cattle. *Theriogenology*, 63: 102-117.
8. Dubuc, J., Duffield, T.F., Leslie, K.E., Walton, J.S. and LeBlanc, S.J. (2011a) Impact of postpartum uterine diseases on milk production and culling in dairy cows. *J. Dairy Sci.*, 94(3): 1339-1346.
9. Plaizier, J.C., King, G.J., Dekkers, J.C. and Lissemore, K. (1997) Estimation of economic values of indices for reproductive performance in dairy herds using computer simulation. *J. Dairy Sci.*, 80(11): 2775-2783.
10. Mateus, L., Costa, L.L.D., Bernardo, F. and Silva, J.R. (2002) Influence of puerperal uterine infection on uterine involution and postpartum ovarian activity in dairy cows. *Reprod. Dom. Anim.*, 37(1): 31-35.
11. Kim, I.H., Na, K.J. and Yang, M.P. (2005) Immune responses during the peripartum period in dairy cows with postpartum endometritis. *J. Reprod. Dev.*, 51: 757-764.
12. Galvão, K.N., Santos, N.R., Galvao, J.S. and Gilbert, R.O. (2011) Association between endometritis and endometrial cytokine expression in postpartum Holstein cows. *Theriogenology*, 76: 290-299.
13. Hammon, D.S., Evjen, I.M., Dhiman, T.R., Goff, J.P. and Walters, J.L. (2006) Neutrophil function and energy status in Holstein cows with uterine health disorders. *Vet. Immunol. Immunopathol.*, 113: 21-29.
14. Humblet, M.F., Guyot, H., Boudry, B., Mbayahi, F., Hanzen, C., Rollin, F. and Godeau, J.M. (2006) Relationship between haptoglobin, serum amyloid A, and clinical status in a survey of dairy herds during a 6-month period. *Vet. Clin. Pathol.*, 35: 188-193.
15. Kovac, G., Popelkova, M., Tkacikova, L., Burdova, O. and Ihnat, O. (2007) Interrelationship between somatic cell count and acute phase proteins in serum and milk of dairy cows. *Acta Vet. Brno.*, 76: 51-57.
16. Chan, J.P.W., Chang, C.C., Chin, C., Hsu, W.L., Liu, W.B. and Chen, T.H. (2010) Association of increased serum acute-phase protein concentrations with reproductive performance in dairy cows with postpartum metritis. *Vet. Clin. Pathol.*, 39(1): 72-78.
17. Huzzey, J.M., Duffield, T.F., LeBlanc, S.J., Veira, D.M., Weary, D.M. and von Keyserlingk, M.A.G. (2009) Short communication: Haptoglobin as an early indicator of metritis. *J. Dairy Sci.*, 92(2): 621-625.
18. Huzzey, J.M., Nydam, D.V., Grant, R.J. and Overton, T.R. (2011) Associations of prepartum plasma cortisol, haptoglobin, fecal cortisol metabolites, and nonesterified fatty acids with postpartum health status in Holstein dairy cows. *J. Dairy Sci.*, 94(12): 5878-5889.
19. Dubuc, J., Duffield, T.F., Leslie, K.E., Walton, J.S. and LeBlanc, S.J. (2010) Risk factors for postpartum uterine diseases in dairy cows. *J. Dairy Sci.*, 93(12): 5764-5771.
20. Eckersall, P.D. and Bell, R. (2010) Acute phase proteins: Biomarkers of infection and inflammation in veterinary medicine. *Vet. J.*, 185(1): 23-27.
21. Ceciliani, F., Ceron, J.J., Eckersall, P.D. and Sauerwein, H. (2012) Acute phase proteins in ruminants. *J. Proteomics*, 75(14): 4207-4231.
22. Gilbert, R.O., Santos, N.R., Galvao, K.N., Brittin, S.B. and Roman, H.B. (2007) The relationship between postpartum uterine bacterial infection (BI) and subclinical endometritis (SE). *J. Dairy Sci.*, 90(1): 469.
23. Beutler, B., Hoebe, K., Du, X. and Ulevitch, R.J. (2003) How we detect microbes and respond to them: Toll-like receptors and their transducers. *J. Leuk. Biol.*, 74: 479-485.
24. Fischer, C., Drillich, M., Odau, S., Heuwieser, W., Einspanier, R. and Gabler, C. (2010) Selected pro-inflammatory factor

transcripts in bovine endometrial epithelial cells are regulated during the oestrous cycle and elevated in case of subclinical or clinical endometritis. *Reprod. Fertil. Dev.,* 22: 818-829.

25. Zerbe, H., Schuberth, H.J., Engelke, F., Frank, J., Klug, E. and Leibold, W. (2003) Development and comparison of *in vivo* and *in vitro* models for endometritis in cows and mares. *Theriogenology,* 60: 209-223.

26. Zerbe, H., Obadnik, C., Leibold, W. and Schuberth, H.J. (2001) Influence of *Escherichia coli* and Arcanobacteriumpyogenes isolated from bovine puerperal uteri on phenotypic and functional properties of neutrophils. *Vet. Microbiol.,* 79: 351-365.

27. Herath, S., Lilly, S.T., Santos, N.R., Gilbert, R.O., Goetze, L., Bryant, C.E., White, J.O., Cronin, J. and Sheldon, I.M. (2009) Expression of genes associated with immunity in the endometrium of cattle with disparate postpartum uterine disease and fertility. *Reprod. Biol. Endocrinol.,* 7: 55.

28. Chapwanya, A., Meade, K.G., Doherty, M.L., Callanan, J.J., Mee, J.F. and O'Farrelly, C. (2009) Histopathological and molecular evaluation of Holstein-Friesian cows postpartum: Toward an improved understanding of uterine innate immunity. *Theriogenology,* 71: 1396-1407.

29. Ishikawa, Y., Nakada, K., Hagiwara, K., Kirisawa, R., Iwai, H., Moriyoshi, M. and Sawamukai, Y. (2004) Changes in interleukin-6 concentration in peripheral blood of pre-and post-partum dairy cattle and its relationship to postpartum reproductive diseases. *J. Vet. Med. Sci.,* 66(11): 1403-1408.

30. Islama, R., Kumar, H., Nandi, S. and Rai, R.B. (2013) Determination of anti-inflammatory cytokine in periparturient cows for prediction of postpartum reproductive diseases. *Theriogenology,* 79: 974-979.

31. Kasimanickam, R.K., Kasimanickam, V.R., Olsen, J.R., Jeffress, E.J., Moore, D.A. and Kastelic, J.P. (2013) Associations among serum pro-and anti-inflammatory cytokines, metabolic mediators, body condition, and uterine disease in postpartum dairy cows. *Reprod. Biol. Endocrinol.,* 11: 103.

32. Sordillo, L.M., Pighetti, G.M. and Davis, M.R. (1995) Enhanced production of bovine tumor necrosis factor-alpha during the periparturientperiod. *Vet. Immunol. Immunopathol.,* 49: 263-270.

33. Trevisi, E., Amadori, M., Bakudila, A.M. and Bertoni, G. (2009) Metabolic changes in dairy cows induced by oral, low-dose interferon-alpha treatment. *J. Anim. Sci.,* 87: 3020-3029.

34. Bradford, B.J., Mamedova, L.K., Minton, J.E., Drouillard, J.S. and Johnson. B.J. (2009) Daily injection of tumor necrosis factor-α increases hepatic triglycerides and alters transcript abundance of metabolic genes in lactating dairy cattle. *J. Nutr.,* 139: 1451-1456.

35. Loor, J.J. and Everts, R.E. (2007) Nutrition-induced ketosis alters metabolic and signaling gene networks in liver of periparturient dairy cows. *Physiol. Genomics.,* 32(1): 105-116.

36. Beam, S.W. and Butler, W.R. (1998) Energy balance, metabolic hormones, and early postpartum follicular development in dairy cows fed prilled lipid. *J. Dairy Sci.,* 81: 121-131.

37. Wathes, D.C., Cheng, Z., Chowdhury, W., Fenwick, M.A., Fitzpatrick, R., Morris, D.G., Patton, J. and Murphy, J.J. (2009) Negative energy balance alters global gene expression and immune responses in the uterus of postpartum dairy cows. *Physiol. Genomics.,* 39: 1-13.

38. Galvao, K.N., Flaminio, M.J.B., Brittin, S.B., Sper, R., Fraga, M., Caixeta, L., Ricci, A., Guard, C.L., Butler, W.R. and Gilbert, R.O. (2010) Association between uterine disease and indicators of neutrophil and systemic energy status in lactating Holstein cows. *J. Dairy Sci.,* 93: 2926-2937.

39. Giuliodori, M.J., Magnasco, R.P., Becu-Villalobos, D., Lacau-Mengido, I.M., Risco, C.A. and De la Sota, R.L. (2013) Clinical endometritis in an Argentinean herd of dairy

cows: Risk factors and reproductive efficiency. *J. Dairy Sci.,* 96(1): 210-218.

40. Bell, M.J. and Roberts, D.J. (2007) The impact of uterine infection on a dairy cow's performance. *Theriogenology,* 68: 1074-1079.

41. Rossi, F., Righi, F., Romanelli, S. and Quarantelli, A. (2008) Reproductive efficiency of dairy cows under negative energy balance conditions. *Ann. Fac. Med. Vet. Parma.,* 28: 173-180.

42. Silva, E., Gaivao, M., Leitao, S., Antibioticro, A. and Costa, L.L. (2008) Blood COX-2 and PGES gene transcription during the peripartum period of dairy cows with normal puerperium or with uterine infection. *Domest. Anim. Endocrinol.,* 35: 314-323.

43. Cairoli, F., Battocchio, M., Veronesi, M.C., Brambilla, D., Conserva, F., Eberini, I., Wait, R. and Gianazza, E. (2006) Serum protein pattern during cow pregnancy: Acute-phase proteins increase in the Peripartum period. *Electrophoresis,* 27: 1617-1625.

44. Petersen, H.H., Nielsen, J.P. and Heegaard, P.M.H. (2004) Application of acute phase protein measurement in veterinary clinical chemistry. *Vet. Res.,* 35: 163-187.

45. Eckersall, P.D. and Conner, J.G. (1988) Bovine and canine acute phase proteins. *Vet. Res.,* 12(2-3): 169-178.

46. Alsemgeest, S.P.M., Kalsbeek, H.C., Wensing, T., Koeman, J.P., Van Ederen, A.M. and Gruys, E. (1994) Concentrations of SAA (SAA) and haptoglobin (Hp) as parameters of inflammatory diseases in cattle. *Vet. Q.,* 16: 21-23.

47. Gruys, E., Ederen, A.M., Alsemgeest, S.P.M., Kalsbeek, H.C. and Wensing, T. (1993) Acute phase protein values in blood of cattle as indicator of animals with pathological process. *Arch. Lebensmittel Hyg.,* 44(5): 107-111.

48. Horadagoda, A., Eckersall, P.D., Hodgson, J.C., Gibbs, H.A. and Moon, G.M. (1994) Immediate responses in serum TNF-α and acute phase protein concentrations to infection with Pasteurella haemolytica A1 in calves. *Res. Vet. Sci.,* 57: 129-132.

49. Horadagoda, N.U., Knox, K.M.G., Gibbs, H.A., Reid, S.W.J., Horadagoda, A., Edwards, S.E.R. and Eckersall, P.D. (1999) Acute phase proteins in cattle: Discrimination between acute and chronic inflammation. *Vet. Rec.,* 144: 437-441.

50. Pyorala, S. (2000) Hirvonen's Thesis on Acute Phase Response in Dairy Cattle. Finnland: University of Helsinki.

51. Murata, H., Shimada, N. and Yoshioka, M. (2004) Current research on acute phase proteins in veterinary diagnosis: An overview. *Vet. J.,* 168: 28-40.

52. Eckersall, P.D., Young, F.J., McComb, C., Hogarth, C.J., Safi, S., Weber, A., McDonald, T., Nolan, A.M. and Fitzpatrick, J.L. (2001) Acute phase proteins in serum and milk from dairy cows with clinical mastitis. *Vet. Rec.,* 148(2): 35-41.

53. Suojala, L., Orro, T., Jarvinen, H., Saatsi, J. and Pyorala, S. (2008) Acute phase response in two consecutive experimentally induced *E. coli* intra-mammary infections in dairy cows. *Acta Vet. Scand.,* 50: 18.

54. Wenz, J.R., Fox, L.K., Muller, F.J., Rinaldi, M., Zeng, R. and Bannerman, D.D. (2010) Factors associated with concentrations of select cytokine and acute phase proteins in dairy cows with naturally occurring clinical mastitis. *J. Dairy Sci.,* 93: 2458-2470.

55. Larsen, T., Rontved, C.M., Ingvartsen, K.L., Vels, L. and Bjerring, M. (2010) Enzyme activity and acute phase proteins in milk utilized as indicators of acute clinical *E. coli* LPS-induced mastitis. *Animal,* 4: 1672-1679.

56. Krakowski, L. and Zdzisińska, B. (2007) Selected cytokines and acute phase proteins in heifers during the ovarian cycle course and in different pregnancy periods. *Bull. Vet. Inst. Pulway.,* 51: 31-36.

57. Smith, B.I., Donovan, G.A., Risco, C., Littell, R., Young, C., Stanker, L.H. and Elliott, J. (1998b) Comparison of various

antibiotic treatments for cows diagnosed with toxic puerperal metritis. *J. Dairy Sci.,* 81(6): 1555-1562.

58. Hirvonen, J., Huszenicza, G., Kulcsar, M. and Pyorala, S., (1999) Acute-phase response in dairy cows with acute postpartum metritis. *Theriogenology,* 51: 1071-1083.

59. Jeremejeva, J., Orro, T., Waldmann, A. and Kask, K. (2012) Treatment of dairy cows with PGF2α or NSAID, in combination with antibiotics, in cases of postpartum uterine inflammation. *Acta Vet. Scand.,* 54: 45.

60. Mordark, R. (2009) Postpartum serum concentration of haptoglobin in cows with fetal membranes retention. *Cattle Pract.,* 17: 100-102.

61. Williams, E.J., Fischer, D.P., Noakes, D.E., England, G.C., Rycroft, A., Dobson, H. and Sheldon, I.M. (2007) The relationship between uterine pathogen growth density and ovarian function in the postpartum dairy cow. *Theriogenology,* 68: 549-559.

62. Baumann, H. and Gauldie, J. (1994) The acute phase response. *Immunol. Today,* 15: 74-80.

63. Regassa, F. and Noakes, D.E. (1999) Acute phase protein response of ewes and the release of PGFM in relation to uterine involution and the presence of intrauterine bacteria. *Vet. Rec.,* 144: 502-506.

64. Sheldon, I.M., Noakes, D.E., Rycroft, A.N. and Dobson, H. (2001) Acute phase protein responses to uterine bacterial contamination in cattle after calving. *Vet. Rec.,* 148(6): 172-175.

65. Heidarpour, M., Mohri, M., Fallah Rad, A.H., Shahreza, F.D. and Mohammadi, M. (2012) Acute-phase protein concentration and metabolic status affect the outcome of treatment in cows with clinical and subclinical endometritis. *Vet. Rec.,* 171: 1-5.

66. Schneider, A., Corrêa, M.N. and Butler, W.R. (2013) Acute phase proteins in Holstein cows diagnosed with uterine infection. *Res. Vet. Sci.,* 95(1): 269-271.

67. Kovac, G., Tothova, C., Nagy, O., Seidel, H. and Konvicna, J. (2009) Acute phase proteins and their relation to energy metabolites in dairy cows during the pre- and postpartal period. *Acta Vet. Brno.,* 78: 441-447.

68. Young, C.R., Eckersall, P.D., Saini, P.K. and Stanker, L. (1995) Validation of immunoassays for bovine haptoglobin. *Vet. Immunol. Immunopathol.,* 49: 1-13.

69. Alsemgeest, S.P.M., Vant Clooster, G.A.E., Van Miert, A.S.J., Hulskamp-Koch, C.K. and Gruys, E. (1996) Primary bovine hepatocytes in the study of cytokine induced acute-phase protein secretion *in vitro. Vet. Immunol. Immunopathol.,* 53: 179-184.

70. Mordak, R. (2008) Usefulness of haptoglobin for monitoring the efficiency of therapy of fetal membrane retention in cows. *Med. Wet.,* 64(4A): 434-443.

71. Chan, J.P., Chu, C.C., Fung, H.P., Chuang, S.T., Lin, Y.C., Chu, R.M. and Lee, S.L. (2004) Serum haptoglobin concentration in cattle. *J. Vet. Med. Sci.,* 66(1): 43-46.

72. Sabedra, D.A. (2012) Thesis on Serum Haptoglobin as an Indicator for Calving Difficulties and Postpartal Diseases in Transition Dairy Cows. An Undergraduate Thesis Submitted to Oregon State University.

73. Burke, C.R., Meier, S., McDougall, S., Compton, C., Mitchell, M. and Roche, J.R. (2010) Relationships between endometritis and metabolic state during the transition period in pasture-grazed dairy cows. *J. Dairy Sci.,* 93: 5363-5373.

74. Huzzey, J.M., Mann, S., Nydam, D.V., Grant, R.J. and Overton, T.R. (2015) Associations of peripartum markers of stress and inflammation with milk yield and reproductive performance in Holstein dairy cows. *Prev. Vet. Med.,* 120(3-4): 291-297.

75. Krausea, A.R.T., Pfeifer, L.F.M., Montagnera, P., Weschenfeldera, M.M., Schweglera, E., Limaa, M.E., Xavierb, E.G., Braunera, C.C., Schmittc, E., Del Pinoa, F.A.B., Martinsa, C.F., Corrêaa, M.N. and Schneidera, A. (2014) Associations between resumption of postpartum ovarian activity, uterine health and

76. Nightingale, C.R., Sellers, M.D. and Ballou, M.A. (2015) Elevated plasma haptoglobin concentrations following parturition are associated with elevated leukocyte responses and decreased subsequent reproductive efficiency in multiparous Holstein dairy cows. *Vet. Immunol. Immunopathol.,* 164: 16-23.

77. Gabler, C., Fischer, C., Drillich, M., Einspanier, R. and Heuwieser, W. (2010) Time-dependent mRNA expression of selected pro-inflammatory factors in the endometrium of primiparous cows postpartum. *Reprod. Biol. Endocrinol.,* 8: 152.

78. Lecchi, C., Avallone, G., Giurovich, M.M., Roccabianca, P. and Ceciliani, F. (2009) Extra hepatic expression of the acute phase protein alpha 1-acid glycoprotein in normal bovine tissues. *Vet. J.,* 180(2): 256-258.

79. Rahman, M.M. and Lecchi, C. (2010) Lipopolysaccharide-binding protein: Local expression in bovine extrahepatic tissues. *Vet. Immunol. Immunopathol.,* 137: 28-35.

80. Ghasemi, F., Gonzalez-Cano, P., Griebel, P.J. and Palmer, C. (2012) Proinflammatory cytokine gene expression in endometrial cytobrush samples harvested from cows with and without subclinical endometritis. *Theriogenology,* 78(7): 1538-1547.

81. Galvao, K.N., Felippe, M.J., Brittin, S.B., Sper, R., Fraga, M., Galvão, J.S., Caixeta, L., Guard, C.L., Ricci, A. and Gilbert, R.O. (2012) Evaluation of cytokine expression by blood monocytes of lactating Holstein cows with or without postpartum uterine disease. *Theriogenology,* 77(2): 356-372.

82. Loyi, T., Kumar, H., Nandi, S., Mathapati, B.S., Patra, M.K. and Pattnaik, B. (2013) Differential expression of pro-inflammatory cytokines in endometrial tissue of buffaloes with clinical and sub-clinical endometritis. *Res. Vet. Sci.,* 94: 336-340.

83. Chapwanya, A., Meade, K.G., Doherty, M.L., Callanan, J.J. and O'Farrellya, C. (2013) Endometrial epithelial cells are potent producers of tracheal antimicrobial peptide and serum amyloid A3 gene expression in response to *E. coli* stimulation. *Vet. Immunol. Immunopathol.,* 151(1-2): 157-162.

84. Heinrich, P.C., Behrmann, I., Muller-Newen, G., Schaper, F. and Graeve, L. (1998) Interleukin-6-type cytokine signalling through the gp130/Jak/STAT pathway. *Biochem. J.,* 334: 297-314.

85. Agrawal, A., Cha-Molstad, H., Samols, D. and Kushner, I. (2003) Over expressed nuclear factor-kappa B can participate in endogenous C-reactive protein induction, and enhances the effects of C/EBP beta and signal transducer and activator of transcription-3. *Immunology,* 108: 539-547.

86. Jensen, L.E. and Whitehead, A.S. (1998) Regulation of serum amyloid A protein expression during the acute-phase response. *Biochem. J.,* 334: 489-503.

87. Betts, J.C., Cheshire, J.K., Akira, S., Kishimoto, T. and Woo, P. (1993) The role of NF-kappa B and NF-IL6 trans activating factors in the synergistic activation of human serum amyloid A gene expression by interleukin-1 and interleukin-6. *J. Biol. Chem.,* 268: 25624-25631.

88. Edbrooke, M.R., Foldi, J., Cheshire, J.K., Li, F., Faulkes, D.J. and Woo, P. (1991) Constitutive and NF-kappa B-like proteins in the regulation of the serum amyloid A gene by interleukin-1. *Cytokine,* 3: 380-388.

89. Lee, Y.M., Miau, L.H., Chang, C.J. and Lee, S.C. (1996) Transcriptional induction of the alpha-1 acid glycoprotein (AGP) gene by synergistic interaction of two alternative activator forms of AGP/enhancer-binding protein (C/EBP beta) and NF-kappa B or Nopp140. *Mol. Cell. Biol.,* 16: 4257-4263.

90. Hagihara, K., Nishikawa, T., Sugantibioticta, Y., Song, J., Isobe, T., Taga, T. and Yoshizaki, K. (2005) Essential role

of STAT3 in cytokine-driven NF-kappaB-mediated serum amyloid A gene expression. *Genes Cells,* 10: 1051-1063.

91. Quinton, L.J., Jones, M.R., Robson, B.E. and Mizgerd, J.P. (2009) Mechanisms of the hepatic acute-phase response during bacterial pneumonia. *Infect. Immu.,* 77: 2417-2426.

92. Bode, J.G., Albrecht, U., Haussinger, D., Heinrich, P.C. and Schaper, F. (2012) Hepatic acute phase proteins-regulation by IL-6-and IL-1-type cytokines involving STAT3 and its crosstalk with NF-kB-dependent signaling. *Eur. J. Cell Biol.,* 91: 496-505.

10

Prevalence of vero toxic *Escherichia coli* in fecal samples of domestic as well as wild ruminants in Mathura districts and Kanpur zoo

Raghavendra Prasad Mishra[1], Udit Jain[1], Basanti Bist[1], Amit Kumar Verma[2] and Ashok Kumar[3]

1. Department of Veterinary Public Health, College of Veterinary Sciences and Animal Husbandry, Pandit Deen Dayal Upadhayay Pashu Chikitsa Vigyan Vishvidhyalaya Ewam Go-Anusandhan Sansthan, Mathura - 281 001, Uttar Pradesh, India; 2. Department of Veterinary Epidemiology and Preventive Medicine, College of Veterinary Sciences and Animal Husbandry, Pandit Deen Dayal Upadhayay Pashu Chikitsa Vigyan Vishvidhyalaya Ewam Go-Anusandhan Sansthan, Mathura - 281 001, Uttar Pradesh, India; 3. Division of Veterinary Public Health, Indian Veterinary Research Institute, Izatnagar, Bareilly, Uttar Pradesh, India.
Corresponding author: Raghavendra Prasad Mishra, e-mail: rmishra523@rediffmail.com,
UJ: druditjain@hotmail.com, BB: vasanti.bist@gmail.com, AKV: drakverma79@gmail.com, AK: ashokakt@rediffmail.com

Abstract

Aim: The present study was planned to reveal the prevalence of verocytotoxigenic *Escherichia coli* (VTEC) in fecal samples of domestic and wild ruminants in Mathura district and Kanpur zoo.

Materials and Methods: A total of 240 fecal samples comprising 60 each of cattle, buffalo, sheep and deer from Mathura districts and Kanpur zoo were screened for the presence of *E. coli* and VTEC genes positive by polymerase chain reaction (PCR).

Result: Out of 240 fecal samples, 212 *E. coli* strains were obtained. All the *E. coli* isolates were screened by PCR to detect virulence genes stx_1, stx_2, *eaeA* and *hlyA*. Of these, 25 isolates were identified as VTEC. The prevalence of VTEC in cattle, buffalo, sheep and deer was found 13.4% (8/60), 13.4% (8/60), 6.67% (4/60) and 8.33% (5/60), respectively.

Conclusion: stx_1, stx_2, *eaeA* and *hlyA* genes were prevalent in VTEC isolates from feces of cattle, buffalo, sheep and deer population of Mathura districts and Kanpur zoo. The presence of VTEC isolates in this region may pose a threat to public health.

Keywords: domestic and wild ruminants, feces, prevalence, polymerase chain reaction, verotoxic *Escherichia coli*.

Introduction

Diarrhea is one of the most common multifactorial diseases of man and animals mainly caused by *Escherichia coli* [1]. *E. coli* is the most common observed gastrointestinal flora of animals and environmental contaminant considered as important foodborne pathogen causing serious complications in man and animals [2-5].

Verocytotoxigenic *E. coli* (VTEC) was the first identified as a distinct group of *E. coli* named as VTEC, which had the ability to produce toxins with profound and irreversible effect on vero cells. VTEC is also termed as shiga-like toxin producing *E. coli* (SLTEC) or shiga toxin producing *E. coli* or STEC. Acronym STEC is derived from the fact that the toxins are shiga like that is similar to those produced by *Shigella dysenteriae* Type 1 [6].

The enterohemorragic *E. coli* belong to the VTEC. VTEC always do not induce clinical signs and are not enterohemorrhagic until addition virulence factor are present like enterohemolysin and adherence factors (intimin). The adherence factor(s) enables the organism to attach to and colonize intestinal mucosal cells [7]. Among VTEC, serotype O157:H7 has been closely associated with the sporadic and clinical outbreaks of hemorrhagic colitis (HC), hemolytic uremic syndrome (HUS) and thrombotic thrombocytopenic purpura (TTP) in human beings [8-10]. Healthy domestic ruminants are recognised as the main natural reservoir of STEC and large game animal may be healthy carriers of STEC [11,12].

Keeping in view the importance of this organism, the present study was planned to reveal the prevalence of VTEC in fecal samples of domestic and wild ruminants in Mathura district and Kanpur zoo.

Materials and Methods

Ethical approval

This work does not require ethical approval because we have collected fecal samples of animals after defecation.

Sampling and isolation of *E. coli*

A total of 240 samples of feces (180 domestic ruminants 60 wild ruminants) were collected from Mathura district and Kanpur zoo. The samples were collected aseptically in UV sterile polythene bags

(Fisher Scientific, UK) and immediately transported to the laboratory under chilled conditions for microbiological analysis. For primary isolation of *E. coli* (VTEC), 10 g of fecal sample were enriched in 90 ml modified trypticase soya broth (mTSB) (Himedia, Mumbai) containing acriflavine (10 mg/ml) to reduce the growth of Gram-positive organism. The method used for collection of materials, and isolation and identification techniques were performed as suggested by the World organization for Animal Health [13]. These samples were incubated at 37°C for 6 h. MacConkey's agar was used as differential media while eosin methylene blue agar (Hi-Media, Mumbai) was used as selective media. Suspected *E. coli* strains were subjected to morphological, cultural and biochemical characterization as per standard methods [14]. A statistical analysis was done as per the standard method [15].

Molecular characterization

Multiplex polymerase chain reaction (pcr) was used for detection of virulent genes (stx_1, stx_2, eaeA, and hlyA) of VTEC. All the *E. coli* isolates were subjected to genomic DNA isolation. The bacterial growth in mTSB broth (HiMedia, Mumbai) was centrifuged at 3000 rpm for 15 min to make the pellet of bacterial cells. These cells were washed twice with phosphate-buffered saline (pH 7.4) to remove any impurity of broth media. Bacterial DNA was extracted by using DNA extraction kit (Genei, Bangalore) as per the manufacturer's protocol. For the PCR reaction, PCR Master Mix solution (Genei, Bangalore) was used. DNA amplification targeted to virulent genes (stx_1, stx_2, eaeA and hlyA) of VTEC was performed using primers on 3 µl of DNA sample in 25 µl reaction mixture [16]. After an initial denaturation step at 95°C for 4 min, 30 amplification cycles were performed, each consisting of 2 min at 94°C, 2 min at 65°C, and 1.5 min at 72°C and followed by a final extension step at 72°C for 2.5 min. After the amplification, amplicons were separated in 1.5% gel in tris acetate EDTA (TAE) buffer at 60 volt for 80 min, stained with 0.5% ethidium bromide solution and visualized under ultraviolet light.

Results and Discussion

Out of 240 fecal samples, a total of 212 *E. coli* strains were obtained (Table-1). All the strains of *E. coli* were screened to detect the presence of VTEC genes using PCR. An overall prevalence of VTEC in ruminants (both wild and domestic) was found to be 10.42% (25/240). The highest prevalence of VTEC was reported in cattle and buffalo 13.4% (8/60) in each followed by sheep 6.67% (4/60) and deer 08.33% (5/60). In cattle, 2 VTEC were found to be positive for stx_1 gene (180 bp) and 6 VTEC for stx_1 and stx_2 (180 bp and 255 bp). In buffalo, 3 VTEC were found positive for stx_1 gene and 5 was positive for stx_1 and stx_2. In sheep, out of 4 VTEC, only one VTEC was having stx_1 gene and 3 VTEC isolates having stx_1 and stx_2 both. In

wild ruminants (deer), out of 5 VTEC, only one was found to be positive for stx_1 gene, one isolates was found to be positive for stx_2 with hlyA (534 bp), one stx_1 with eaeA (384 bp) and two VTEC have stx_2, eaeA and hlyA genes. Two *E. coli* strains were found having eaeA with hlyA genes, i.e., lacking stx gene and they may be enteropathogenic.

In the previous study, the prevalence of VTEC in sheep, cattle and buffalo were reported as 4.81% [17], 7.4% [18] and 8.9% [19], respectively. However, the prevalence of VTEC in higher level was reported by previous workers as the prevalence of VTEC was 16.66% [20], 18% [21] and 18.47% [22]. In contrast, investigations have shown a higher detection rate of 46% [23] in fecal samples of cattle and buffalo. Lower isolation rate, i.e. 9% [24]. Isolation rate as low as 1.0% has also been reported [25]. In deer previously reported, the prevalence of VTEC 9.3% [26], 16.2% [27] and 16.5% [28], which likely similar as present finding. These hazardous strains of *E. coli* have been given immense attention due to their involvement in serious illnesses like HC (bloody diarrhea, HC), HUS and TTP in human [29-31]. The low infective dose, unusual acid tolerance and close association with ruminants have made VTEC a serious global zoonotic problem of great public health significance. VTEC can be present in the intestinal tract of a wide range of domestic and wild animals and ruminants (sheep, goats, cattle, buffalo and deer) [32-36], especially cattle and buffalo are considered as a major reservoir for VTEC [37,38].

Conclusion

The presence of VTEC in feces causes fecal contamination of water, and also contaminates other food sources, thus depicts a dangerous picture regarding human and animal health safety because water is essential for the survival of every living being. Constant monitoring and surveillances program to keep a record of the prevalence from time to time is needed, and proper hygienic measure may reduce the chance of infection.

Authors' Contributions

UJ, BB and AKV designed and planned this research work. RPM collected the samples and executed the isolation and biochemical work. UJ monitored the isolation, biochemical characterization. RPM and UJ was involved in the molecular characterization experiment. Manuscript was drafted and revised by AK, BB & RPM under the guidance of UJ. All authors read and approved the final manuscript.

Acknowledgements

The authors are highly thankful to Indian Council of Agricultural Research, New Delhi and Dean, College of Veterinary Science and Animal Husbandry, Uttar Pradesh Pandit Deen Dayal Upadhayay Pashu Chikitsa Vigyan Vishvidhyalaya

Table-1: Details of sample collection and prevalence of *E. coli* and VTEC in fecal sample.

Sources*	Place of collection	Number of sample collected	Percentage of *E. coli*	No. of VTEC isolates	Percentage of VTEC
Cattle	DDD farm DUVASU, Mathura	35	85.7 (30/35)	7	20
	Gaushalas of Vrindavan	15	93.4 (14/15)	1	6.67
	TVCC Kothari	10	90 (9/10)	0	0
Buffalo	DDD farm DUVASU, Mathura	40	95.6 (38/40)	8	20
	TVCC Kothari	20	90 (18/20)	0	0
Sheep	Sheep farm DUVASU, Mathura	30	86.7 (26/30)	2	6.67
	Sheep farm, farah	20	80 (16/20)	1	5
	Aurangabad	10	70 (7/10)	1	10
Deer	Kanpur Zoo	30	86.7 (26/30)	2	6.66
	Ramanreti	30	93.4 (28/30)	3	10
Total		240	88.5 (212/240)	25	10.41 (25/240)

$p < 0.05$, VTEC=Verocytotoxigenic *Escherichia coli*, *E. coli=Escherichia coli*

Ewam Go-Anusandhan Sansthan (DUVASU), Mathura, Uttar Pradesh, India for providing necessary funds and facilities to carry out the investigations.

Competing Interests

The authors declare that they have no competing interests.

References

1. Kumar, A., Verma, A.K., Sharma, A.K. and Rahal, A. (2013) Presence of extended spectrum Beta-lactamases producing alpha hemolytic *Escherichia coli* in yellow-wattled Lapwing (*Vanellus malabaricus*). *Asian J. Anim. Sci.*, 7(2): 64-69.

2. Mailk, S., Kumar, A., Verma, A.K., Gupta, M.K., Sharma, S.D., Sharma, A.K. and Rahal, A. (2013) Incidence and drug resistance pattern of collibacillosis in cattle and buffalo calves in Western Uttar Pradesh in India. *J. Anim. Health Prod.*, 1(1): 15-19.

3. Dhama, K., Rajagunalan, S., Chakraborty, S., Verma, A.K., Kumar, A., Tiwari, R. and Kapoor, S. (2013) Food-borne pathogens of animal origin-diagnosis, prevention and control and their zoonotic significance - A review. *Pak. J. Biol. Sci.*, 16(20): 1076-1085.

4. Kumar, A., Verma, A.K., Malik, S., Gupta, M.K., Sharma, A. and Rahal, A. (2014) Occurrence of extended spectrum beta-lactamases producing alpha hemolytic *Escherichia coli* in neonatal diarrhea. *Pak. J. Biol. Sci.*, 17(1): 109-113.

5. Anita, Kumar, A., Verma, A.K., Gupta, M.K. and Rahal, A. (2014) Multi drug resistant pathogenic *Escherichia coli* in water sources and Yamuna River in and around Mathura, India. *Pak. J. Biol. Sci.*, 17(4): 540-544.

6. O'Brien, A.D. and Holmes, R.K. (1987) Shiga and Shiga-like toxins. *Microbiol. Rev.*, 51: 206-220.

7. Hiruta, N., Murase, T. and Okamura, N. (2001) An outbreak of diarrhoea due to multiple antimicrobial resistant Shiga toxin producine *E.coli* O26:H7 ina nursery. *Epidemiol. Infect.*, 127: 221-227.

8. Croxen, M.A. and Finlay, B.B. (2010) Molecular mechanisms of *Escherichia coli* pathogenicity *Nat. Rev. Microbiol.*, 8: 26-38.

9. Gyles, C.M. and Fairbrother, J.M. (2010) *Escherichia coli* In: Gyles, C.L., Prescott, J.F., Thoen, C.O., editors. Pathogenesis of Bacterial Infections in Animals. Blackwell Publishing, Ames, p267-308.

10. Sanchez, S., Sanchez, D.S., Martinez, R., Llorente, M.T., Herrera-Leon, S. and Vidal, D. (2013) The new allelic variantof the subtilase cytotoxin (sub AB₂) is common among Shiga toxin producing *Escherichia coli* strains from large animals and their meat and meat products. *Vet. Microbiol.*, 166: 645-649.

11. Diaz, S., Vidal, D., Herrera-Leon, S. and Sanchez, S. (2011) Sorbitol-fermenting, b-glucuronidase-positive, Shiga toxin negative *Escherichia coli* O157:H7 in free-ranging red deer in South-Central Spain. *Foodborne Pathog. Dis.*, 8: 1313-1315.

12. Sanchez, S., Martnez, R., Garca, A., Vidal, D., Blanco, J., Blanco, M., Blanco, J.E., Mora, A., Herrera-Leon, S., Echeita, A., Alonso, J.M. and Rey, J. (2010) Detection and characterization of O157:H7 and non-O157 Shiga toxin producing *Escherichia coli* in wild boars. *Vet. Microbiol.*, 143: 420-423.

13. OIE. (2004) Verocytotoxigenic *Escherichia coli*. In: Word Organization for Animal Health, Pairs manual of Diagnostic Tests and Vaccines for Terrestrial Animals. 5th ed. OIE, Paris.

14. Ewing, W.H. (1986) The genus *Escherichia*. In: Edwards, P.R., Ewing, W.H., editors. Edwards and Ewing's identification of Entero Bacteriaceae. 4th ed. Elsevier Science Publishing Co., Inc., NewYork. p93-122.

15. Snecedor, G.W. and Cochran, W.G. (1994) In: Statistical Methods. 8th ed. IOWA State University Press, Ames, IOWA.

16. Paton, A.W. and Paton, J.C. (1998) Detection and characterization of shiga toxigenic *Escherichia coli* by using multiplex PCR Assays for stx_1, stx_2, eaeA, enterohemorrhagic *E. coli* hlyA, rfb O111, and rfb O157 J. C. Microbial, February. p598-602.

17. Chattopadhyay, U.K., Gupta, S. and Dutta, S. (2003) Search for Shiga toxin producing *Escherichia coli* (STEC) including O157:H7 strains in and around Kolkata. *Indian J. Med. Microbiol.*, 21: 17-20.

18. Cobbold, R.N., Rice, D.H., Szymanski, M., Call, D.R. and Hancock, D.D. (2004) Comparison of Shiga - Toxigenic *Escherichia coli* prevalences among dairy, feedlot and cow calf herds in Washington State. *Appl. Environ. Microbiol.*, 70: 4375-4378.

19. Eriksson, E., Aspon, A., Gunnarsson, A. and Vagsholm, I. (2005) Prevalence of verotoxin producing *Escherichia coli* (VTEC) O157 in Swedish dairy herds. *Epidemiol. Infect.*, 133: 349-358.

20. Parul, Bist, B., Sharma, B. and Manjula. (2014) Prevalence of verotoxin producing *Escherichia coli* non O157 in diarrhoeic and healthy calves. One Health: Harnesting biotechnology for addressing veterinary and biomedical concerns on food safety, zoonoses and environment sustainability.12th Annual Conference of IAVPHS, Guwahati, India. p245-246.

21. Rogerie, F., Marecat, A., Gambade, S., Dupond, F., Beaubois, P. and Lange, M. (2001) Characterization of Shiga toxin producing *E. coli* and O157 serotype isolated in France from healthy domestic cattle. *Int. J. Food Microbiol.*, 63: 217-223.

22. Rabin, B. (1999) Prevalence of verotoxic *Escherichia coli* in man animals, food and pulic health significance. M. V. Sc Thesis, Deemed University, IVRI, Izatnagar.

23. Kobayashi, H., Shimada, J., Nakazawa, M., Morozumi, T., Pohjanvirta, T., Pelkonen, S. and Yamamoto, K. (2001) Prevalence and characteristics of Shiga toxin-producing *Escherichia coli* from healthy cattle in Japan. *Appl. Environ. Microbiol.*, 67: 484-489.

24. Blanco, M., Blanco, J., Blanco, J.E. and Ramos, J. (1993) Enterotoxigenic, verotoxigenic and necrotoxigenic *Escherichia coli* isolated from cattle in Spain. *Am. J. Vet. Res.*, 54: 1446-1451.

25. Khurana, P. and Kumar, A. (2005) Occurance of vero-toxic *E. coli* in faeces and milk of cattle. *Harayana Vet.*, 44: 83-85.

26. Bardiau, M., Gregoire, F., Muylaert, A., Nahayo, A., Duprez, J.N., Mainil, J. and Linden, A. (2010) Enteropathogenic (EPEC), enterohaemorragic (EHEC) and verotoxigenic (VTEC) *Escherichia coli* in wild cervids. *J. Appl. Microbiol.*, 109(6): 2214-2222.

27. Hiroshi, A., Sou-ichi, M., Toshikazu, S., Teizo, T., Hisao, K., Tetsuya, I. and Kouichi, T. (2013) Detection and genetical characterization of Shiga toxin-producing Escherichia coli from wild deer. *Microbiol. Immunol.*, 42(12): 815-822.

28. Sanchez, S., Martínez, R., Rey, J., García, A., Blanco, J., Blanco, M., Blanco, J.E., Mora, A., Herrera-León, S., Echeita, A. and Alonso, J.M. (2010) Pheno-genotypic characterisation of *Escherichia coli* O157:H7 isolates from domestic and wild ruminants. *Vet. Microbiol.*, 142(3-4): 445-9.

29. Scotland, S.M., Willshaw, G.A., Smith, H.R. and Rowe, B. (1987) Properties of strains of *Escherichia coli* belonging to serogroup 0157 with special reference to production of Verocytotoxins VT1 and VT2. *Epidemiol. Infect.*, 99: 613-624.

30. Karmali, M.A. (1989) Infection by verocytotoxin-producing *Escherichia coli. Clin. Microbiol. Rev.*, 2: 15-38.

31. Wani, S.A., Bhat, M.A., Samanta, I., Ishaq, S.M., Ashraff, M.A. and Buchh, A.S. (2004) Epidemiology of diarrhoea caused by rota virus and *Escherichia coli* in lambs in Kashmir Valley, India. *Small Rumin. Res.*, 52: 145-153.

32. Beutin, L., Geier, D., Zimmerman, S. and Karch, H. (1995) Virulence markers of Shiga-like toxin-producing *E. coli* strains from healthy domestic animals of different species. *J. Clin. Microbiol.*, 33: 631-635.

33. Chapman, P.A. and Siddons, C.A. (1997) A comparison of immunomagnetic separation and direct culture for the isolation of verocytotoxin-producing *Escherichia coli* O157 from cases of bloody diarrhoea, non-bloody diarrhoea and asymptomatic contacts. *J. Med. Microbiol.*, 44: 267-271.

34. Johnson, R.P., Clarke, R.C. and Gyles, C.L. (1996) Growing concerns and recent outbreaks involving non-O157:H7 serotypes of verotoxigenic *Escherichia coli. J. Food Protect.*, 59: 1112-1122.

35. Schouten, J.M., van de Giessen, A.W., Frankena, K., De Jong, M.C.M. and Graat, E.A.M. (2005) *Escherichia coli* O157 prevalence in dutch poultry, pig finishing and veal herds and risk factors in dutch veal herds. *Prev. Vet. Med.*, 70: 1-15.

36. Oporto, B., Esteban, J.I., Aduriz, G., Juste, R.A. and Hurtado, A. (2008) *Escherichia coli* O157:H7 and non-O157 Shiga toxin-producing *E. coli* in healthy cattle, sheep and swine herds in Northern Spain. *Zoonoses Public Health.*, 55(2): 73-81.

37. Mainil, J. (1999) Shiga/verocytotoxins and Shiga/verotoxigenic *Escherichia coli* in animals. *Vet. Res.*, 30: 235-257.

38. Krause, G., Zimmermann, S. and Beutin, L. (2005) Investigation of domestic animals and pets as a reservoir for intimin - (eae) gene positive *Escherichia coli* types. *Vet. Microbiol.*, 106: 87-95.

11

Utilization of carrageenan, citric acid and cinnamon oil as an edible coating of chicken fillets to prolong its shelf life under refrigeration conditions

Anshul Kumar Khare, Robinson J. J. Abraham, V. Appa Rao and R. Narendra Babu

Department of Livestock Products Technology (Meat Science), Madras Veterinary College, Tamil Nadu Veterinary and Animal Sciences University, Chennai - 600 007, Tamil Nadu, India.
Corresponding author: Anshul Kumar Khare, e-mail: akksagar@gmail.com,
RJJA: robinson@tanuvas.org.in, VAR: varao1966@yahoo.com, RNB: nbabu@tanuvas.org.in

Abstract

Aim: The present study was conducted to determine efficacy of edible coating of carrageenan and cinnamon oil to enhance the shelf life of chicken meat stored under refrigeration conditions.

Materials and Methods: Chicken breast was coated with carrageenan and cinnamon oil by three methods of application *viz.*, spraying brushing and dipping. The coated meat was evaluated for drip loss, pH, thiobarbituric acid number (TBA), tyrosine value (TV), extract release volume (ERV), Warner-Bratzler shear force value (WBSFV), instrumental color, microbiological, and sensory qualities as per standard procedures.

Results: There was a significant difference observed for physicochemical parameters (pH, TBA, TV, ERV, drip loss and WBSFV) and microbiological analysis between storage periods in all the samples and between the control and treatments throughout the storage period but samples did not differed significantly for hunter color scores. However, there was no significant difference among three methods of application throughout the storage period though dipping had a lower rate of increase. A progressive decline in mean sensory scores was recorded along with the increase in storage time.

Conclusion: The carrageenan and cinnamon edible coating was found to be a good alternative to enhance the shelf life of chicken meat under refrigeration conditions. It was also observed from study that dipping method of the application had comparatively higher shelf life than other methods of application.

Keywords: carrageenan, chicken breast/fillets, cinnamon oil, edible coating, spraying/brushing/dipping.

Introduction

Poultry breast (fillets) is a very popular food commodity and its consumption has increased over the last decades in Indian subcontinent. Broiler meat production in India is nearly 2.47 million tonnes [1] with growth rate of 6%. Exports of poultry products are currently 5,56,698 millon tonnes worth about Rs. 6512.1 millions with a growth rate of 7%. [2]. The processed meat industry is growing even much faster, at about 20%.

With the proliferation of different sources of media and use of these information media for education and awareness on transfer of technologies on good quality complete proteinaceous foods, consumption of animal origin foods are increasing. To have essential amino acids in the diet of human beings, supply of about 20-25% of total daily protein needs to be made through good quality proteinaceous foods of animal origin.

However, under Indian conditions meat and meat products are also prone to lipid oxidation because of high ambient temperature and lack of cold chain which eventually leads to spoilage of meat products [3]. Therefore, development of conditions such as edible coating could be a good option that can increase the shelf life of meat and its product. Edible coatings have been particularly considered in food preservation, because of their capability for improving global food quality by preventing quality loss such as shrinkage, oxidative off-flavors, microbial contamination, and discoloration in meat and meat products [4]. The edible coating is also defined as thin layers of edible materials, are usually applied as a liquid of varying viscosity to the surface of food product by spraying, dipping, brushing or other methods. Polysaccharides, proteins, and lipids are the main polymeric ingredients used to produce edible coating [5,6]. Polysaccharides are similar to hydrophilic materials; their polarity determines their poor barrier to water vapor as well as sensitive to moisture, which affects their functional properties [7]. Carrageenan, a naturally occurring anionic sulfated linear polysaccharides extracted from certain red seaweed [8] of the Rhodophyceae family. Carrageenan can function as a bulking agent, carrier, emulsifier, gelling agent, glazing agent, humectants, stabilizer, or thickener [9].

Cinnamon (*Cinnamomum zeylanicum* or *Cinnamomum verum*) belongs to the Lauraceae family and is an importanttraditional herbal medicine that is widely distributed in China,Vietnam, Sri Lanka, Madagascar, Seychelles and India [10]. It contains large quantities of terpenes andaromatic compounds specifically, cinnamaldehyde [11]. It is used worldwide as a food additive, flavoring agent and hasgood antioxidant and antimicrobial potential and it is considered "Generally Recognized as Safe (GRAS)" by US Food and Drug Administration [12-15]. The possibility of incorporating active compounds (antimicrobials, antioxidants, nutraceuticals, flavors, colorants) in polymeric matrices is one of the main advantages of coatings [16].

Citric acid is a hydroxy tricarboxylic acid produced naturally by various plants. It is water soluble, approved for direct addition to multiple foods, is affirmed as GRAS and is approved for use in the manufacture of fresh and processed meats and poultry at concentrations specific to its purpose. It has antimicrobial as well as tenderizing effect in meat and meat products [17]. The literature related to the application of hydrocolloids such as carrageenan and essential oil such as cinnamon oil as edible coating is very scanty and also no previous literature available regarding comparative study of three methods of application *viz.* spraying, brushing and dipping of coating chicken fillets. Carrageenan, citric acid, and cinnamon oil coating showed antimicrobial and antioxidant activity. Therefore, this study provides innovative and novel approach for extending shelf life of chicken meat under refrigeration conditions and this study also helpful to determine suitable method of application of coating among three methods *viz.* spraying, brushing and dipping.

The aim of this study was to evaluate the efficiency of edible coating of carrageenan incorporated with citric acid and cinnamon oil on the shelf life of chicken fillets stored under refrigerated conditions and also to select suitable method of application out of three methods *viz.* spraying, brushing and dipping.

Materials and Methods

Ethical approval

Permission of Animal Ethics Committee of Madras Veterinary College was taken for slaughter of experimental birds.

Source of meat

Meat samples required for the experiments were obtained from broilers slaughtered as per standard procedure in the experimental slaughterhouse of Department of Livestock Products Technology (Meat Science) at Madras Veterinary College, Chennai-7, Tamil Nadu. The breast portion of the dressed carcasses (boneless skinless breast) after removal of all separable connective tissues, fat, skin, fascia, and blood vessels were used for edible coating. Analytical grade chemicals and media, required for analyzing

the coated meat were procured from standard firms like SRL, Fisher Scientific, CDH, HiMedia, Sigma-Aldrich, etc. Cinnamon bark oil was procured from Plant Lipids Pvt. Cochin, Kerala.

Preparation of coating solution

A coating solution was prepared by adding carrageenan and potassium chloride (1%) in ratio of 4:1 and citric acid was added at a level of 0.5% w/v and coating solution is heated at 60°C. This coating solution was followed with 0.05% cinnamon oil addition and proper mixing (carrageenan citric acid and cinnamon oil were selected on the basis of preliminary trials and previous literature available) and then divided into three parts 100 ml each for each for spraying and brushing and rest of 800 ml for dipping. pH of the coating solution were 7.56 (without citric acid) and citric acid incorporated coating solution had pH of 3.88-4.

Methods of application

Spraying

Spraying was performed using hand sprayer, 50-100 ml coating solution was filled in sprayer then it was uniformly sprayed all over the breast (500-600 g). After deboning, spraying was also done on the back side which remained unsprayed.

Brushing

Boneless skinless breast (500-600 g) was brushed with coating solution (50 ml) using brush (4 cm×2 cm) uniformly and once after deboning on the remaining part.

Dipping

Dipping was done in a vessel containing 700-800 ml of coating solution. In this vessel, breast is dipped for 30 s after that draining of coating solution from breast was done for 30 s.

Packaging of coated meat

The meat was deboned and 60 g of meat packaged separately for control, spraying, brushing, and dipping stored under refrigeration temperature at 4±1°C (Samsung, India).Low-density polyethylene and polyester propylene laminated plastic bags of 200 Gauge in natural color were procured from reputed firms (Jeyam Plastics, Chennai) and used for aerobic packaging of coated chicken meat. 5 g (control and three treatments) of meat was packed separately in small lockable polythene bags (10 g size) for microbiological analysis. The coated meat samples were drawn at alternate days (1st, 3rd, 5th, and 7th) and analyzed for various physicochemical, microbiological and sensory attributes. Economics of coating solution was also estimated (Table-1).

Analytical procedures

The pH of chicken meat was determined [18] with digital pH meter equipped with a combined glass electrode (Digisun Electronics System Model

No. 2001). The estimation of water-holding capacity (WHC) of the coated chicken meat samples were carried out by adopting the filter paper press method recommended by Grau and Hamm [19,20] with slight modifications. A extract release volume (ERV) was determined by modified method of Pearson [21]. Drip loss was estimated as per the method outlined by Somers et al., [22]. Tyrosine value (TV) and thiobarbituric acid (TBA) value were determined by the modified method by Strange et al., 1977 [23]. The ability to scavenge 1, 1 diphenyl-2picrylhydrazyl radical by added antioxidants in coating solution (Table-2) was estimated following the method of Khare et al., [24] with slight modifications. The polyphenol content (Table-2) was quantified by Folin–Ciocalteau's reagent and was expressed as gallic acid equivalents [24]. Warner-Bratzler shear force value (WBSFV) of frozen chicken breast meat was determined using Warner-Bratzler shear (G.R. Electric Manufacturing Co., Manhattan, USA). Color changes were measured using a MiniScan XE Spectrophotometer (Hunter Associates Laboratory, Reston, Virginia, USA), standard plate counts (SPC) in the samples were enumerated following the methods as described by American Public Health Association [25]. A six-member experienced panel of judges consisting of faculty and postgraduate students of Madras Veterinary College, Chennai-7 evaluated the samples for the attributes of color, odor and general appearance using 9 points descriptive scale [26] for color and general appearance while 10 point scale for odor.

Statistical analysis

Data were analyzed statistically on "SPSS-16.0" software package as per standard methods [27]. Samples were drawn for each parameter, and the experiment was replicated six times (n=6). Sensory evaluation was performed by a panel of six trained panelist. Data were subjected to one-way analysis of variance, homogeneity test and Duncan's multiple range test for comparing the means to find the effects between treatment and between storage periods.

Table-1: Economics of coating of chicken breast meat with carrageenan and cinnamon oil coating solution.

Characteristics	Carrageenan
Quantity/breast (500-600 g)	50-100 ml (S/B) 600 ml (D)
Name of company	HiMedia
Cost of pack	Rs. 690/100 g
Cost of coating solution	Rs. 7/100 ml (max)

S=Spraying, B=Brushing, D=Dipping - Methods of application of coating solution

Table-2: DPPH and total phenolic content of coating solution.

DPPH (% scavenging activity)	32.68
Total phenolics (gallic acid equivalent mg/g)	0.93

DPPH=1, 1 diphenyl-2picrylhydrazyl

Results and Discussion
Physico-chemical parameters
pH

There was no significant difference (p>0.05) in pH values in between the treatments during 1st and 3rd day of storage, whereas a significant difference (p<0.05) was observed during 5th and 7th day of storage (Table-3). There was highly significant increase (p<0.01) in pH with increase in storage period in all the samples. Control samples had the highest values followed by spraying, brushing, and dipping throughout storage period. Coated meat samples had comparatively lower values than control. This might be attributed to the addition of citric acid in coating solution. Similar, increase in pH during storage period was reported by Sinhamahapatra et al., [28] in broiler carcasses dipped and sprayed with decontaminants (lactic acid, acidified sodium chlorite [ASC] solution and chlorine solution). However, Petrou et al., [29] observed no significant difference in pH of chicken fillets dipped in chitosan and oregano oil throughout storage period.

ERV

ERV is an important indicator of spoilage in meat and its value decreases with storage period. During the initial days of storage, there was no significant difference (p>0.05) in between the treatments. The ERV values decreased significantly (p<0.01) with increase in storage period irrespective of different methods of application. Pearson [21] revealed that meat could be considered acceptable provided that the ERV is at least 17 ml. The ERV value of control was well below the acceptable limit during 3rd day of storage. However, spraying, brushing, and dipping samples had ≤ 17 ml value during 5th day of storage (Table-3). Dipping could be better method of application due to more viscous nature of carrageenan which coats the chicken breast effectively. These results were in agreement with Kandeepan and Biswas [30] who indicated that ERV values continuously decreased during refrigerated storage (23.5 ml on 0th day to 14.3 ml on 7th day) in buffalo meat. The decrease in ERV values could be attributed to increase in microbial count [31]. However, Sinhamahapatra et al., [28] observed that spraying and dipping of chicken meat with various decontaminants (lactic acid, ASC solution and chlorine solution) did not cause any significant change in ERV values during storage.

WHC

There was a highly significant (p<0.01) difference in WHC between storage period in all the samples and WHC decreased significantly with storage period. However, no significant difference was observed in between the treatments in all the storage days except on the 3rd day (Table-3). Coated meat sample had comparatively higher WHC compared to uncoated meat which could be attributed to lower moisture loss by application of carrageenan and addition of citric

Table-3: Mean±SE values of physico-chemical properties (pH, ERV and water holding capacity, TBA, TV, drip loss and WBSFV) of carrageenan, potassium chloride, citric acid, and cinnamon oil coated chicken meat stored at 4±1°C.

Days	Methods of application				
	Control	Spraying	Brushing	Dipping	F value
pH					
1st	5.82±0.06[aA]	5.91±0.08[aA]	5.88±0.04[aA]	5.94±0.05[aA]	0.68[NS]
3rd	6.10±0.13[bA]	6.04±0.08[aA]	5.96±0.05[aA]	5.95±0.09[aA]	1.20[NS]
5th	6.15±0.09[bB]	6.28±0.07[bB]	6.16±0.04[bAB]	6.03±0.03[abA]	4.62*
7th	6.59±0.07[cC]	6.38±0.04[bBC]	6.29±0.07[bAB]	6.20±0.04[bA]	6.26**
F value	11.66**	9.54**	12.29**	4.26*	
ERV					
1st	18.25±0.48[cA]	20.33±0.82[cB]	19.25±0.17[cAB]	20.00±0.55[bB]	2.76[NS]
3rd	15.42±0.78[bA]	18.42±0.37[bB]	18.33±0.49[bB]	19.67±0.85[bB]	7.54**
5th	14.42±0.58[abA]	15.83±0.78[aAB]	16.92±0.54[aB]	17.25±0.91[aB]	3.15*
7th	12.75±0.48[aA]	14.00±0.46[aB]	14.00±0.46[aC]	16.33±0.17[aC]	21.92**
F value	15.14**	18.95**	26.96**	6.88**	
WHC					
1st	1.72±0.09[aA]	1.70±0.16[aA]	1.97±0.21[aA]	2.07±0.09[aA]	1.53[NS]
3rd	2.13±0.08[bA]	2.13±0.14[bB]	2.25±0.17[bB]	2.10±0.26[aB]	1.66**
5th	2.48±0.07[cA]	2.30±0.05[bcA]	2.50±0.17[bcA]	2.32±0.19[aA]	0.62[NS]
7th	2.70±0.14[cA]	2.60±0.08[cA]	2.80±0.25[cA]	3.03±0.13[bA]	1.29[NS]
F valve	18.34**	9.77**	3.03**	6.21**	
TBA number					
1st	0.05±0.009[aB]	0.02±0.003[aA]	0.03±0.006[aA]	0.02±0.005[aA]	4.15*
3rd	0.09±0.015[bB]	0.05±0.004[bA]	0.05±0.003[abA]	0.05±0.008[bA]	5.53**
5th	0.10±0.007[bcB]	0.06±0.007[cA]	0.07±0.010[bAB]	0.08±0.012[bcAB]	0.39[NS]
7th	0.13±0.005[cB]	0.09±0.006[dA]	0.11±0.020[aAB]	0.09±0.003[cA]	2.71[NS]
F value	0.264**	25.228**	8.539**	16.133**	
TV (mg/100 g)					
1st	2.84±0.30[aB]	2.50±0.16[aAB]	1.93±0.19[aA]	2.16±0.22[aAB]	3.140*
3rd	3.97±0.26[bB]	2.27±0.15[aA]	2.43±0.17[aA]	3.37±0.24[bB]	14.234**
5th	4.64±0.28[bB]	4.00±0.27[bcAB]	3.52±0.26[bA]	3.17±0.26[bA]	5.640**
7th	4.80±0.27[bC]	4.57±0.19[cBC]	4.07±0.20[bAB]	3.59±0.19[bA]	6.136**
F value	10.35**	15.812**	16.74**	14.66**	
Drip loss (%)					
1st	3.45±0.15[aB]	3.00±0.09[aAB]	3.22±0.12[aAB]	2.94±0.19[aA]	2.52[NS]
3rd	4.57±0.21[bAB]	5.38±0.41[bB]	4.49±0.29[bAB]	4.44±0.19[bA]	2.35[NS]
5th	5.61±0.25[cA]	6.05±0.19[cA]	6.29±0.22[cAB]	6.66±0.16[cB]	3.26*
7th	7.33±0.07[dB]	6.35±0.14[dA]	6.80±0.09[cAB]	7.34±0.58[cB]	4.33*
F value	78.313**	75.47**	69.85**	26.70**	
WBSF (kg/cm²)					
1st	0.87±0.06[aC]	0.56±0.02[aA]	0.88±0.02[aB]	0.71±0.06[aC]	10.99**
3rd	1.02±0.05[abB]	0.69±0.03[abA]	1.05±0.02[bB]	0.73±0.06[aA]	16.78**
5th	1.08±0.07[bB]	0.74±0.04[bA]	1.06±0.05[bA]	0.82±0.06[aB]	9.07**
7th	1.18±0.05[bC]	0.83±0.05[bA]	1.18±0.02[cC]	1.01±0.05[bB]	12.39**
F value	4.83*	14.73**	9.32**	5.27**	

Means bearing different superscript between rows a, b, c and between columns A, B, C differs significantly (p<0.05), *Indicates significant value (p<0.05); **Highly significant value (p<0.01). NS=Non significant, ERV=Extract release volume, WHC=Water holding capacity, TBA=Thiobarbituric acid, TV=Tyrosine value, WBSFV=Warner-Bratzler shear force value, SE=Standard error

acid in coating solution which leads to decrease in pH. The results in the present study were in agreement with Ayadi et al., [32] who revealed higher WHC in carrageenan added turkey meat sausages. Gault [33] proposed that the increased WHC of beef muscle at lower pH values was due to the increase in the net positive charges on the protein molecules and the osmotic pressure exerted by the presence of large amounts of organic acids to decrease pH. WHC of muscle foods increases when the pH is below the isoelectric point of the major myofibrillar proteins [33,34].

TBA number

The TBA test has been widely used to estimate the extent of lipid oxidation in meat and meat products [35]. TBA value increased significantly with storage period in all the samples and during initial days of storage (Figure-1) there was highly significant difference in between control and treatments. However, no significant difference was observed during the 5th and 7th day of storage (Table-3). Coated meat irrespective of the methods of the application had slightly lower values than control samples. These results were in agreement with Wu et al., [36] who opined that coating of precooked beef patties with carrageenan lowered the TBA values compared to control suggesting that the oxidation of precooked beef patties may be controlled to some extent by hydrocolloids like carrageenan.

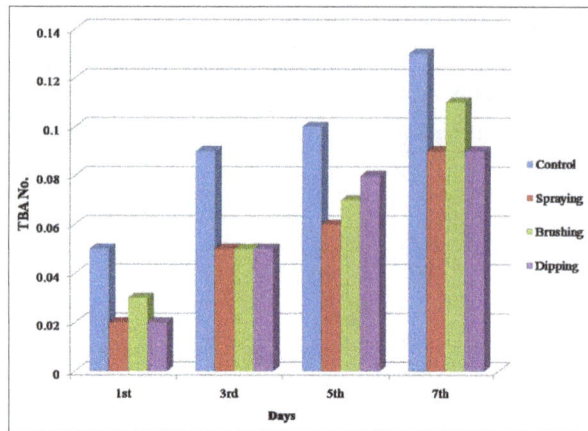

Figure-1: Thiobarbituric acid values of carrageenan, potassium chloride, citric acid, and cinnamon oil coated chicken meat stored at 4±1°C.

Lower TBA values of coated meat might be attributed to the synergistic effect of carrageenan, cinnamon and citric acid on lipid peroxidation. These findings were in agreement with Pikul et al., [37] who demonstrated a significant decrease in TBA values of various meats incorporated with butylated hydroxyanisole. Sheikh Dalia [38] also revealed lower TBA values in chicken breast meat coated with gum Arabic and plantago throughout the entire storage period of 21-day under refrigeration temperature. The result in the present study was in agreement with Qiu et al., [39] who found lower TBA values in samples incorporated with chitosan, citric acid and licorice extract in Japanese fish fillets. Kamel [40] studied effect of mango kernel and cactus peel as edible coating on chicken breast meat and concluded that 25% cactus peels and 0.8% mango kernel showed the lowest TBA value of 0.421 mg malondialdehyde/kg compared to 1.30 mg malondialdehyde/kg in control after 2 weeks of storage

TV

The degree of autolysis and bacterial proteolysis in meat can be measured as TV which actually determines the quantity of amino acids, i.e., tyrosine and tryptophan present in an extract of meat. In the present study, TV increased significantly ($p < 0.05$) with storage period and dipping samples showed the lowest TV followed by spraying and brushing while control had highest values (Table-3). Increase in TV of the control and treatment sample during storage period might be due to the increased microbial load and enhanced production of proteolytic enzymes in the late logarithmic phase of microbial growth; causing autolysis and bacterial proteolysis [41]. The results of the present study could be collated with the observation of Pearson [21], Strange et al., [20]. The lower values in treatments could be attributed to antimicrobial activity of cinnamon oil and citric acid. Similar results were observed in duck patties stored at ambient and refrigeration temperature where TV increased significantly with storage period [42].

Drip loss

There was no significant difference ($p > 0.05$) in drip loss in between the treatments during 1st and 3rd day of storage. However, control had higher values than treatments throughout the storage period. During 5th and 7th day of storage, there was significant ($p < 0.05$) difference was observed in between the treatments (Table-3). Kester and Fennema [43] reported similar results with polysaccharide coating such as carrageenan which act as a moisture barrier when applied in food products such as meat. The results were also in agreement with Pearce and Lavers [44] who observed lower drip loss and higher shelf life in carrageenan dipped meat compared to uncoated meat. Drip loss increased significantly ($p < 0.01$) throughout the storage period. This could be due to degradation of the protein resulting in expulsion of water that is expelled from intermyofibrillar spaces leading to drip. This result was in agreement with Lesiak et al., [45] who found that longer the storage period greater the drip loss. Lee et al., [46] also reported that broiler meat aged for 6 day had higher drip loss than that aged for 1 day. In the present study, at 5th day of storage control samples had slightly lower value than treatments which could be due to high water loss during earlier storage period. However, at the end of the storage period (7th day) control and dipping had the highest values followed by spraying and brushing. Lower drip losses in treatment could be attributed to antimicrobial activity of citric acid and cinnamon oil and its synergistic effect with carrageenan which had moisture barrier property/or reducing moisture loss.

WBSFV

There was a significant difference ($p < 0.05$) in WBSF between the storage period and also in between the treatments. WBSFV increased significantly ($p < 0.01$) with storage period, control had higher values followed by brushing, dipping and spraying (Table-3). WBSFV is inversely related to tenderness of meat. Lower WBSFV in treatment could be due to citric acid incorporation in coating solution. Komoltri and Pakdeechanuan [47] also observed lower shear force value in Golek chicken marinated with citric acid. Ke et al., [48] suggested that tenderness is related to the pH of the muscle. They reported that Warner-Bratzler shear force decreased as muscle pH lowered to 3.52, and then shear force significantly increased as the pH was buffered back to pH 5.26. Many researchers have observed that the tenderness of muscle increased when the pH is below the isoelectric point of the major myofibrillar proteins [33,34].

Instrumental/hunter color

There was no significant difference in color between the storage periods, whereas a significant difference was observed in between the treatment during 1st and 3rd day of storage. Similar results were revealed by Machado de Melo et al., [49] in refrigerated chicken meat in contact with cellulose acetate-based film incorporated with rosemary essential oil (20% and 50%, v/w) they found control samples and film incorporated with 50% rosemary essential oil had no significant variation with respect to the L*, a* and b* values between storage days and treatments. Coated meat sample had higher L* value than uncoated/ control sample. The results were in contradiction to those reported by Tyburcy and Kozyra [50] who found lower L* value in carrageenan coated sausages. Chouliara et al., [51] reported a decrease in L* parameter values in chicken breast meat with storage time in samples containing 0.1 ml/100 g oregano oil. There was no significant difference (p>0.05) in redness a* value observed between the treatments and between the storage period except on 3rd day (Table-4). This might be due to antioxidant activity of cinnamon oil which prevent lipid oxidation and change in pigment color. Keokamnerd et al., [52] reported a decrease in a* value in ground chicken meat during 12 days of storage. These results are in agreement with those of Rodríguez-Calleja et al., [53] who found that a combination of high hydrostatic pressure, a commercial liquid antimicrobial edible coating and MAP did not affect color acceptability of chicken breast fillets. There was no significant difference between storage period and between treatments in yellowness value. There was a significant difference (p<0.05) in yellowness value between the treatments during the 3rd day of storage. Coated meat samples revealed higher values

than control which could be due to addition of cinnamon oil. This was in agreement with Lu et al., [54] who also found higher yellowness value in fish fillets treated with cinnamon oil. Giatrakou et al., [55] reported that b* (yellowness) values were varied with no specific pattern produced by any of the treatments (combination of thyme oil and chitosan) in a poultry product.

Total color change (delta-E) value had significant (p<0.05) difference during 1st and 3rd day of storage. Control had lower value than treatments due to higher L* and b* value in treated samples. However, no significant difference (p>0.05) was observed during 5th and 7th day of storage (Table-4).

Microbiological quality

SPC (log_{10}cfu/gm)

There was highly significant difference (p<0.01) in SPC between the treatments and in between storage period (Figure-2). During initial day of storage control had significantly (p<0.01) higher values compared to treatment. However, no significant difference was observed in between treatments during the 1st day and SPC increased significantly (p<0.01) with storage period in all the samples (Table-5).

SPC value on the 3rd day in control sample was 6.74 log_{10}cfu/g and it was very close to the maximum permissible limit of 7 log_{10}cfu/g total viable count (TVC) for good quality fresh poultry meat as prescribed by ICMSF [56]. However, all other samples

Table-4: Mean±SE values of instrumental/hunter color of carrageenan, potassium chloride, citric acid, and cinnamon oil coated chicken meat stored at 4±1°C.

Days	Methods of application				
	Control	Spraying	Brushing	Dipping	F value
L*value					
1st	56.93±1.15[aA]	61.49±1.34[aB]	62.30±1.05[aB]	62.94±1.24[aB]	5.14**
3rd	59.38±1.35[aA]	60.53±1.61[aB]	62.25±1.06[aB]	61.62±1.54[aB]	0.81**
5th	59.79±1.32[aA]	62.54±0.85[aA]	61.57±1.10[aA]	61.58±1.22[aA]	1.01[NS]
7th	60.02±1.63[aA]	61.48±1.31[aA]	63.27±0.75[aA]	62.89±1.46[aA]	1.23[NS]
F value	11.66**	9.54**	12.29**	4.26*	
a* value					
1st	18.25±0.48[cA]	20.33±0.82[cB]	19.25±0.17[cAB]	20.00±0.55[bB]	2.76[NS]
3rd	15.42±0.78[bA]	18.42±0.37[bB]	18.33±0.49[bB]	19.67±0.85[bB]	7.54**
5th	14.42±0.58[abA]	15.83±0.78[aAB]	16.92±0.54[aB]	17.25±0.91[aB]	3.15*
7th	12.75±0.48[aA]	14.00±0.46[aB]	14.00±0.46[aC]	16.33±0.17[aC]	21.92**
F value	15.14**	18.95**	26.96**	6.88**	
b* value					
1st	1.72±0.09[aA]	1.70±0.16[aA]	1.97±0.21[aA]	2.07±0.09[aA]	1.53[NS]
3rd	2.13±0.08[bA]	2.13±0.14[bB]	2.25±0.17[bB]	2.10±0.26[aB]	1.66**
5th	2.48±0.07[cA]	2.30±0.05[bcA]	2.50±0.17[bcA]	2.32±0.19[aA]	0.62[NS]
7th	2.70±0.14[cA]	2.60±0.08[cA]	2.80±0.25[cA]	3.03±0.13[bA]	1.29[NS]
F value	18.34**	9.77**	3.03**	6.21**	
ΔE value					
1st	58.54±1.90[aA]	64.49±1.12[aB]	65.06±1.09[aB]	65.48±1.24[aB]	5.60**
3rd	62.74±1.09[bA]	63.51±1.42[aB]	65.46±0.91[aB]	64.64±1.64[aB]	4.21**
5th	63.56±1.34[bA]	64.95±0.93[aA]	64.79±0.85[aA]	65.08±1.29[aA]	0.39[NS]
7th	62.96±1.09[bA]	64.62±1.59[aAB]	66.24±0.72[aAB]	66.88±1.08[aB]	2.27[NS]
F value	2.71[NS]	0.23[NS]	0.486[NS]	0.530[NS]	

Means bearing different superscript between rows a, b, c and between columns A, B, C differs significantly (p<0.05), *Indicates significant value (p<0.05); ** Highly significant value (p<0.01). NS=Non significant, SE=Standard error, L*-Lightness, a*-redness, b*-yellowness and ΔE value-Total color change

Table-5: Mean±SE values of SPC ($\log_{10}$ cfu/g) of carrageenan, potassium chloride, citric acid, and cinnamon oil coated chicken meat stored at 4±1°C.

Days	Methods of application				
	Control	Spraying	Brushing	Dipping	F value
SPC ($\log_{10}$ cfu/g)					
1st	4.66±0.30[aB]	3.16±0.10[aA]	3.31±0.14[aA]	3.15±0.09[aA]	16.84**
3rd	6.74±0.21[bC]	5.44±0.26[bB]	4.73±0.20[bAB]	4.23±0.10[bA]	19.44**
5th	8.29±0.10[cB]	7.64±0.24[cA]	7.00±0.23[cA]	6.88±0.31[cA]	6.52**
7th	8.72±0.12[cB]	7.81±0.27[cA]	7.85±0.28[dAB]	7.83±0.23[dA]	3.76*
F value	86.21**	91.83**	93.09**	113.76**	

Means bearing different superscript between rows a, b, c and between columns A, B, C differs significantly (p<0.05), *Indicates significant value (p<0.05); **Highly significant value (p<0.01). NS=Non significant, SPC=Standard plate count

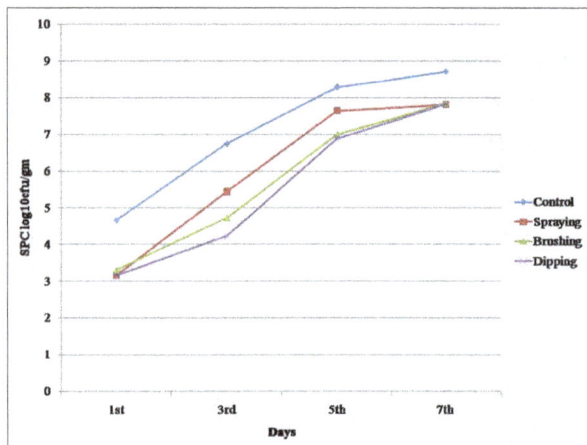

Figure-2: Standard plate count ($\log_{10}$cfu/g) of carrageenan, potassium chloride, citric acid, and cinnamon oil coated chicken meat stored at 4±1°C.

reached approxiamtely 7 $\log_{10}$cfu/g on 5th day of storage and all the samples exceeded the limit on 7th day of storage. Dipping sample had lower value throughout storage period than brushing and spraying. This might be attributed to antimicrobial activity of cinnamon and more viscous nature of carrageenan. Cinnamon oils contain high concentrations of trans-cinnamaldehyde, a well-known antimicrobial compound [57], and also contain linalool, eugenol and other phenolic compounds. Previous studies have also identified trans-cinnamaldehyde as the major antibacterial constituent of cinnamon oil [14].Similar results were revealed by Ojagh et al., [58] in rainbow trout (Oncorhynchus mykiss) coated with chitosan (Ch) and cinnamon oil (Ch + C) under refrigerated storage (4±1°C) for a period of 16-day and found that coated sample exhibited good quality characteristics (lower microbial load) and higher shelf life.

Seol et al., [59] also revealed the carrageenan film incorporated with ovotransferrin and ethylenediaminetetraacetic acid had antimicrobial activity than carrageenan alone and they found that chicken breast meat wrapped with carrageenan reached 7 $\log_{10}$cfu/g on 7th day while treatments had nearly 5.23-6.91 $\log_{10}$cfu/g. Similarly, Shojaee-Aliabadi et al., [60] observed that k-carrageenan film incorporated with plant essential oil had antimicrobial activity against most of the pathogenic microorganism.

Olaimat et al., [61] concluded that κ-Carrageenan/chitosan-based coatings containing 50 or 100 µl/g containing allyl isothiocyanate (AITC) reduced viable Campylobacter jejuni to undetectable levels on chicken breast after 5 day at 4°C, while 25 µl/g AITC or 200-300 mg/g mustard extract in coatings reduced C. jejuni numbers by 1.75-2.78 $\log_{10}$cfu/g.

Sensory attributes

Color scores decreased significantly (p<0.01) with storage period in all the samples and there was highly significant difference was observed between the storage period in all the samples and between samples throughout storage period (Figure-3a). Coated meat samples had higher color score than control, and this was in accordance with Cierach et al., [62] who found higher color scores in carrageenan added sausages than control samples. On the last day of storage, all the samples had lowest values which might be attributed to higher microbial load which lead to change in color from pink to pale pink.

Odor scores were not significant (p>0.05) during initial and final day of storage (Figure-3b). However, highly significant difference was observed during 3rd and 5th day of storage. Odor score reached unacceptable score on 3rd day in control sample while on 5th day in other treatments. At the end of storage (7th day) no significant difference (p>0.05) was observed in odor score which could be correlated to higher bacterial load which leads to the production of sulfurous compounds/off odor. Similar results were obtained by Baston and Barna [63] who compared sensory scores (three point scale) of raw chicken leg and breast at refrigerated storage and revealed that after 1 week of storage breast meat had odor, skin color and slime formation score of 1.3, 2 and 2.3 while leg meat had 1.9, 2.3 and 2.2, respectively.

The antioxidant, antimicrobial and gas barrier effects by coating have been shown to minimize the oxidative effects, prolonging the product shelf life while maintaining quality. Mexis et al., [64] reported that chicken meat treated with citrus extract and control had shelf life of 6 and 4 days, respectively, based on sensory scores and microbiological analysis. Del Rio et al., [65] reported an increase in shelf life by 2 days for chicken legs after treatment with a solution of 2 ml citric acid/100 ml.

There was highly significant difference (p<0.01) was observed in general appearance scores (Figure-3c) in between the treatments throughout the storage period and between storage period in all the samples.

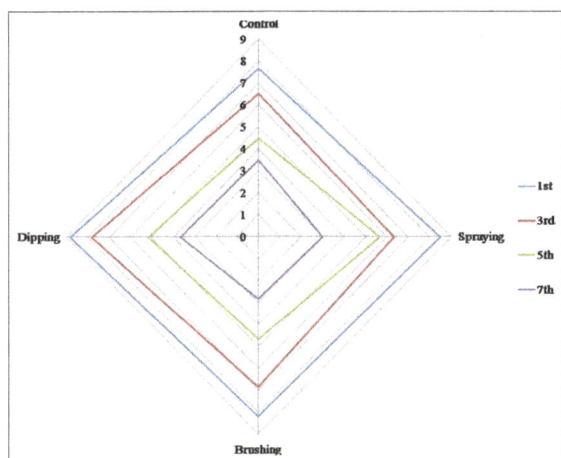

Figure-3a: Sensory attributes (color) of carrageenan, potassium chloride, citric acid, and cinnamon oil coated chicken meat stored at 4±1°C.

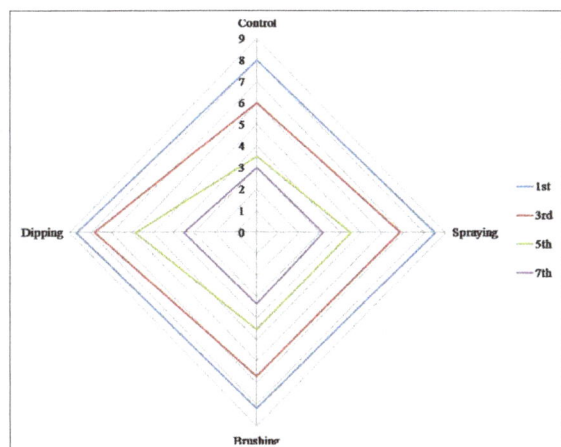

Figure-3b: Sensory attributes (odor) of carrageenan, potassium chloride, citric acid, and cinnamon oil coated chicken meat stored at 4±1°C.

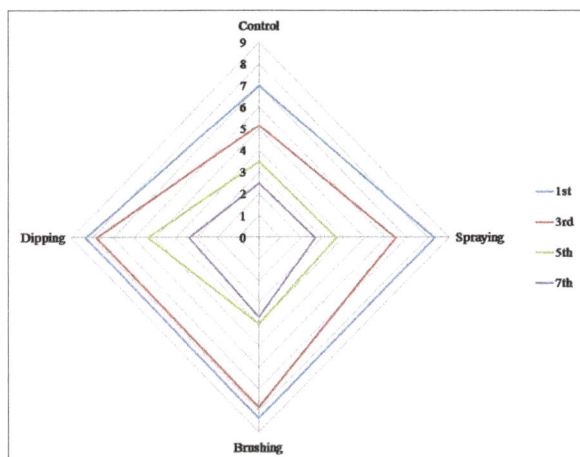

Figure-3c: Sensory attributes (general appearance) of carrageenan, potassium chloride, citric acid, and cinnamon oil coated chicken meat stored at 4±1°C.

It decreased significantly with storage period. During 7th day of storage, there was no significant difference in between the treatments. Control had the lowest score followed by spraying, brushing and dipping sample throughout storage period. Data obtained from sensory panelist were in agreement with microbiological (TVC) quality results.

Conclusion

The edible coating of carrageenan, cinnamon oil and citric acid can be used to enhance shelf life of chicken meat under chilled condition and dipping method is comparatively better than other methods of application.

Authors' Contributions

The study is the major component of the special problem of first author AKK. RJJA provided the guidelines during the work and corrected manuscript. VAR and RNB assisted in solving technical issues during program of work preparation and also give valuable suggestions throughout study. All the authors have read and approved the final manuscript.

Acknowledgments

We extend our sincere gratitude to Madras Veterinary College, (Tamil Nadu Veterinary and Animal Sciences University), Chennai for providing necessary facilities and funds to carry out this work.

Competing Interests

The authors declare that they have no competing interests.

References

1. FAO. (2012) Available from: http://www.fao.org/docrep/015/i2490e/i2490e00.htm. Accessed on 19-11-2015.
2. Available from: http://www.apeda.gov.in/apedawebsite/six_head_product/animal.htm. Accessed on 25-02-2015.
3. Kandeepan, G., Anjaneyulu, A.S.R., Kondaiah, N. and Mendiratta, S.K. (2010) Quality of buffalo meat Keema at refrigerator temperature. *Afr. J. Food Sci.,* 4(6): 410-417.
4. Falguera, V., Quintero, J.P., Jimenez, A., Munoz, J.A. and Ibarz, A. (2011) Edible films and coatings: Structures, active functions, trends and their use. *Trends Food Sci. Technol.,* 22: 292-303.
5. Dhanapal, A., Sasikala, P., Rajamani, L., Kavitha, V., Yazhini, G. and Banu, M.S. (2012) Edible films from polysaccharides. *Food Sci. Q. Manag.,* 3: 9-17.
6. Sánchez-González, L., Cháfer, M., Chiralt, A. and González-Martínez, C. (2010) Physical properties of edible chitosan films containing bergamot essential oil and their inhibitory action on *Penicillium italicum. Carbohyd. Polym.,* 82: 277-283.
7. Codex Alimentarius Commission. (2010) GSFA Online: Food Additive Details, Carrageenan. Available from: http://www.codexalimentarius.net/gsfaonline/additives/details.html?id=49 Accessed on 25-02-2015.
8. Janjarasskul, T. and Krochta, J.M. (2010) Edible packaging materials. *Annu. Rev. Food Sci. Technol.,*1: 415-148.
9. Prajapati, V.D., Maheriya, P.M., Jani, G.K. and Solanki, H.K. (2014) Carrageenan: A natural seaweed polysaccharide and its applications. *Carbohyd. Polym.,* 105: 97-112.
10. Li, Y.Q., Kong, D.X. and Wu, H. (2013) Analysis and evaluation of essential oil components of cinnamon barks

using GC-MS and FTIR spectroscopy. *Ind. Crop Prod.*, 41: 269-278.

11. China Pharmacopeia Commission. (2010) Pharmacopoeia of the People's Republic of China. Chinese Medical Science and Technology Press, Beijing, China. p163-127.

12. Tzortzakis, N.G. (2009) Impact of cinnamon oil-enrichment on microbial spoilage of fresh produce. *Innov. Food Sci. Emerg.*, 10: 97-102.

13. Du, H. and Li, H. (2008) Antioxidant effect of cassia essential oil on deep-fried beef during the frying process. *Meat Sci.*, 78: 461-468.

14. Ouattara, B., Simard, R.E., Holley, R.A., Piette, G.J.P. and Begin, A. (1997) Antibacterial activity of selected fatty acids and essential oils against six meat spoilage organisms. *Int. J. Food Microbiol.*, 37(2-3): 155-162.

15. Shan, B., Cai, Y., Brooks, J.D. and Corke, H. (2007) Antibacterial properties and major bioactive components of cinnamon stick (*Cinnamomum burmannii*): Activity against foodborne pathogenic bacteria. *J. Agric. Food Chem.*, 55(14): 5484-5490.

16. Sánchez-González, L., Vargas, M., Gonzalez Martinez, C., Chiralt, A. and Cháfer, M. (2011) Use of essential oils in bioactive edible coatings. CRC *Food Eng.*, 3: 1-16.

17. USDA-FSIS. (2010) Safe and suitable ingredients used in the production of meat andpoultryproducts.Directive7120.1, Rev. 2. Available from: http://www.fsis.usda.gov/OPPDE/rdad/FSISDirectives/7120.1Rev2.pdf. Accessed on 11-01-2015.

18. Trout, E.S., Hunt, M.C., Johson, D.E, Clans, J.R., Castner, C.L. and Kroff, D.H. (1992) Characteristics of low fat ground beef containing texture modifying ingredients. *J. Food Sci.*, 57(1): 19-24.

19. Grau, R. and Hamm, R. (1953) Water. In: Price, J.F. and Scheweigert, B.S., editors. The Science of Meat and Meat Products. 2nd ed. W.H. Freemen and Company, San Francisco. p186-189.

20. Grau, R. and Hamm, R. (1957) In biochemistry of meat hydration. *Adv. Food Res.*, 10: 356-359.

21. Pearson, D. (1968) Application of chemical methods for the assessment of beef quality methods related to protein breakdown. *J. Sci. Food Agric.*, 19(7): 366-369.

22. Somers, C., Tarrant, O.V. and Sherington, J. (1985) Evaluation of some objective methods of measuring pork quality. *Meat Sci.*, 15: 63-76.

23. Strange, E.D., Benedict, R.C., Smith, J.L. and Swift, C.E. (1977) Evaluation of rapid tests for monitoring the alterations in meat quality during storage. *J. Food Prot.*, 40: 843-847.

24. Khare, A.K., Biswas, A.K. and Sahoo, J. (2014) Comparison study of chitosan, EDTA, eugenol and peppermint oil for antioxidant and antimicrobial potentials in chicken noodles and their effect on color and oxidative stability at ambient temperature storage. *Food Sci. Technol.*, 55: 286-293.

25. APHA. (1984) Compendium of Methods for Microbiological Examination of Foods. 2nd ed. American Public Health Association, Washington, DC.

26. Keeton, J.T. (1983) Effect of fat and sodium chloride and phosphate levels on the chemical and sensory properties of pork patties. *J. Food Sci.*, 48(3): 878-881.

27. Snedecor, G.W. and Cochran, W.G. (1994) Statistical Methods. 8th ed. The Iowa State University Press Ames, Iowa, USA.

28. Sinhamahapatra, M., Biswas, S., Das, A.K. and Bhattacharyya, D. (2004) Comparative study of different surface decontaminants on chicken quality. *Br. Poultr. Sci.*, 45(5): 624-630.

29. Petrou, S., Tsiraki, M., Giatrakou, V. and Savvaidis, I.N. (2012) Chitosan dipping or oregano oil treatments, singly or combined on modified atmosphere packaged chicken breast meat. *Int. J. Food Microbiol.*, 156: 264-271.

30. Kandeepan, G. and Biswas, S. (2007) Effect of low temperature preservation on quality and shelf-life of buffalo meat. *Am. J. Food Technol.*, 2(3): 126-135.

31. James, M.J. (1966) Response of the extract-release volume and water-holding capacity phenomena to microbiologically spoiled beef and aged beef. *Appl. Microbiol.*, 14(4): 492-496.

32. Ayadi, M.A., Kechaou, A., Makni, I. and Attia, H. (2009) Influence of carrageenan additionon turkey meat sausages properties. *J. Food Eng.*, 93(3): 278-283.

33. Gault, N.F.S. (1985) The relationship between water holding capacity and cook meat tenderness in some beef muscles as influenced by acidic conditions below the ultimate pH. *Meat Sci.*, 15(1): 15-30.

34. Rao, M. and Gault, N.F.S. (1989) The influence of fibre-type composition and associated biochemical characteristics on the acid buffering capacities of several beef muscles. *Meat Sci.*, 26: 5-18.

35. Gheisari, H.R. (2011) Correlation between acid, TBA, peroxide and iodine values, catalase and glutathione peroxidase activities of chicken, cattle and camel meat during refrigerated storage. *Vet. World*, 4(4): 153-157.

36. Wu, Y., Rhim, J.W., Weller, C.L., Hamouz, F., Cuppett, S. and Schnepf, M. (2000) Moisture loss and lipid oxidation for precooked beef patties store in edible coatings and films. *J. Food Sci.*, 65: 300-304.

37. Pikul, J., Leszcynski, D.E., Niewiarowicz, A. and Kummerow, F.A. (1984) Lipid oxidation in chicken breast and leg meat after sequential treatments of frozen storage, cooking, refrigerated storage and reheating. *J. Food Technol.*, 19: 575-580.

38. Sheikh Dalia, M.E. (2014) Efficiency of using Arabic gum and plantago seeds mucilage as edible coating for chicken boneless breast. *Food Sci. Q. Manag.*, 32: 28-33.

39. Qiu, X., Chen, S., Liu, G. and Yang, Q. (2014) Quality enhancement in the Japanese sea bass (*Lateolabrax japonicas*) fillets stored at 4°C by chitosan coating incorporated with citric acid or licorice extract. *Food Chem.*, 162: 156-160.

40. Kamel, S.M. (2014) Utilization of cactus dear peels mucilage as an edible coating of chicken meat to prolong its shelf life. *Food Sci. Q. Manag.*, 28: 71-77.

41. Dainty, R.H., Shaw, B.G., Boer, K.A. and Scheps, E.S.J. (1975) Protein changes caused by bacterial growth on beef. *J. Appl. Bacteriol.*, 39(1): 73-81.

42. Biswas, S., Chakraborty, A., Patra, G. and Dhargupta, A. (2011) Quality and acceptability of duck patties stored at ambient and refrigeration temperature. *Int. J. Livest. Prod.*, 1(1): 1-6.

43. Kester, J.J. and Fennema, O. (1986) Edible films and coatings: A review. *Food Technol.*, 40: 47-59.

44. Pearce, J.A. and Lavers, C.G. (1949) Frozen storage of poultry. V. Effects of some processing factors on quality. *Can. J. Res.*, 27: 253-265.

45. Lesiak, M.T., Olson, D.G., Lesiak, C.A. and Ahn, D.U. (1996) Effects of postmortem temperature and time in water-holding capacity of hot-boned turkey breast and thigh muscle. *Meat Sci.*, 43(1): 51-60.

46. Lee, Y.S., Owens, C.M. and Meullenet, J.F. (2009) Changes in tenderness, color, and water holding capacity of broiler breast meat during post deboning aging. *J. Food Sci.*, 74(8): 449-454.

47. Komoltri, P. and Pakdeechanuan, P. (2012) Effects of marinating ingredients on physicochemical, microstructural and sensory properties of Golek chicken. *Int. Food Res. J.*, 19(4): 1449-1455.

48. Ke, S., Huang, Y., Decker, E.A. and Hultin, H.O. (2009) Impact of citric acid on the tenderness, microstructure and oxidative stability of beef muscle. *Meat Sci.*, 82: 113-118.

49. Machado de Melo, A.A., Geraldine, R.M., Araujo Silveira, M.F., Torres, M.C.L., Rezende, C.S.M., Fernandes, T.H. and Oliveira, A.N. (2012) Microbiological quality and other characteristics of refrigerated chicken

meat in contact with cellulose acetate-based film incorporated with rosemary essential oil. *Braz. J. Microbiol.*, 43(4): 1419-1427.

50. Tyburcy, A. and Kozyra, D. (2010) Effects of composite surface coating and pre-drying on the properties of Kabanosy dry sausage. *Meat Sci.*, 86(2): 405-410.

51. Chouliara, E., Badeka, A., Savvaidis, I. and Kontominas, M.G. (2008) Combined effect of irradiation and modified atmosphere packaging on shelf life extension of chicken breast meat: Microbiological, chemical and sensory changes. *Eur. Food Res. Technol.*, 226(4): 877-888.

52. Keokamnerd, T., Acton, J.C., Han, I.Y. and Dawson, P.L. (2008) Effect of commercial rosemary oleoresin preparations on ground chicken thigh meat quality packaged in a high-oxygen atmosphere. *Poultr. Sci.*, 87: 170-179.

53. Rodríguez-Calleja, J.M., Cruz-Romero, M.C., O'Sallivan, M.G., García-López, M.L. and Kelly, J.P. (2012) High-pressure-based hurdle strategy to extend the shelf-life of fresh chicken fillets. *Food Control.*, 25: 516-524.

54. Lu, F., Liu, D.H., Ye, X.Q., Wei, Y.X. and Liu, F. (2010) Alginate calcium coating incorporating nisin and EDTA maintains the quality of fresh northern snakehead (*Channa argus*) fillets stored at 4°C. *J. Sci. Food Agric.*, 89: 848-854.

55. Giatrakou, V., Ntzimani, A., Zwietering, M. and Savvaidis, I.N. (2010) Combined chitosan thyme treatments with modified atmosphere packaging on a Greek ready-to-cook (RTC) poultry product. *J. Food Prot.*, 73: 663-669.

56. ICMSF (International Commission on Microbiological Specifications for Foods). (1986) Microorganisms in Foods. 2. Sampling for Microbiological Analysis: Principles and Scientific Applications. 2nd ed. University of Toronto Press, Toronto.

57. Shan, B.E., Yoshida, Y., Sugiura, T. and Yamashita, U. (1999) Stimulating activity of Chinese medicinal herbs on human lymphocytes *in vitro*. *Int. J. Immunopharmacol.*, 21: 149-159.

58. Ojagh, S.M., Rezaei, M., Razavi, S.H. and Hosseini, S.M.H. (2010) Effect of chitosan coatings enriched with cinnamon oil on the quality of refrigerated rainbow trout. *Food Chem.*, 120: 1193-1198.

59. Seol, K.H., Lim, D.G., Jang, A., Jo, C. and Lee, M. (2009) Antimicrobial effect of κ-carrageenan-based edible film containing ovotransferrin in fresh chicken breast stored at 5°C. *Meat Sci.*, 83(3): 479-483.

60. Shojaee-Aliabadi, S., Hosseini, H., Mohammadifar, M.A., Mohammadi, A., Ghasemlou, M. and Ojagh, S.M. (2013) Characterization of antioxidant antimicrobial j-carrageenan films containing Satureja hortensis essential oil. *Int. J. Biol. Macromol.*, 52(1): 116-124.

61. Olaimat, A.N., Fang, Y. and Holley, R.A. (2014) Inhibition of campylobacter jejuni on fresh chicken breasts by κ-carrageenan/chitosan-based coatings containing allyl isothiocyanate or deodorized oriental mustard extract. *Int. J. Food Microbiol.*, 187:77-82.

62. Cierach, M., Modzelewska-Kapituła, M. and Szaciło, K. (2009) The influence of carrageenan on the properties of low-fat frankfurters. *Meat Sci.*, 82(3): 295-299.

63. Baston, O. and Barna, O. (2010) Raw Chicken Leg and breast sensory evaluation. *Ann. Food Sci. Technol.*, 11(1): 50-53.

64. Mexis, S.F., Chouliara, E. and Kontominas, M.G. (2012) Shelf life extension of ground meat using an oxygen absorber and a citrus extract. *Food Sci. Technol.*, 49: 21-27.

65. Del Rio, E., Muriente, R., Prieto, M., Alosnso-Calleja, C. and Capite. R. (2007) Effectiveness of trisodium phosphate, acidified sodium chlorite, citric acid and peroxyacids against pathogenic bacteria on poultry during refrigerated storage. *J. Food Prot.*,70(9): 2063-2071.

12

Evaluation of *Emblica officinalis* fruit powder as a growth promoter in commercial broiler chickens

A. P. Patel[1], S. R. Bhagwat[1], M. M. Pawar[1], K. B. Prajapati[2], H. D. Chauhan[3] and R. B. Makwana[3]

1. Department of Animal Nutrition, College of Veterinary Science and Animal Husbandry, Sardarkrushinagar Dantiwada Agricultural University, Banaskantha, Gujarat, India; 2. Livestock Research Station, Sardarkrushinagar Dantiwada Agricultural University, Banaskantha, Gujarat, India; 3. Department of Livestock Production and Management, College of Veterinary Science and Animal Husbandry, Sardarkrushinagar Dantiwada Agricultural University, Banaskantha, Gujarat, India.
Corresponding author: M. M. Pawar, e-mail: mahespawar@gmail.com,
APP: ashokveti@gmail.com, SRB: shekhar.bhagwat@gmail.com, KBP: Kbprajapati.savita@gmail.com,
HDC: Hdchauhan1970@rediffmail.com, RBM: rinkeshvets@gmail.com

Abstract

Aim: The present study was conducted to evaluate the dietary addition of *Emblica officinalis* (Amla) fruit powder as a growth promoter in commercial broiler chickens.

Materials and Methods: An experiment was conducted on 135 commercial broiler chicks (Ven-Cobb 400 strain) divided into three groups with three replicates of 15 chicks each. Three treatment groups were as follows – T_1: Basal diet as per BIS standards; T_2: Basal diet supplemented with 0.4% of *E. officinalis* fruit powder; and T_3: Basal diet supplemented with 0.8% of *E. officinalis* fruit powder.

Results: The average body weights at the end of the 6th week were significantly higher ($p<0.05$) in groups T_2 and T_3 compared to group T_1. Feed intake, feed conversion ratio and feed cost per kg live weight production were similar among the treatment groups. The net profit per bird was the highest in group T_2 (Rs. 19.22/bird) followed by group T_3 (Rs. 17.86/bird) and the lowest in group T_1 (Rs. 14.61/bird).

Conclusion: Based on the results of the present study, it was concluded that dietary addition of *E. officinalis* (Amla) fruit powder had a positive effect on growth performance and net profit per bird in commercial broiler chickens.

Keywords: broiler chickens, *Emblica officinalis*, feed conversion ratio, growth performance.

Introduction

Growth promoters are chemical and biological substances which are added to diet with the aim to improve the growth, utilization of nutrients and in this way realize better production and financial results. Their positive effect can be expressed through better appetite, improved body weight and feed conversion ratio (FCR), stimulation of the immune system and increased vitality, regulation of the intestinal microflora, etc. In any case, expected results of the use of these additives are increased financial returns over the cost of production. Furthermore, due to ban on the use of antibiotic growth promoters in poultry, herbal preparations have been tried as feed additives as an alternative to antibiotics to increase feed efficiency and growth rate in broiler chickens [1].

In the last decade, herbal feed additives have attracted the attention of scientists as useful resource for improving productivity. Besides, these herbs are natural component and do not have any side effects like residues in meat products. Amla (*Emblica officinalis*) fruit powder is one of the herbs which have potential to boost broiler production. Amla is extensively cultivated all over India. The fruits of the plants are used in Ayurveda as a potant rasayana (revitalisers, biological response modifiers) in which the amla was added as anti-stress agent. Phyto-chemical analysis of amla fruit powder provided evidence of presence of the medicinally important bioactive compounds which can be exploited beneficially to improve productivity in broilers.

Emblica officinalis (Amla) is one of the richest sources of ascorbic acid, minerals, amino acids, tannins, and phenolic compounds [2]. Rapid growth rate in commercial broilers accelerate the metabolic rate and make them vulnerable to oxidative stress owing to increased free radical generation [3]. Gallic acid and tannic acids are the phenolic acids present in *E. officinalis* contribute to the antioxidant activity, in addition, to ascorbic acid [4]. Therefore, the present study was conducted to evaluate the dietary addition of *E. officinalis* (Amla) fruit powder as a growth promoter in commercial broiler chickens.

Materials and Methods

Ethical approval

This research was carried out after approval of Institutional Animal Ethics Committee of College of Veterinary Science and Animal Husbandry, Sardarkrushinagar Dantiwada Agricultural University, Gujarat.

Experimental design

A total of 1351-day-old unsexed broiler chicks (Ven-Cobb 400 strain) purchased from a local hatchery were weighed and randomly assigned to one of three treatments with three replicates of 15 chicks based on a completely randomized design. Three treatments were as follows – T_1: Basal diet as per BIS standards; T_2: Basal diet supplemented with 0.4% of E. officinalis fruit powder; and T_3: Basal diet supplemented with 0.8% of E. officinalis fruit powder.

Feeding and management procedures

Broilers were raised on deep litter housing system for 6 weeks. Feed and water were provided ad libitum throughout the experiment. Broilers were fed in three phases, viz., pre-starter (0-10 days), starter (11-21 days), and finisher (22-42 days) ration as per BIS [5] specifications. Chicks were individually weighed at weekly intervals. Feed consumption and FCR (FCR=feed intake/weight gain) were calculated at weekly intervals. Mortality was recorded daily. The feed cost-economics of broiler production in different treatment groups was calculated based on the current market price of various particulars.

Chemical and statistical analysis

The ingredients and chemical composition of basal diet used during experimental feeding are given in Table-1. Samples of feeds were milled to pass through a 1mm sieve and then analyzed for the chemical composition according to standard procedures of the AOAC [6] methods. The experimental data were statistically analyzed using SPSS software (version 16.0, SPSS Inc., Chicago, USA) as per procedures of Snedecor and Cocharan [7]. The significant differences among the tested means were tested with Duncan's multiple range test [8], and significance was declared at $p < 0.05$.

Results and Discussion

Growth performance

The data on growth performance is presented in Table-2. The average body weights of the birds at the end of the 6th week were higher ($p < 0.05$) in groups T_2 (2186.00±19.48 g) and T_3 (2170.60±14.62 g) compared to group T_1 (2076.30±22.27 g). In the present study, the birds supplemented with E. officinalis fruit powder at the rate of 0.4% and 0.8% had higher ($p < 0.05$) overall body weights and weekly body weight gain at the end of 6th week compared to un-supplemented group. The higher body weights observed in E. officinalis supplemented groups may

Table-1: Ingredients and chemical composition of basal diet used during experimental feeding.

Attributes	Pre-starter	Starter	Finisher
Ingredients (%)			
Yellow maize	51.28	52.05	57.00
Soybean meal	40.21	38.43	33.03
Vegetable oil	4.56	5.6	6.38
Dicalcium phosphate	1.93	1.97	1.71
Common salt	0.35	0.35	0.35
Limestone	0.97	1.01	0.93
Maduramycine	0.05	0.05	0.05
Lipocare[1]	0.10	0.10	0.10
L-lysine	0.17	0.15	0.14
DL-methionine	0.15	0.15	0.07
Vitamin premix[2]	0.05	0.05	0.05
Mineral premix[3]	0.20	0.20	0.20
Total	100.02	100.01	100.01
Nutrient composition (%)			
Dry matter	94.63	94.71	94.32
Crude protein	23.21	21.64	19.62
Ether extract	2.75	3.46	4.20
Crude fiber	4.98	5.03	5.01
Total ash	5.72	6.63	5.07
ME (kcal/kg)	2998.2	3075.1	3185.6

[1]Lecithin treated with co-enzyme, [2]Provides per kg of diet: 12,500 IU vitamin A; 2500 IU vitamin D_3; 12 mg vitamin E; 1.5 mg vitamin K; 1.5 mg vitamin B_1; 5 mg; vitamin B_2; 2 mg vitamin B_6, 15 mcg vitamin B_{12}; 15 mg niacin, 10 mg pantothenic acid and 0.5 mg folic acid, [3]Provides per kg of diet: 50 mg iron; 10 mg copper; 80 mg zinc; 80 mg manganese; 1 mg iodine and 0.2 mg selenium. ME: Metabolizable energy

be attributed to anabolic and antioxidant effect of ascorbic acid, gallic acid and tannic acids present in E. officinalis [9]. Similar findings were reported by Maini et al. [10], Patil et al. [11], Kumari et al. [12] Patil et al. [13]. In another studies, Sujatha et al. [14] and Kumar et al. [15] reported increase in body weight when birds were supplemented with polyherbal feed premix containing E. officinalis.

Feed intake and FCR

Feed intake and FCR were non-significant ($p > 0.05$) among the treatment groups (Table-3). Dietary supplementation of E. officinalis at both levels (0.4% and 0.8%) did not have any adverse ($p = 0.307$) effect on feed intake in broilers. Our findings are in agreement with prior studies [15,16] which demonstrated that supplementation of E. officinalis had no effect of feed intake and FCR. In contrast Patil et al. [13] reported that significant increase in feed intake when birds were supplemented with either E. officinalis fruit powder alone or in form of poly-herb.

Return over feedcost

The cost of feed per kilogram of live weight production was similar among the treatment groups(Table-4). The profit per bird was the highest ($p < 0.05$) in group T_2 (Rs. 19.22/bird) followed by group T_3 (Rs. 17.86/bird) and lowest in group T_1 (Rs. 14.61/bird). The higher net profit per bird in E. officinalis supplemented groups attributed to higher

Table-2: Average weekly body weights (g/bird) and body weight gain (g) of broiler chicks under different treatment groups.

Weeks	Treatments			Significance
	T_1	T_2	T_3	
Average weekly body weights (g/bird)				
Day old	47.04±0.56	46.22±0.36	46.71±0.47	NS
I	129.49±2.48	131.93±2.35	130.47±1.59	NS
II	394.36[a]±5.53	425.38[b]±6.62	423.34[b]±3.48	0.012*
III	699.73[a]±8.48	776.76[b]±13.97	750.32[b]±6.07	0.016*
IV	1101.50[a]±14.58	1176.80[b]±17.15	1152.60[b]±10.99	0.032*
V	1583.20[a]±20.43	1653.90[b]±25.13	1642.20[b]±11.74	0.027*
VI	2076.30[a]±22.27	2186.00[b]±19.48	2170.60[b]±14.62	0.003**
Average weekly weight gain (g)				
I	82.4±2.41	85.7±2.33	83.8±1.56	NS
II	265.5[a]±5.92	293.4[b]±6.79	293.1[b]±3.69	0.009**
III	305.4[a]±8.13	351.4[b]±14.72	327.0[ab]±5.98	0.026*
IV	403.2±12.96	400.0±19.01	402.3±11.49	NS
V	481.7±22.33	470.7±24.48	489.6±13.27	NS
VI	493.1±25.45	532.1±25.55	528.4±11.07	NS
0-VI	2029.3[a]±22.33	2139.7[b]±19.43	2123.8[b]±14.56	0.002**

[a,b,c]Means bearing different superscripts in a row differ significantly (*$p<0.05$; **$p<0.01$)

Table-3: Average weekly feed intake (g/bird) and FCR in broilers under different treatment groups.

Weeks	Treatments			Significance
	T_1	T_2	T_3	
Average weekly feed intake (g/bird)				
I	113.9±3.12	116.1±1.12	114.0±0.45	NS
II	396.5±9.23	419.6±11.58	416.4±4.07	NS
III	501.6[a]±9.45	536.5[b]±1.18	510.0[a]±4.53	0.016*
IV	693.3±3.10	693.0±6.10	697.3±5.61	NS
V	898.5±19.30	855.2±42.34	880.8±18.74	NS
VI	1018.2[a]±15.60	1087.9[b]±7.77	1071.0[b]±11.83	0.018*
0-VI	3622.1±38.54	3708.4±45.34	3689.4±26.89	NS
Average weekly FCR				
I	1.38±0.03	1.36±0.05	1.36±0.04	NS
II	1.49±0.04	1.43±0.01	1.42±0.01	NS
III	1.64[b]±0.01	1.53[a]±0.04	1.56[a]±0.01	0.034*
IV	1.72±0.01	1.73±0.02	1.73±0.02	NS
V	1.86±0.02	1.82±0.03	1.80±0.01	NS
VI	2.06±0.03	2.05±0.01	2.03±0.01	NS
0-VI	1.80±0.02	1.75±0.02	1.74±0.01	NS

[a,b,c]Means bearing different superscripts in a row differ significantly ($p<0.05$). FCR=Feed conversion ratio

Table-4: Economics of broiler production and mortality in different treatment groups.

Particulars	Treatments		
	T_1	T_2	T_3
Feed cost/kg live weight production (Rs.)	45.36	44.51	45.00
Net profit/bird (Rs.)	14.61	19.22	17.86
Mortality (%)	4.44	2.22	2.22

body weights compared to the un-supplemented group and similar feed intakes among all the treatment groups.

Mortality

The mortality was 4.4%, 2.2% and 2.2% in T_1, T_2 and T_3 groups, respectively (Table-3). The data indicated that the percent mortality is well within the normal limit, i.e., below 5%. However, the percent mortality in *E. officinalis* fruit powder supplemented groups (T_2 and T_3) were lower indicating better livability of birds as compared to T_1 group, which may be due to immune-modulatory property of bioactive compounds present in *E. officinalis*. Similarly, Kumar and Singh [17] reported that mortality was reduced in birds supplemented with either *E. officinalis* fruit powder or its mixture with other herbs.

Conclusion

Results indicated that dietary addition of *E. officinalis* (Amla) fruit powder at the rate of 0.4% and 0.8% had higher growth rate and net profit per bird in commercial broiler chickens. Though *E. officinalis* supplementation had shown positive response in the present study, but it needs to be tested at different supplemental levels and in different ration compositions to get the best results.

Authors' Contributions

SRB and MMP designed and supervised the experiment. APP carried out the experimental work.

RBM carried out laboratory analysis of feed samples. MMP, KBP and HDC did the data analysis and drafted the manuscript. All authors read and approved the final manuscript.

Acknowledgments

The authors acknowledge the facilities and financial support provided for the present study from Director of Research, Sardarkrushinagar Dantiwada Agricultural University, Sardarkrushinagar, Banaskantha, Gujarat, India.

Competing Interests

The authors declare that they have no competing interests.

References

1. Toghyani, M., Tavalaeian, E., Landy, N., Ghalamkari, Z. and Radnezhad, H. (2011) Efficiency of different levels of *Saturej hortensis L.* (Savoery) in comparison with an antibiotic growth promoter on performance, carcass traits, immune responses and serum biochemical parameters in broiler chickens. *Afr. J. Biotechnol.,* 10: 13318-13323.
2. Yokozawa, T., Kim, Y.H., Kim, J.H., Tanaka, T., Sugino, H., Okubo, T., Chichu, D. and Juneja, R.L. (2007) Amla (*Emblica officinalis* Gaertn) attenuates age related renal dysfunction by oxidative stress. *J. Agric. Food Chem.,* 55: 7744-7752.
3. Feng, J., Zhang, M., Zheng, S., Xie, P. and Ma, A. (2008) Effects of high temperature on multiple parameters of broilers *in vitro* and *in vivo. Poult. Sci.,* 87: 2133-2139.
4. Suresh Kumar, G., Nayak, H., Shylaja, M.D. and Salimath, P.V. (2006) Free and bound phenolic antioxidants in Amla (*Emblica officinalis*) and turmeric (*Curcuma longa*). *J. Food Compos. Anal.,* 19: 446-452.
5. BIS. (1992) Indian Standards: Poultry Feed Specifications. 4th Revision. Bureau of Indian Standards, New Delhi.
6. AOAC. (1995) Association of Official Analytical Chemists. Official Methods of Analysis. 16th ed. Association of Official Analytical Chemists, Washington, DC, USA.
7. Snedecor, G.W. and Cocharan, W.G. (1989) Statistical Methods. 8th ed. Affiliated East West Press Pvt. Ltd., New Delhi, India.
8. Duncan, D.B. (1955) Multiple range and multiple F tests. *Biometrics,* 11: 1-42.
9. McDowell, L.R., editor. (1989) Vitamins in Animal Nutrition. Comparative Aspects to Human Nutrition. Vitamin A and E. Academic Press, London. p93-131.
10. Maini, S., Rastogi, S.K., Korde, J.P., Arun, M.K. and Shukla, K.K. (2007) Evaluation of oxidative stress and amelioration through certain antioxidants in broilers during summer. *J. Poult. Sci.,* 44: 339-347.
11. Patil, R.G., Kulkarni, A.N., Bhutkar S.S. and Korake, R.L. (2012) Effect of different feeding levels of *Emblica officinalis* (Amla) on performance of broilers. *Res. J. Anim. Husbandry Dairy Sci.,* 3:102-04.
12. Kumari, M., Wadhwa, D., Sharma, V.K. and Sharma, A. (2012) Effect of Amla (*Emblica officinalis*) pomace feeding on growth performance of commercial broilers. *Indian J. Anim. Nutr.,* 29: 388-392.
13. Patil, A.S., Wankhede, S.M. and Kale, V.R. (2014) Effect of *Emblica officinalis* (Amla) and vitamin E addition in diet on growth performance of broiler chicken reared under nutritional stress. *Indian J. Anim. Nutr.,* 31: 389-392.
14. Sujatha, V., Korde, J.P., Rastogi, S.K., Maini, S., Ravikanth, K. and Rekhe, D.S. (2010) Amelioration of heat stress induced disturbances of the antioxidant defense system in broilers. *J. Vet. Med. Anim. Health,* 2:18-28.
15. Kumar, M., Sharma, R.K., Chaudhari, M. and Jakhar, A. (2013) Effect of Indian gooseberry and multi-enzyme supplementation on the performance of broilers during hot weather. *Haryana Vet.,* 52: 66-68.
16. Sanjyal, S. and Sapkota, S. (2011) Supplementation of broilers diet with different sources of growth promoters. *Nepal J. Sci. Technol.,* 12: 41-50.
17. Kumar, M. and Singh, K.C.P. (2005) Effect of supplementation of herbal product on the production potential of chickens. In: XXII Annual Conference of IPSA and National Symposium, 02-04 February, Hyderabad, India. p69.

13

Studies of the macroscopic and microscopic morphology (hippocampus) of brain in Vencobb broiler

Shailesh Kumar Gupta[1], Kumaresh Behera[1], C. R. Pradhan[1], Arun Kumar Mandal[2], Kamdev Sethy[3], Dayanidhi Behera[1] and Kuladip Prakash Shinde[4]

1. Department of Livestock Production and Management, College of Veterinary Sciences and Animal Husbandry, Bhubaneswar - 751 003, Odisha, India; 2. Department of Veterinary Anatomy and Histology, College of Veterinary Sciences and Animal Husbandry, Bhubaneswar - 751 003, Odisha, India; 3. Department of Animal Nutrition, College of Veterinary Sciences and Animal Husbandry, Bhubaneswar - 751 003, Odisha, India; 4. Livestock Production Management Section, ICAR - National Dairy Research Institute (NDRI), Karnal - 132 001, Haryana, India.
Corresponding author: Shailesh Kumar Gupta, e-mail: sgshailesh786@gmail.com,
KB: kumaresh.behera@gmail.com, CRP: pradhancr@gmail.com, AKM: arunmandal_2005yahoo.com,
KS: babuivri@gmail.com, DB: phddaya@gmail.com, KPS: kuls164@gmail.com

Abstract

Aim: The aim of this study was to study the anatomy of different parts of brain and histology of hippocampus of Vencobb broiler chicken.

Materials and Methods: A 12 adult experimental birds were sacrificed by cervical dislocation. After separation of the brain, gross anatomy features were studied. Brain tissue was fixed in 10% buffered neutral formalin for 2-3 days, and then routine dehydration process in ascending grades of ethyl alcohol was done. After xylene cleaning, paraffin impregnation was prepared. Paraffin blocks were cut, and slides were stained by Harris hematoxylin and eosin. Photography was carried out both under lower (×10) and higher (×40) magnifications.

Results: The brain structure (dorsal view) of Vencobb bird resembled the outline of a playing card symbol of a "spade." The brain subdivisions are cerebrum, cerebellum, and medulla oblongata. Cerebrum was devoid of usual convolutions (elevations), gyri, depressions (grooves), and sulci. The cerebral hemispheres were tightly apposed along a median sulcus called interhemispheric fissure and cerebrum and cerebellum were separated by a small transverse fissure. The olfactory bulb was small structures, and the pineal body was clearly visible. The optic lobes were partially hidden under cerebral hemispheres, but laterally, it was large, prominent rounded or spherical bodies of the midbrain. The hippocampal area appeared as dorso-medial protrusion. Different types of neurons were distinguished in the hippocampus were pyramidal neurons, pyramidal-like neurons, and multipolar neurons, etc. There was rich vascularization in the form of blood capillaries throughout the hippocampus.

Conclusion: Cerebrum was pear shaped and largest part of the brain. Cerebrum hemisphere was smooth devoid of convolutions, gyri, and depressions, but in the surface of cerebellum, there was the presence of a number of transverse depression (grooves) and sulci subdividing into many folds. Olfactory bulb was poorly developed, whereas optic lobes were rounded and large. The exact boundary line of the hippocampus was not discernable. In hippocampus histology, two categories of neuron local circuit neurons and projection neurons, high vascularization and epididymal lining of lateral ventricle were observed. Hippocampal neurons were comparatively larger without any distinct layers. The afferent neurons projected to the medium septum.

Keywords: capillaries, hemisphere, hippocampus, neurons, Vencobb broiler.

Introduction

Avian brain research was started in the early 20th century. Brain research in birds is important for bird's welfare and knowledge about the nervous system function, physiology, anatomical development, and behavior. The cognitive ability of a species might be due its total number of brain neurons [1]. Large brains might have evolved as an adaptation to cope with novel or altered conditions. The large optic lobes in avian species can be attributed to the fact that the birds have a very well-developed sense of vision [2]. There is wide variation in brain morphology among different birds. The brain was hour-glass shape and large in the white crested polish chicken and cerebellum, hippocampus, septum, and olfactory bulb were well developed [3]. Smaller birds tend to have round and avian-type brains, whereas larger birds show elongated and reptilian-type brains [4]. Sturnus vulgaris birds showed that the cerebral is an oval shape with the absence of gyrus and sulcus, with right and left cerebral hemisphere separated by medium fissure, whereas another transverse fissure situated between cerebral and cerebellum [5]. The cerebral cortex of the domestic fowls is similar to that of the Pekin Duck and African ostrich [6].

The role of the avian hippocampus in spatial learning, memory, cognitive, and navigation is well established. Five fields were recognized in the hippocampal complex: Medial and lateral hippocampus, parahippocampal area, central field of the parahippocampal area, and crescent field [7]. Several types of local circuit neurons (LC) beside the three types of projection neurons: Pyramidal, pyramidal-like, and multipolar neuron have been described in domestic chicks [8]. In case of strawberry finch, *Estrada amandava* birds several types of neurons present in the hippocampal complex on the basis of differential dendritic tree pattern [7].

Till today little work has been published regarding anatomical and histological study of brain in birds. So the present study was designed to investigate the macroscopic and microscopic morphology (hippocampus) of brain in Vencobb broiler. This work will help to find more information related to brain in Vencobb broiler.

Materials and Methods

Ethical approval

The present retrospective study was duly approved by the Institutional Animal Ethics Committee (IAEC), OUAT, College of Veterinary Science and Animal Husbandry, Bhubaneswar, Odisha-751003.

Sample collection and staining

About 12, day old Vencobb chicks were obtained from Eastern Hatchery, Bhubaneswar, Odisha, India. Birds were reared up to 8 weeks with standard housing, feeding, vaccination, and management system. Adult birds (8 weeks) were slaughtered by cervical dislocation. The head of the birds under study was carefully separated at the level of second cervical vertebrae. Immediately, the separated head of these birds was taken to the laboratory of the Department of Veterinary Anatomy and Histology. The cranial cavity was cut open very carefully with the help of forceps, scissors, and scalpel. The meanings covering of the brain and its attachment with cranial bones was cut followed by serving of anterior/rostral attachment of olfactory lobes and optic nerves at the level of optic chiasma on the ventral surface of the brain; the intact brain was removed from the cranial cavity. After the collection, the brain samples were cleaned (washed) in normal saline solution then the gross anatomical study was done. Small tissue pieces were collected from dorsomedial (DM) part of each cerebral hemisphere through the transverse section; the representative tissue pieces were immediately fixed in 10% buffered neutral formalin for 2-3 days before tissue processing. The tissue pieces were washed under slow running tap water for an overnight period, followed by routine dehydration process in ascending grades of ethyl alcohol (70% → 80% → 90% → absolute

alcohol) for 45 min to one hour in each change. Thereafter, the tissue was cleared in two changes of xylene (4-5 h in each) followed by paraffin impregnation in a thermostatically controlled oven to prepare the paraffin blocks. The trimmed paraffin blocks were cut with the help of a semi-motorized rotary microtome (Leica RM 2245™) to obtain 5-7 µm thick serial paraffin section. The tissue sections were mounted on clean, grease free, albumenized glass slides. After air drying, the slides were kept on a slide drier for better fixation of the section. Finally, the desired slides with tissue section were stained by Harris hematoxylin and eosin as per the standard method [9]. Photography was carried out from the selected fields both under lower (×10) and higher (×40) magnifications under (Leica DM 2500, Germany) microscope.

Results and Discussion

Gross anatomical study of brain

After careful removal of meninges covering, the gross anatomical features of the brain were observed. The general appearance of the brain (dorsally) resembled the outline of a playing card symbol of a "spade." The finding on the shape of brain corroborates well with the observations in barn owl [2], in locally bred chicken [10], and in migratory bird [5]. They mentioned that the general shape of the avian brain was more or less triangular or pear shaped. The brain consisted of three major subdivisions: Cerebrum, cerebellum, and medulla oblongata. The cerebrum was pear shaped or obtuse triangle like in Vencobb birds (Figure-1). Cerebrum was well developed and the largest part of the brain in experimental birds. These observations are in accordance with the reports in both white crested polish chickens and uncrested chicken breeds [3]. Cerebrum comprised two symmetrical cerebral hemispheres (right and left) (Figures-1 and 2). The cerebral hemisphere shape is an important determining factor for the shape of the entire brain. Even

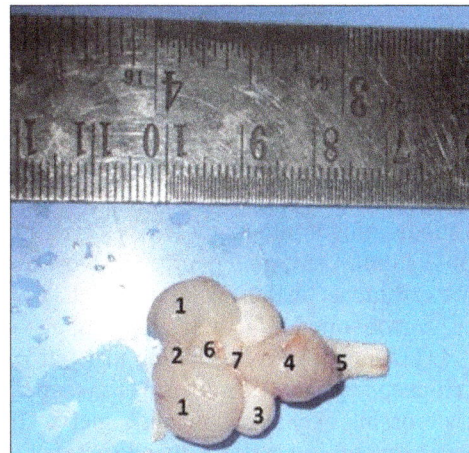

Figure-1: Dorsal view of brain showing different gross anatomical parts (1) Cerebral Hemisphere, (2) Interhemispheric Fissure, (3) Optic Lobe, (4) Cerebellum, (5) Medulla Oblongata, (6) Pineal body, (7) Transverse Fissure.

it may vary with shape and size of the large eye and orbit [4]. The dorsal surface of the cerebral hemispheres was moderately convex and more or less smooth contoured as it was devoid of usual convolutions (elevations), gyri, depressions (grooves), and sulci. The finding corroborates well with finding in Sturnus vulgaris birds [5]. Caudal part of each hemisphere gradually became much wider than its narrow rostral (anterior) tip. The cerebral hemispheres were tightly apposed along a median sulcus called interhemispheric fissure. The cerebrum and cerebellum were separated by a small transverse fissure similar as the previous finding (Figure-1) [5]. The olfactory bulbs were relatively small structures of poorly developed rhinencephalon at the rostral pole of the hemispheres. Because of its intimate connection with olfactory nerve (neurons), the olfactory bulbs in many specimens appeared distorted during collection. On either side of the interhemispheric (longitudinal) fissure was a slight enlargement called sagittal eminence (Wulst), (Figure-1) whose lateral curved margin was demarcated from the rest of the hemispheric surface by an indistinct groove (vallecula). The sagittal eminence became flattened and continued to the caudal (posterior) pole of the hemisphere. However, the presence of indistinct groove (vallecula) and relatively small sagittal eminence was in contrary in ostrich [6] and barn owl [2], who observed very large wulst and distinct vallecula in the brain. The entire optic lobes were not visible on dorsal view. The optic lobes were partially hidden under cerebral hemispheres (Figure-1). However, these optic lobes, i.e. tectum were very large, prominent rounded or spherical bodies of the midbrain on the lateral view. The finding was corroborated well with the previous observations [11]. A small pineal body was clearly visible at the posterior end of the interhemispheric fissure (Figure-1). The cerebellum was large, laterally compressed, wedge-shaped structure posterior to cerebrum that formed the major part of the hindbrain (rhombencephalon). Both the anterior and posterior ends were comparatively narrower than its middle part (Figure-1). The presence of large cerebellum was in contrary to the observation in swifts and falcons birds as they have small cerebellum [12]. The cerebellum extended a backward covering the most part of the medulla oblongata. The surface of the cerebellum presented a number of transverse grooves (sulci) subdividing it into many folds (folia).

On ventral view, the poorly developed olfactory lobes (rhinencephalon) were observed. The finding was corroborated well with the previous observations [11] and contrary to finding in white crested polish chicken [3]. The optic chiasma (X-shaped point of criss-crossing/exchange of optic nerve fibers), which was present just posterior diencephalon (hypothalamus and its connection with pituitary gland/hypophysis) (Figure-2). However, none of the brain specimens showed intact hypophysis and its attachment. A transverse section was made through the posterior 1/3rd part of both the cerebral hemispheres to locate the hippocampus in respect to the respective lateral ventricle. The hippocampal area appeared as DM protrusion/elevation into the narrow, slit-like lateral ventricle on either side (Figure-3). However, the exact boundary line of the hippocampus was not discernable as earlier has been reports [13].

Histology of hippocampus

Our prime focus of the histological study was hippocampus and adjacent associated structure (lateral ventricle), i.e. hippocampal formation. Hippocampus was separated from the rest of the hemisphere by the presence of a narrow slit-like lateral ventricle (Figure-3). The hippocampal area protruded above the lateral ventricle was subdivided into 3 parts: Dorsolateral, DM, and ventricle (V) (Figure-4). The topographical location (in respect to lateral ventricle) of the hippocampus and its three subdivisions are exactly same as earlier reports in barn owl [2] in laying hens [14], in strawberry finch [7], and in different avian species [13].

Histomorphologically, two broad categories of neurons populated the hippocampus: The projection

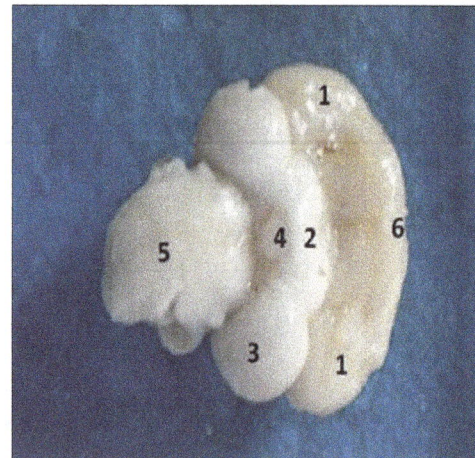

Figure-2: Ventral view of brain showing different gross anatomical parts. (1) Cerebral hemisphere, (2) Optic chiasma, (3) Optic lobe, (4) Hypothalamus, (5) Medulla oblongata, (6) Olfactory bulb.

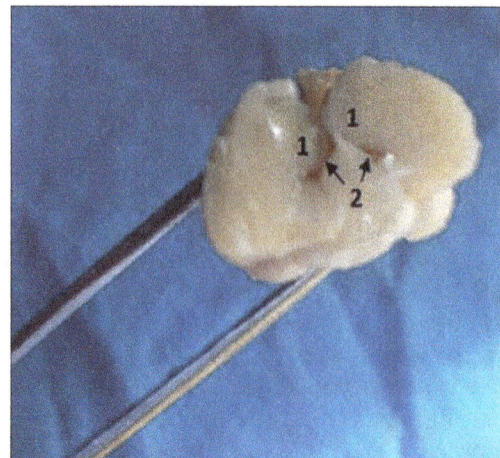

Figure-3: Transverse section of brain. (1) Hippocampus, (2) Lateral Ventricle.

neurons and the LC. Hippocampal neurons in this study did not reveal any distinct cell layer as earlier observed in barn owl [2]. Three visible cell layers in the hippocampus of strawberry finch observed using special Cresyl Violet and Golgi (silver impregnation) staining [7]. They were even able to observe other cell population such as mono and bitufted neurons and radial glial cells in hippocampus. The projection neurons were the predominant cell group included different subtypes: Pyramidal neurons (P), pyramidal-like neurons (PL), and multipolar neurons (M) (Figure-5). Similar neuronal cell types were identified in different birds [2,7,8]. The pyramidal neurons were characterized by their unique pyramidal or triangular shaped medium to the large cell body (soma) with single, thick apical dendrite facing toward piamater (surface). The appearance shape and size of "pyramidal-like cells" were very similar to the pyramidal neurons with poorly developed apical dendrites and the axon facing the lateral ventricle. The multipolar neurons showed 4-5 thick dendrite branches toward different directions after their origin from medium to large sites soma (cell body). Their axons were usually oriented toward the ventricular surface (Figure-5). The LC had small to medium size ovoid perikarya (cell body) and were interspersed with other types of neurons of the hippocampus. The cells were almost like multipolar or even bipolar neurons in appearance (Figure-5). Some of these cells were close/adjacent to pyramidal and multipolar neurons. The axons of the projection neurons joined to form the fiber bundle running parallel to the lateral ventricle. Similar hippocampal projections were studied earlier by several workers in different species of birds [7,8]. These are efferent (outgoing) neuronal projections from the hippocampus to the median septum [7]. Previously, it was reported that hippocampal efferent projections extend also to the hypothalamus and even directly to cerebellum [15]. Other general histological features of the hippocampus in the current study, i.e. high vascularization in the form of capillaries (C) throughout the hippocampus and ependymal lining of lateral ventricle were also reported previously [2] (Figure-6). In our study, the hippocampal neurons appeared comparatively larger (cell body size) under high magnification.

Conclusion

In conclusion, cerebrum was pear shaped and largest part of the brain. Cerebral hemispheres were smooth without convolutions (elevations), gyri, depressions (grooves), and sulci, but in the surface of cerebellum, there was the presence of a number of transverse depressions (grooves) and sulci subdividing into many folds. Olfactory bulb was poorly developed, whereas optic lobes were rounded and large in size. Hippocampus appeared as DM protrusion, but the exact boundary line of the hippocampus was not discernable as previous reports. In histological studies,

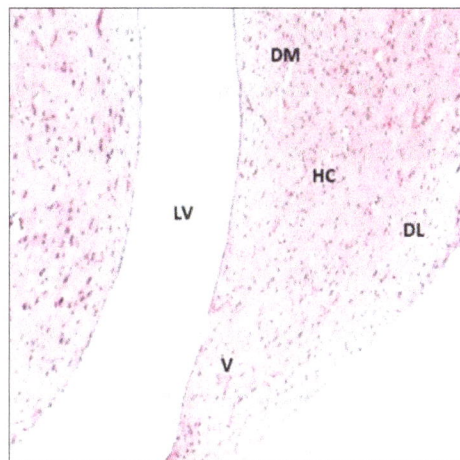

Figure-4: Cross section of hippocampus (HC) & adjacent Lateral Ventricle (LV) (H & E ×100). (DL) Dorso-lateral, (DM) Dorso-medial, (V) Ventral.

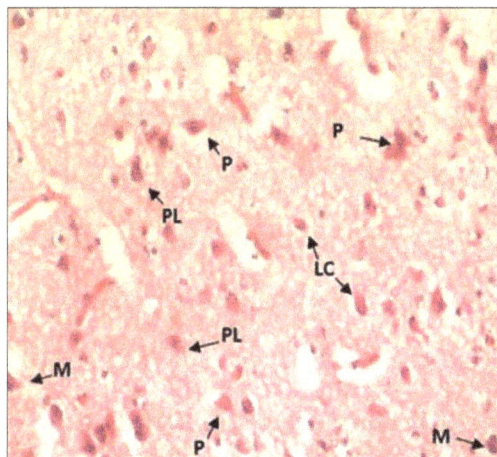

Figure-5: Cross section of hippocampus (H & E ×400) showing different types of neurons. (P) Pyramidal, (M) Multipolar, (PL) Pyramidal like cells, (LC) Local circuit neuron).

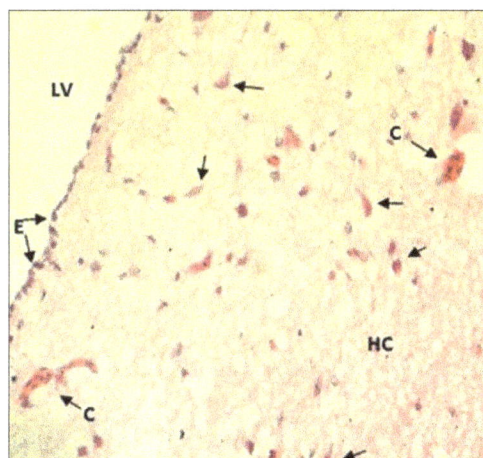

Figure-6: Cross section of hippocampus (HC) (H & E ×400) showing (arrows) Neurons, (C) Capillaries and (E) Ependyma, (LV) Lining of the lateral ventricle.

two categories of neuron LC and projection neurons (P, PL, and M), high vascularization and epididymal lining of lateral ventricle were observed. Hippocampal neurons are comparatively larger in size without any distinct layers. The afferent neurons projected to the medium septum. Further study may be directed to the use of more advanced techniques for tissue section preparation and staining of the brain tissue.

Authors' Contributions

SKG, KB, and CRP designed the plan of work. AKM, SKG, and KB performed laboratory investigation. KS and DB helped in the laboratory investigations. SKG, KB, AKM, and KPS participated in draft and revision of the manuscript. All authors read and approved the final manuscript.

Acknowledgments

The authors are thankful to the staff of Department of Veterinary Anatomy and Histology at College of Veterinary Sciences and Animal Husbandry, Orissa University of Agriculture and Technology, Bhubaneswar, Odisha-751003.

Competing Interests

The authors declare that they have no competing interests.

References

1. Herculano-Houzel, S. (2011) Brains matter, bodies may be not: The case for examining neuron numbers irrespective of body size. *Ann. N.Y. Acad. Sci.*, 1225: 191-199.
2. Abd-Alrahman, S.A. (2012) Morphological and histological study of the cerebrum in a nocturnal bird species (Barn Owl) *Tyto alba. Ibn Al-Haitham J. Pure Appl. Sci.*, 25(3): 73-87.
3. Frahm, H.D. and Rehkamper, G. (1998) Allometric comparison of the brain and brain structures in the white crested polish chicken with uncrested domestic chicken. *Brain Behav. Evol.*, 52: 292-307.
4. Kawabe, S., Shimokawa, T., Miki, H., Matsuda, S. and Endo, H. (2013) Variation in avian brain shape: Relationship with size and orbital shape. *J. Anat.*, 223(5): 495-508.
5. Dhage, S.A., Shehan, N.A., Ali, S.A. and Aziz, F.H. (2013) Anatomical and histological study of cerebral in *Sturnus vulgaris. Bas. J. Vet. Res.*, 12(2): 221-227.
6. Peng, K., Feng, Y., Zhang, G., Liu, H. and Song, H. (2010) Anatomical study of the brain of the African ostrich. *Turk. J. Vet. Anim. Sci.*, 34(3): 235-241.
7. Srivastava, U.C., Chand, P. and Maurya, R.C. (2007) Cytoarchitectonic organization and morphology of the cells of hippocampal complex in Strawberry Finch, *Estrilda amandava. Cell. Mol. Biol.*, 53(5): 103-120.
8. Tombol, T., Davies, D.C., Németh, A., Alpár, A. and Sebestény, T. (2000) A Golgi and a combined Golgi/GABA immunogold study of local circuit neurons in the homing pigeon hippocampus. *Anat. Embryol.*, 201: 181-196.
9. Bancroft, J.D., Stevens, A. and Turner, D.R. (1996) Theory and Practice of Histological Techniques. 4th ed. Churchill Livingstone, New York. p99-112.
10. Batah, A.L., Ghaje, M.S. and Aziz, S.N. (2012) Anatomical and Histological study for the brain of the locally breed chicken. *J. Thi-Qar Sci.*, 3(3): 47-53.
11. Husband, S. and Shimizu, T. (1999) Evolution of the avian visual system. Available from: http://www.luna.cas.usf. edu/~husband/evolve/default.htm.
12. Sultan, F. (2005) Why some bird brains are larger than others. *Curr. Biol.*, 15: 649-650.
13. Krebs, J.R., Clayton, N.S., Healy, S.D., Cristol, D.A., Patel, S.N. and Jolliffe, A.R. (1996) The ecology of the avian brain: Food-storing memory and the hippocampus. *Int. J. Avian Sci.*, 138(1): 34-46.
14. Patzke, N., Ocklenburg, S., vanderStaay, F.J., Gunturkun, O. and Manns, M. (2009) Consequences of different housing conditions on brain morphology in laying hens. *J. Chem. Neuroanat.*, 37: 141-148.
15. Liu, X., Ramirez, S., Pang, P.T., Puryear, C.B., Govindarajan, A., Deisseroth, K. and Tonegawa, S. (2012) Optogenetic stimulation of a hippocampal engram activates fear memory recall. *Nature*, 484: 381-385.

14

Isolation, antibiogram and pathogenicity of *Salmonella* spp. recovered from slaughtered food animals in Nagpur region of Central India

D. G. Kalambhe, N. N. Zade, S. P. Chaudhari, S. V. Shinde, W. Khan and A. R. Patil

Department of Veterinary Public Health, Nagpur Veterinary College, Nagpur, Maharashtra, India.
Corresponding author: D. G. Kalambhe, e-mail: drdeepalikalambhe@gmail.com,
NNZ: n_zade@rediffmail.com, SPC: sandeep_vph@gmail.com, SVS: shilpi_shri5@rediffmail.com,
WK: waqar_khan73@rediffmail.com, ARP: drarchanavph@gmail.com

Abstract

Aim: To determine the prevalence, antibiogram and pathogenicity of *Salmonella* spp. in the common food animals slaughtered for consumption purpose at government approved slaughter houses located in and around Nagpur region during a period of 2010-2012.

Materials and Methods: A total of 400 samples comprising 50 each of blood and meat from each slaughtered male cattle, buffaloes, pigs and goats were collected. Isolation was done by pre-enrichment in buffered peptone water and enrichment in Rappaport-Vassiliadis broth with subsequent selective plating onto xylose lysine deoxycholate agar. Presumptive *Salmonella* colonies were biochemically confirmed and analyzed for pathogenicity by hemolysin production and Congo red dye binding assay (CRDA). An antibiotic sensitivity test was performed to assess the antibiotic resistance pattern of the isolates.

Results: A total of 10 isolates of *Salmonella* spp. from meat (3 from cattle, 1 from buffaloes and 6 from pigs) with an overall prevalence of 5% among food animals was recorded. No isolation was reported from any blood samples. Pathogenicity assays revealed 100% and 80% positivity for CRDA and hemolytic activity, respectively. Antimicrobial sensitivity test showed multi-drug resistance. The overall resistance of 50% was noted for trimethoprim followed by ampicillin (20%). A maximum sensitivity (80%) was reported to gentamycin followed by 40% each to ampicillin and trimethoprim, 30% to amikacin and 10% to kanamycin.

Conclusion: The presence of multidrug resistant and potentially pathogenic *Salmonella* spp. in slaughtered food animals in Nagpur region can be a matter of concern for public health.

Keywords: antibiogram, Congo red binding assay, food animals, hemolysis, *Salmonella* Typhimurium.

Introduction

Salmonella is a genus within the Enterobacteriaceae family distributed worldwide, can cause serious disease in both humans and animals. Their pathogenic potential and abilities to harbor and spread resistance pose tremendous medical, public health and economic problems affecting animals and humans [1]. Outbreaks in animals are a zoonotic threat, but due to limited surveillance performed in animals it is difficult to identify human outbreaks that corresponds closely to an outbreak in a single animal species [2].

Pathogenicity of *Salmonella* has been widely studied with the *in-vivo* method of production of enterotoxin in rabbit using rabbit illial loop test. However, this test has certain limitations, *viz.*, use of live animals and animal ethical issues. Assay such as Congo red (CR) binding test could prove a good alternative to *in-vivo* tests.

Although there is a plethora of information regarding pathogenesis and molecular biology of *Salmonella* spp., there is a paucity of information concerning the prevalence and incidence that serotypes associated with foodborne disease. About 80% of typhoid fever cases accounts from Bangladesh, China, India, Indonesia, Laos, Nepal, Pakistan, or Vietnam infecting roughly 21.6 million people and kills about 200,000 people every year [3].

Due to the high significance of *Salmonella* pathogen from public health point of view, the present work was aimed to determine the prevalence, antibiogram and pathogenicity of *Salmonella* in common food animals slaughtered in and around Nagpur region.

Materials and Methods

Ethical approval

Sampling and experiments have been carried out as per the guidelines laid down by the Institutional Ethical Committee and in accordance with local laws and regulations.

Collection, transportation and isolation of samples

A total of 400 samples comprising 50 each of blood and meat samples from 50 each slaughtered male cattle, buffaloes, pigs and goats were collected from the government approved slaughter houses in and around Nagpur region. The purpose of selecting these food animals was that they were commonly preferred for consumption in the region. Moreover, the study relating to the prevalence of *Salmonella* among these food animals intended for consumption purposes was highly lacking in the region. The meat (approximately 50 g) and blood samples (15 ml) were collected aseptically in sterile polyethylene sachet and in sterilized test tubes, respectively, and were transported to the laboratory by maintaining cold chain inside an insulated box containing ice packs. Samples were immediately processed for isolation on arrival to the laboratory.

Meat samples each weighing 10 g were added with diluent (sterilized nine-salt solution [NSS]) and homogenized aseptically in stomacher blender (LabMed, UK), from this homogenized solution 1 ml was transferred to 9 ml buffered peptone water (BPW) similarly, the blood clots were inoculated into 9 ml BPW broth and incubated at 37°C for 24 h. After incubation, the inoculums from the respective pre-enriched broth were transferred to the second step enrichment media, i.e., Rappaport-Vassiliadis enrichment (RV) broth and further incubated at 44°C for 24 h. The enriched inoculums from RV broth were streaked onto xylose lysine deoxycholate (XLD) agar and incubated at 37°C for 24 h. Translucent colonies with typical black center were considered to be *Salmonella* (Plate-1). Each time along with the test samples standard *Salmonella* Typhimurium (MTCC-98) was processed as a reference positive culture and sterile NSS was used as a negative control.

The presumptive *Salmonella* colonies were subjected to Gram-staining which revealed the organisms as Gram-negative cocobacillary rods. Further, the Gram-negative organisms were subjected to biochemical characterization, sugar fermentation, *in-vitro* pathogenicity tests and antibiotic susceptibility.

Isolates were biochemically characterized by urease, triple sugar iron (Plate-2), methyl red, Voges–Proskauer, indole, citrate, nitrate, malonate utilization tests and carbohydrates fermentation reaction using lactose, sucrose, salicin, adonitol, glucose, dulcitol, inositol, sorbitol sugars (Table-1).

Antibiotic sensitivity test

Antibiotic sensitivity of *Salmonella* isolates to various antibiotics and therapeutic agents *viz.*, ampicillin (A) (10 mcg/unit), gentamicin (G) (5 mcg/unit), kanamycin (K) (30 mcg/unit), amikacin (Ak) (30 mcg/unit), and trimethoprim (Tr) (5 mcg/unit) was studied by agar disc diffusion method. Briefly, the overnight incubated cultures were spread evenly onto the brain heart infusion (BHI) agar plates by sterile swabs. The antibiotic disc was then placed with the help of sterile forceps onto the agar plates and incubated at 37°C for 24 h. The characterization of strains as sensitive, moderately sensitive and resistant was based on the size of zones of the inhibition

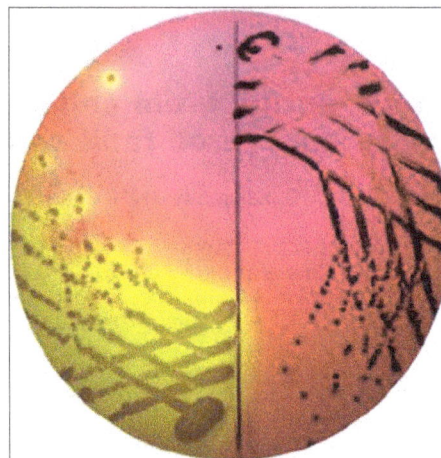

Plate-1: Characteristics colonies of *Salmonella* isolates on xylose lysine deoxycholate agar.

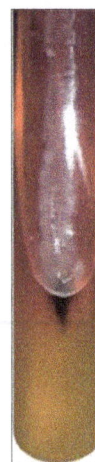

Plate-2: Typical pattern of *Salmonella* on triple sugar iron agar.

Table-1: Biochemical characteristics of isolates.

Characteristics	Reaction
Gram's-staining	Gram-negative, coccobacillary rods
Acid and gas from carbohydrates	
Lactose	−ve
Sucrose	−ve
Salicin	−ve
Adonitol	−ve
Glucose	+ve
Dulcitol	+ve
Inositol	±ve
Sorbitol	+ve
Methyl red	+ve
Voges–Proskauer test	−ve
Indole	−ve
Citrate	+ve
Nitrate	+ve
Urease	−ve
Malonate utilization	−ve
TSI	+ve (pink slope, yellow butt and H_2S production indicated by blackening)

around each disc according to manufactures instruction (Hi-media, Mumbai).

In-vitro pathogenicity tests

Further pathogenicity was determined by applying *in-vitro* pathogenicity tests *viz.*; hemolysin production and CR binding assay.

Hemolysis on sheep blood agar (SBA)

Detection of hemolysin production was conducted on 5% SBA. Defibrinated sheep blood was used for the preparation of 5% SBA plates. Freshly grown broth cultures were streaked onto the blood agar plates and incubated at 37°C for 24 h. Zone of hemolysis around the colonies was identified as α-hemolysis and accordingly the isolate was designated as pathogenic (Table-2 and Plate-3).

CR binding assay

The ability of the isolates to bind CR dye was evaluated by streaking freshly grown culture onto the CR BHI agar plates (0.003%) and incubating at 37°C for 24-48 h. The positive results were indicated by the formation of typical brick red colonies. The evaluation of the pathogenicity as +++, ++ and + was done based on intensity of brick red color development in colonies (Table-2 and Plate-4).

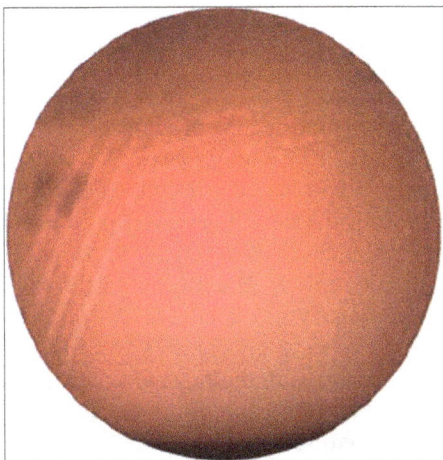

Plate-3: Hemolysin production of *Salmonella* isolate on sheep blood agar.

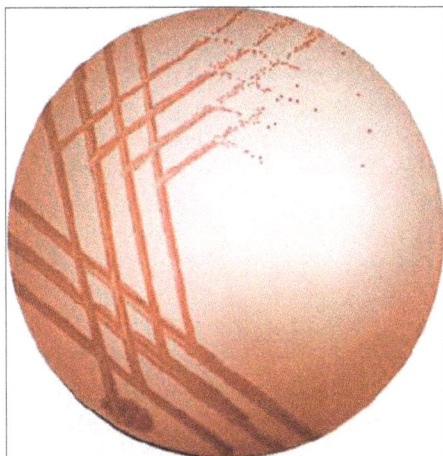

Plate-4: Typical (brick red) colonies Congo red agar.

Results

Isolation, biochemical characteristics, and pathogenicity of the isolates

In the present investigation, a total of 400 samples (comprising 50 each of meat and blood) from respective slaughtered cattle male animals, buffalo, goat and pig (50 each) were screened for studying the prevalence, pathogenicity and antibiogram of *Salmonella* spp.

Of 400 samples, 10 meat (three beef, one buffalo beef, zero chevon and six pork) samples were assumed as *Salmonella* based on their colony characteristics and biochemical profile (Table-1 and Plates-1 and 2). However, none of the chevon and blood sample from any food animals was found to be positive for *Salmonella* spp. Cent percent beef and buffalo beef isolates turned positive for hemolysin production and CR binding assay, whereas 66.66% and 100% pork samples revealed positivity for hemolysin and CR binding assay (Tables-2 and 3 and Plates-2 and 3).

Antibiotic sensitivity patterns

Out of total 10 isolates screened for antimicrobial sensitivity test against five antibiotics, five isolates were found to be resistant for trimethoprim, whereas resistance against ampicillin was observed among two isolates registering resistance of 50% and 20%, respectively. The moderate sensitivity of 90% was reported for kanamycin followed by amikacin (70%), ampicillin (40%), gentamycin (20%), and trimethoprim (10%). A maximum sensitivity (80%) was reported to gentamycin followed by 40% each to ampicillin and trimethoprim, 30% to amikacin and 10% to kanamycin (Table-4).

Discussion

The results of the present investigation, i.e., 6% *Salmonella* prevalence in beef and 2% in carabeef were comparable to the findings of 7.7% from minced beef from supermarkets in Addis Ababa, 9% prevalence from raw beef samples reported from Ethiopia [4] and 4.2% prevalence in slaughtered cattle reported

Table-2: Pathogenicity of the isolates.

Species	Cattle	Buffalo	Goat	Pig
Total positive samples				
Meat	03	01	00	06
Pathogenicity (%)				
Hemolysis	100	100	00	66.66
Cong red binding	100	100	00	100

Table-3: Isolation of *Salmonella* from meat and blood.

Species	Cattle	Buffalo	Goat	Pig
Total samples				
Meat	50	50	50	50
Blood	50	50	50	50
Total positive samples				
Meat	03	01	00	06
Blood	00	00	00	00

Table-4: Antibiotic sensitivity patterns.

Antibiotics	Cattle (3 isolates)			Buffalo (1 isolates)			Pig (6 isolates)			Total isolates (10)		
	R	MS	S	R	MS	S	R	MS	S	R (%)	MS (%)	S (%)
A	00	02	01	00	01	00	02	01	03	02 (20)	04 (40)	04 (40)
G	00	01	02	00	00	00	00	01	06	00	02 (20)	08 (80)
K	00	03	00	00	01	00	00	05	01	00	09 (90)	01 (10)
Ak	00	03	00	00	00	01	00	04	02	00	07 (70)	03 (30)
Tr	02	00	01	00	01	00	03	00	03	05 (50)	01 (10)	04 (40)

R=Resistant, MS=Moderately sensitive, S=Sensitive, A=Ampicillin, G=Gentamicin, K=Kanamycin, Ak=Amikacin, Tr=Trimethoprim

in Ethiopia [5]. In a study conducted at Washington *Salmonella*, contamination rate in beef cattle carcasses was in the range of 0.2-21.5% [6]. However, an overall 6% *Salmonella* prevalence among beef samples in the current work was higher than those reported as 4% (02/50) in fecal samples from diarrheic young animal, from Telangana, Chennai, Maharashtra, Goa, Uttar Pradesh, and Rajasthan. The workers attributed the reason for lower prevalence in young animals and absences of *Salmonella* in bovine and equine samples to the limited number of samples included in the study [7]. Obtained higher prevalence in the present study could be due to the actual prevalence of *Salmonella* in cattle itself or it may be due to the unhygienic conditions in the slaughter house while dressing and handling the carcasses leading to the cross-contamination of the meat samples.

The prevalence of 2% in buffaloes beef is on the lower side when compared with the findings of the prevalence of *Salmonella* as 13.5% (5/37) in various meat samples including buffalo beef from the local meat market of Kathmandu [8]. The study from Anand, (Gujarat) India recorded (10.66%) prevalence of *Salmonella* spp. in raw buffalo meat and offals *viz.* liver, lung, muscle, intestine, and ground beef [9]. However, other worker isolated 8% (4/50) *Salmonella* organisms from buffalo meat samples from Laos (Japan) [10]. The results of the current work, however are comparable with the findings of (4.0%) prevalence in beef samples in Bareilly city, Izatnagar, India using cultural and polymerase chain reaction method [11].

Due to paucity of work done particularly in buffaloes and carabeef in the region, it is bit difficult to compare our results with the other works on the prevalence of *Salmonella* in buffaloes from the same region. However, when compared with work on raw meat conducted by Maharjan *et al.* and Kshirsagar *et al.* [8,9] who recorded 13.5% and 8% prevalence, respectively, the lower prevalence rates in the present investigation might be attributed to the actual less occurrence of the pathogen in the host [12]. The reason for the prevalence obtained in the present work could be attributed to the fact that transportation of the samples for 24 h might have despaired cold chain resulting into overgrowth of contaminants with suppression of *Salmonella*.

Although none of the samples (chevon or blood) were positive for *Salmonella*, in this study. This result

is, however, in accordance with the study conducted to assess the microbiological quality and prevalence of *Salmonella* spp. in goat carcasses slaughtered at retail shops of Parbhani city, Maharashtra where zero prevalence of *Salmonella* in goat samples was recorded [13]. A study from Anand, Gujarat recorded the incidence of *Salmonella* in chevon as (3.57%) [14]. Results of present finding also goes in parallel with the finding from Mumbai wherein workers reported the absence of *Salmonella* in mutton samples [15]. Another study from Jammu revealed 3.12% prevalence of *Salmonella* spp. in chevon using standard plate count [16]. Among the findings of the other workers 3% *Salmonella* prevalence was reported in goats slaughtered at Ethiopia [17], 3.3% (1/31) prevalence was reported in chevon samples of local meat market in Kathmandu, Nepal [8]. Further, a study at Washington has reported the prevalence of *Salmonella* in the range of 1-18.8% in goats [6].

The observations of present study differ from the works done in the other parts of India wherein, 17.6% prevalence of *Salmonella* was recorded in goats slaughtered at Bareilly (North India) and 38.33% *Salmonella* in chevon at Wardha district of Maharashtra, respectively [18,19].

The differences in the reported prevalence could be associated with the sampling procedures, type of sample, transportation of samples, isolation techniques or the actual difference in the occurrence and distribution of *Salmonella* in the study population itself.

The report of 12% prevalence of *Salmonella* in pork in present study is higher compared to the 8.6% prevalence of *Salmonella* in pigs in the Tarai region of Uttarakhand, India [20] and the 8% (6/75) obtained prevalence of *Salmonella* in the pork samples collected from the markets of Nigeria [21]. However, the results are comparable with 16.4% (9/55) positivity for *Salmonella* in 55 pork samples in Ethiopia [22].

The variation could be attributed to the differences in the geographic location and the sanitary conditions of the slaughterhouses from where the samples are collected.

This can also be explained on the fact that these studies are based on the fecal carriage and rectum/intestinal contents harboring pathogen. There was a general observation that accidental rupture of rectum or intestine, entry of pathogen may lead to contamination of carcass [23] and accidental rupture of intestine during slaughtering is major cause for carcass contamination, as an experiment on use of rectal bag at abattoir were found to reduce the bacterial load of *Yersinia enterocolitica* to 2% [24]. The present investigation confirms reservoir status of the pigs as compared to other food animals in this geographical area. Further, the observation also alarms public health significance of pork with respect to *Salmonella* in this region.

An overall prevalence of *Salmonella* in 6% food animals in current study is comparable with the findings of 5% (15/300) *Salmonella* positive samples (pork, chicken, chevon, beef, carabeef and mutton) from the municipal slaughter houses and the retail meat shops from Hyderabad Karnataka region of Karnataka state, India [25]. Thus, the findings of present work highlight the contamination of the meat with *Salmonella,* alarming the public health risk thus necessitate the strict measures for the proper maintenance of slaughterhouses in the region.

In this study, an attempt was made to determine the pathogenicity of obtained *Salmonella isolates* by CR binding assay and hemolysin assays which yielded results in acceptance with [26-28]. Findings on the hemolytic strains of *Salmonella* observed is in agreement with a study of hemolysin pattern of *Salmonella gallinarum* in poultry reporting multiplicity in the hemolysin production among the pathogenic strain [26]. The observation of 80% hemolytic isolates in the present study is in complete agreement with the findings of a study which employed CR binding test and hemolysin production test to determine virulence of *Salmonella* Typhimurium isolates from calves and human samples and observed 81.81% hemolytic strains from calves, however, it is in partial agreement with cent percent CR binding isolates in present study against the 75% reported in the above-mentioned study [26].

The observation of antibiogram in this study could be compared with previous study conducted in this region on foods of animal origin where workers reported 80% sensitivity to gentamycin [29]. The sensitivity in the findings can be attributed to the similar geographical area of study wherein perpetuation of the strain of pathogen of same clonal origin cannot be denied [29]. The results of the present study differs from the reports obtained from Bareilly India, wherein, workers observed most strains were resistant to streptomycin (84.8%) followed by kanamycin (58.7%), gentamicin (52.2%), ampicillin (50%), and oxytetracycline (50%). Few strains were resistant to cefotaxime (2.2%), amoxicillin (2.2%) and newer fluoroquinolones (6.5%) [30]. However, variation among the sensitivity for amikacin, ampicillin and trimethoprim the tune of 80% and 13.3% in the present study can be contributed by possible variation in serotype isolated in both the studies as the workers used MacConkey and *Salmonella*-Shigella agar for isolation while XLD was used in this study.

Conclusion

An overall 5% prevalence of *Salmonella* among the food animals reported in present study was low, but the fact of the presence of multidrug resistant and potentially pathogenic *Salmonella* in food animals of Nagpur region cannot be ruled out which can be a matter of concern from public health point of view. Further, there is a need of conducting such study in the region on a regular basis to asses and compare the past and present status of this zoonotic pathogen in the foods of animal origin in the region in order secure animal and public health.

Authors' Contributions

DGK as a MVSc student conducted the work. NNZ and SPC guided and supervised the research work. WK edited and selected photographs needed for the work. SVS and ARP participated in analysis of samples. All authors read and approved the final manuscript.

Acknowledgments

The authors are thankful to all the staffs of Department of Veterinary Public Health, Nagpur for their help in the study and also to Maharashtra Animal and Fishery Sciences University, Nagpur, Maharashtra, India and ICAR for financial support for carrying the present work.

Competing Interests

The authors declare that they have no competing interests.

References

1. Pegues, D.A., Oh, M.E. and Miller, S.I. (2005) *Salmonella* species, including *Salmonella* Typhi. In: Mandel, G.L., Bennett, J.E., Dolin, R., editors. Mandell, Douglas and Bennett's Principles and Practice of Infectious Diseases. 6th ed. Elsevier Churchill Livingstone, New York. p2636-2654.
2. Baker, M.G., Thorns, C., Lopez, L.D., Garrett, N.K. and Nikol, C.M. (2007) A recurring Salmonellosis epidemic in New Zealand linked to contact with sheep. *Epidemiol. Infect.*, 135: 76-83.
3. World Health Organization. (2006) 6th International Conference on Typhoid Fever and other Salmonellosis, Geneva.
4. Nyeleti, C., Molla, B., Hilderbandt, G. and Kleer, J. (2000) The prevalence and distribution of *Salmonella* in slaughter cattle, slaughterhouse personnel and minced beef in Addis Ababa, Ethiopia. *Bull. Anim. Health Prod. Afr.*, 48: 19-24.
5. Molla, B., Alemayehmu, D. and Salah, W. (1997-2002) Sources and distribution of *Salmonella* serotypes isolated from food animals, slaughterhouse personnel and retail meat products in Ethiopia, 2003. *Ethiop. J. Health Dev.*, 17: 63-70.
6. D'Aoust, J.Y. (1989) *Salmonella*. In: Doyle, M.P., editor. Foodborne Bacterial Pathogens. Marcel Dekker Inc., New York.
7. Nair, A., Balasaravanan, T., Malik, S.V.S., Mohan, V., Kumar, M., Vergis, J. and Deepak, B.R. (2015) Isolation

and identification of *Salmonella* from diarrheagenic infants and young animals, sewage waste and fresh vegetables. *Vet. World*, 8(5): 669-673.

8. Maharjan, M., Joshi, V., Joshi, D.D. and Manandhar, P. (2006) Trends in the study of disease agents. *Ann N Y Acad. Sci.*, 1081: 249-256.

9. Kshirsagar, D.P., Singh, S., Brahmbhatt, M.N. and Nayak, J.B. (2014) Isolation and molecular characterization of virulence-associated genes of *Salmonella* from buffalo meat samples in Western region of India. *Israel J. Vet. Med.*, 69(4): 228-233.

10. Boonmar, S., Markvichitr, K., Chaunchom, S., Chanda, C. and Bangtrakulnonth, A. (2008) *Salmonella* prevalence in slaughtered buffaloes and pigs and antimicrobial susceptibility of isolates in Vientiane, Lao People's Democratic Republic. *J. Vet. Med. Sci.*, 70: 1345-1348.

11. Khan, J.A., Rathore, R.S., Khan, S. and Ahmad, I. (2013). Prevalence, characterization and detection of *Salmonella* spp. from various meat sources. *Adv. Anim. Vet. Sci.*, 1(1S): 4-8.

12. Arslan, S. and Ayla, E. (2010) Occurrence and antimicrobial resistance profile of *Salmonella* species in retail meat products. *J. Food Prot.*, 73(9): 10-63.

13. Rathod, K.S., Ambadkar, R.K., Zanjad, P.N., Deshmukh, V.V. and Raziuddin, M. (2004) Microbiological quality of chevon sold in Parbhani City. *J. V.P.H.*, 2: 19-22.

14. Makwana, P.P., Nayak, J.B., Brahmbhatt, M.N. and Chaudhary, J.H. (2015) Detection of *Salmonella* spp. from chevon, mutton and its environment in retail meat shops in Anand city (Gujarat), India. *Vet. World*, 8(3): 388-392.

15. Shashidhar, R., Srivastava, I. and Bandekar, J.R. (2011) Quantification of *Salmonella* in food samples from India using the MINI-MSRV MPN and modified MINI-MSRV MPN methods. *J. Food Sci.*, 76(8): M564-M567.

16. Arvind, K., Khajuria, P. and Kaur, M. (2011) Tracking of pathogenic and spoilage microbes in mutton and chevon processing in retail markets of Jammu. *Indian J. Small Rumin.*, 17(1): 74-77.

17. Wassie, M.A. (2004) A cross-sectional study on *Salmonella* in apparently healthy slaughtered sheep and goats at Addis Ababa and Modjo abattoirs, Ethiopia. Master thesis, Addis Ababa University, Faculty of Veterinary Medicine, Debre Zeit, Ethiopia.

18. Chandra, M., Singh, B.R., Shankar, H., Agarwal, M., Agarwal, R.K., Sharma, G. and Babu, N. (2007) Prevalence of *Salmonella* antibodies among goats slaughtered for chevon in Bareilly (northern India). *Prev. Vet. Med.*, 80: 1-8.

19. Moon, A.H. (2011) Studies on: Prevalence and antibiogram of *Salmonella* species of polluted meat origin. *Asiatic J. Biotechnol. Resour.*, 2(04): 447-453.

20. Kumar, T., Rajora, V.S. and Arora, N. (2013) Prevalence of *Salmonella* in pigs and broilers in the Tarai region of Uttarakhand, India. *Indian J. Med. Microbiol.*, 32(1): 99-101.

21. Yemisi, A., Alli Oyebode, T., Margaret, A. and Justina, J. (2011) Prevalence of *Arcobacter*, *Escherichia coli*, *Staphylococcus aureus* and *Salmonella* species in retail raw chicken, pork, beef and goat meat in Osogbo, Nigeria. *Sierra Leone J. Biomed. Res.*, 3(1): 8-12.

22. Ejeta, G., Molla, B., Alemayehu, D. and Muckle, A. (2004) *Salmonella* serotypes isolated from minced meat beef, mutton and pork in Addis Ababa, Ethiopia. *Rev. Med. Vet.*, 155(11): 547-551.

23. Letellier, A., Messier, S. and Quessy, S. (1999) Prevalence of *Salmonella* spp. and *Yersinia enterocolitica* in finishing Swine at Canadian abattoirs. *J. Food Prot.*, 62(1): 22-25.

24. Andreshel, J.K., Sorensen, R. and Glensbjerg, M. (1991) Aspects of the epidemiology of *Yersinia enterocolitica*: A review. *Int. J. Food Microbiol.*, 13(3): 231-237.

25. Kumara, P., Rao, J., Haribabuc, Y. and Manjunath, D. (2014) Microbiological quality of meat collected from municipal slaughter houses and retail meat shops from Hyderabad Karnataka region, India. *APCBEE Proc.*, 8: 364-369.

26. El-Taib, K.A. (2011) Studies on virulence characters of *Salmonella* Typhimurium isolated from animal and human. *Rep. Opin.*, 3(7): 37-43.

27. Agrawal, M., Chandra, M., Sharma, G. and Singh, B.R. (2005) A study on virulence markers of Indian strain of *Salmonella* Enterica subspecies enterica serovar Paratyphi B from foods of animal origin. *J. Food Sci. Technol.*, 42: 66-79.

28. Tiwari, R.P., Deol, K., Rishi, P. and Grewal, J.S. (2002) Factors affecting haemolysin production and Congo red binding in *Salmonella* Enterica serovar Typhimurium DT 98. *J. Med. Microbiol.*, 51: 50.

29. Zade, N.N. and Karpe, A.G. (2010) Final scheme report on characterization of plasmid DNA of the bacteria from foods of animal origin. A Report Submitted to Indian Council of Agriculture Research, New Delhi. p11.

30. Singh, B.R., Agarwal, M., Chandra, M., Verma, M., Sharma, G., Verma, J.C. and Singh, V.P. (2010) Plasmid profile and drug resistance pattern of zoonotic *Salmonella* isolates from Indian buffaloes. *J. Infect. Dev. Ctries.*, 4(8): 477-483.

15

Effect of washing on the post-thaw quality of cryopreserved ram epididymal spermatozoa

Touqeer Ahmed, Rafiqul Islam, Farooz Ahmad Lone and Asloob Ahmad Malik

Division of Animal Reproduction, Gynaecology and Obstetrics, Faculty of Veterinary Sciences and Animal Husbandry, Sher-e-Kashmir University of Agricultural Sciences & Technology of Kashmir, Shuhama, Alusteng, Srinagar, Jammu & Kashmir, India.
Corresponding author: Touqeer Ahmed, e-mail: touqeer_taz@yahoo.co.in,
RI: rafiqvet@gmail.com, FAL: dr.farooz462@gmail.com, AAM: malikasloob@gmail.com

Abstract

Aim: The aim of the study was to evaluate the effect of washing on the post-thaw quality of ram cauda epididymal spermatozoa (P1: Unwashed, P2: Washed).

Materials and Methods: Fresh testicles of adult healthy slaughtered rams were collected and transported to the laboratory in an ice chest, where they were weighed, and cauda epididymides were separated. These cauda epididymides were used for recovery of spermatozoa in tris-citric acid fructose buffer by incision method. Spermatozoa samples showing ≥70% progressive motility were pooled and processed further. The mean values (±standard error) of various parameters such as the percentage of sperm motility, live sperm, intact acrosome, and hypo-osmotic swelling test (HOST) reacted spermatozoa were recorded.

Results: In this experiment, the percent sperm motility, live spermatozoa, and intact acrosome both at pre-freeze and post-thaw were higher (p>0.05) in P1 than P2. However, the post-thaw percent HOST reacted spermatozoa was slightly higher (p>0.05) for P2 than P1.

Conclusion: Washing of cauda epididymal spermatozoa has no significant adverse effect on the quality during cryopreservation. Therefore, this processing method can be applied wherever necessary before the extension of the recovered spermatozoa sample in different ram extenders.

Keywords: cauda epididymis, centrifugation, processing, ram, spermatozoa, washing.

Introduction

The use of cryopreserved sperm in assisted reproductive techniques has become an indispensable tool for breeding management in domestic animals [1]. So, being an important technique semen cryopreservation is used for the application of assisted reproduction such as artificial insemination and *in vitro* fertilization, which contribute to increased production and genetic selection [2]. However, during cryopreservation massive ultrastructural, biochemical, and functional damages occur on the spermatozoa due to the stress and temperature changes, which result in decreased motility and viability of the spermatozoa leading to decreased fertility, which are the main drawbacks of this technique [3,4].

Several researchers have studied the effect of different washing solutions and centrifugations regimes in different species to find out a proper method for improving the quality of cryopreserved semen. In buck semen cryopreservation, the centrifugation regimes and washing solutions used were 600 ×*g* for 10 min with Krebs–Ringer phosphate plus sodium citrate [5], 1200 ×*g* for 15 min with tris-citric acid glucose (TCG) buffer [6], 1500 ×*g* for 10 min with TCG [7], and 1000 ×*g* for 10 min with Ringer's lactate [8]. Earlier studies on the influence of different centrifugation regimes (400, 800, 1600, and 2400 ×*g*) on boar spermatozoa have reported that the use of short-term centrifugation with a relative high g-force (2400 ×*g* for 3 min) caused a positive effect on its cryo-survival [9]. Webb and Dean [10] described that post-thaw motility of frozen stallion sperm was not different between centrifugation treatments (700 ×*g* for 15 min, 600 ×*g* for 12 min, and 400 ×*g* for 7 min). Sarıozkan *et al.* [8] described that a high fertility rate, with or without centrifugation/washing, buck semen could be achieved with the Bioxcell extender.

Therefore, the results presented in the literature about washing of spermatozoa are quite variable [11] and studies evaluating the effects of washing or centrifugation on the cryopreservation of cauda epididymal spermatozoa are still very limited. Hence, to overcome this variability, the researchers should work to reach a consensus that generally addresses accepted practices for the effects of centrifugation in cauda epididymal sperm cryopreservation. Therefore, this study was carried out to study the effect of washing on the quality of cauda epididymal spermatozoa before freezing and after thawing.

Materials and Methods

Ethical approval

No ethical approval was necessary to pursue this work, because no live animal was involved while carrying out the whole study. Samples were collected from government approved slaughter house.

Extender used

Tris-citric acid fructose (TCF) egg yolk extender was used for the extension of the spermatozoa and the effect of washing of spermatozoa on post-thaw quality was evaluated.

Collection of testicles

About 18 intact testicles of freshly slaughtered adult healthy rams were collected from government approved abattoir in Rainawari Srinagar city. They were then transported to the semen processing laboratory at Sperm station, Frozen semen project, Ranbirbagh, Ganderbal, in an ice chest, where further processing of these testicles and recovery of spermatozoa was done.

Processing of testicles

In the laboratory, the testicles were cleaned by removing the additional tissues. Then, biometric measurements of the testicles were done, including testicular, whole epididymal and cauda epididymal weight, on an electronic balance. All the values obtained from the above procedure were recorded simultaneously.

Collection of spermatozoa

The spermatozoa were recovered from the cauda epididymis in tris buffer (Table-1) using incision method [12,13].

Initial evaluation of spermatozoa

After recovery of the spermatozoa from the cauda epididymis in petri-dish, the concentration and progressive motility of each sample were determined. The concentration was determined using a photometer (IMV-France). Then, the progressive motility was determined [14], and samples showing motility ≥70% were pooled and subsequently divided into two aliquots.

Washing of spermatozoa

Two aliquots were made from the pooled cauda epididymal spermatozoa. Spermatozoa of one aliquot (P2) were washed (centrifuged) twice using tris buffer, and the other aliquot (P1) was extended without washing (control). The centrifugation of P2 was carried out at 855 g for 10 min in centrifuge machine (REMI Laboratory R4C, Maharashtra, India). After centrifugation, the supernatant was discarded, and the remaining spermatozoa were diluted with TCF extender.

Extension of the sample

Each aliquot was extended in TCF egg yolk extender (Table-2) [15].

Quality parameters of extended spermatozoa

The quality of the extended cauda epididymal sperm samples was evaluated for percent progressive

Table-1: Composition of TCF buffer.

Ingredients	Quantity
Tris (hydroxyl methylamino methane)	3.028 g
Citric acid monohydrate	1.70 g
Fructose	1.25 g
Distilled Water ad	100 ml

TCF=Tris-citric acid fructose

Table-2: Composition of TCF extender.

Ingredients	Quantity
TCF buffer	72 ml
Glycerol	8 ml
Egg yolk	20 ml
Penicillin G sodium	80000 i.u
Streptomycin sulfate	100 mg

TCF=Tris-citric acid fructose

motility. Then, live sperm percentage was determined using Eosin–Nigrosin differential staining technique as per standard procedures [16], the percentage of intact acrosome was estimated using standard Giemsa staining technique [17] and hypo-osmotic swelling test (HOST) was carried out as per Vasquez et al. [18].

Preservation of the sample

Six cauda epididymal sperm samples from both groups that showed ≥70% motility were extended. The extended semen was filled and sealed in French mini straws (0.25 ml) and subsequently printed, in automatic filling sealing and printing machine (IMV-France). The straws were then equilibrated at 4°C for 4 h. The equilibrated straws were subjected to rapid vapor freezing in Biological Programmable Freezer, and finally, the frozen straws were placed into liquid nitrogen and stored in cryocans until further post-thaw analysis.

Post-thaw analysis

The frozen semen straws were thawed in warm water at 37°C for 15 s, and the post-thaw quality of each sample was determined by the parameters and procedures already discussed.

Statistical analysis

The data obtained in the study were analyzed statistically using t-test. The data pertaining to sperm quality between pre-freeze and post-thaw were compared by paired samples t-test with the help of statistical software SPSS version 16. The level of significance was set at $p < 0.05$. The data are presented in the tables as mean±standrad error of mean.

Results

The mean weight (g) of the testicles utilized for recovery of spermatozoa in this study was 128.67±4.69 (116.60-140.73). The average weight (g) of the whole epididymis was 17.48±1.14 (14.54-20.43) and that of cauda epididymis was 8.35±0.21 (7.82-8.89). The mean spermatozoa concentration (million/ml) of the pooled sample was 1333±142.71 (966.16-1699.84). The recovery of the spermatozoa from the cauda epididymides was done in TCF buffer. Each of the 6 pooled samples was obtained from the spermatozoa recovered from three cauda epididymides. Each pool was divided into two aliquots, out of which, one aliquot was extended without washing (P1), and another was washed using TCF buffer (P2). Both the aliquots were extended in TCF extender and cryopreserved.

Sperm motility

The percent sperm motility at pre-freeze was higher (p>0.05) for P1 (77.50±1.12) than P2 (75.00±1.82). At post-thaw, the percent sperm motility was also higher (p>0.05) for P1 (53.33±3.07) than P2 (40.00±6.45). The percentage of sperm motility for both the processing methods (P1 and P2) decreased significantly (p>0.05) from pre-freeze to post-thaw (Table-3).

Live sperm percentage

The live sperm percentage was higher (p>0.05) for unwashed (P1) cauda epididymal spermatozoa both at pre-freeze and post-thaw than washed sample (P2). The post-thaw live sperm percentage was 65.96±4.79 and 54.98±9.12 for P1 and P2, respectively. The live sperm percentage decreased significantly (p>0.05) from pre-freeze to post-thaw for both the processing methods (Table-3).

Percent intact acrosome

The intact acrosome percentage did not differ significantly (p>0.05) between the processing methods (P1 and P2) both at pre-freeze and post-thaw. However, the intact acrosome percentage was higher (p>0.05) in P1 (74.63±4.96) than P2 (70.89±6.45) at post-thaw. The intact acrosome percentage also declined significantly (p>0.05) from pre-freeze to post-thaw (Table-3).

HOST reacted spermatozoa

The percentage of HOST reacted spermatozoa did not differ significantly (p>0.05) between the processing methods (P1 and P2) both at pre-freeze and post-thaw. However, the percentage of HOST reacted spermatozoa declined significantly (p>0.05) from pre-freeze to post-thaw (Table-3).

Discussion

In the wild, threatened or endangered species of animals may die unexpectedly, either naturally or due to poaching. Recovery and cryopreservation of the epididymal spermatozoa would be one useful way to rescue the germplasm of these dead and valuable animals, and then use them to preserve endangered species. However, cryopreservation causes ultrastructural, biochemical, and functional damages on spermatozoa due to the processing stress and temperature changes resulting in decreased motility and viability with the subsequent decrease in its fertility potential. Studies on the effects of washing with an isotonic buffer using centrifugation on cauda epididymal spermatozoa during cryopreservation are still very limited. Moreover, the results presented in the literature are quite variable. Hence, to overcome this variability, the researchers should endeavor to reach a consensus on the effects of centrifugation on the cauda epididymal spermatozoa during cryopreservation. Therefore, this experiment was carried out to analyze the effects of washing on the quality of cauda epididymal spermatozoa at post-thaw.

The mean percent sperm motility, viable spermatozoa, and intact acrosome were slightly higher (p>0.05) for the unwashed sample, i.e. sample without centrifugation (P1) both at pre-freeze and post-thaw than the washed spermatozoa (P2). Similarly, Hoogewijs et al. [19] also reported no overall effect of centrifugation for the percentage of membrane-intact sperm cells, percentage acrosome-intact sperm cells, total motility, and progressive motility. The percentage of HOST reacted spermatozoa was higher (p>0.05) at pre-freeze; however, at post-thaw, the figure was higher (p>0.05) in the case of washed spermatozoa. The figures for the quality parameters were within the acceptable limit for both the processing methods. The slightly lower percentage of sperm motility, live sperm, and intact acrosome in the P2 at pre-freeze might be due to the stress occurred in the spermatozoa owing to the double centrifugation immediately after recovery and before extension in the final extender and cryopreservation and same has been reflected

Table-3: Quality parameters in washed and unwashed sperm samples at pre-freeze and post-thaw (mean±SEM).

Parameters (%)	Processing methods	Pre-freeze	Post-thaw
Sperm motility	Unwashed (P1)**	77.50±1.12[a]	53.33±3.07[b]
	Washed (P2)**	75.00±1.82[a]	40.00±6.45[b]
	Overall**	76.25±1.09[a]	46.67±3.96[b]
Live sperm	Unwashed (P1)**	83.06±1.23[a]	65.96±4.79[b]
	Washed (P2)**	81.57±1.12[a]	54.98±9.12[b]
	Overall**	82.31±0.83[a]	60.47±5.18[b]
Intact acrosome	Unwashed (P1)**	92.38±0.83[a]	74.63±4.96[b]
	Washed (P2)**	90.59±0.87[a]	70.89±6.45[b]
	Overall**	91.49±0.64[a]	72.76±3.92[b]
HOST reacted spermatozoa	Unwashed (P1)**	86.36±0.87[a]	57.16±2.72[b]
	Washed (P2)**	84.87±0.37[a]	59.95±2.73[b]
	Overall**	85.62±0.50[a]	58.55±1.88[b]

Means with different superscripts in a row (a,b) differ significantly (**p<0.01). HOST=Hypo-osmotic swelling test, SEM=Standard error of mean during the post-thaw. These results are in agreement with the findings of Lone *et al.* [13] in ram epididymal spermatozoa and Islam *et al.* [20] in case of washed goat spermatozoa after holding. Washing of ram spermatozoa is also known to cause damage to the plasma membrane and the acrosome [21].

Decrease in sperm motility of ejaculated goat spermatozoa owing to double centrifugation after holding at 24°C for 1, 3, and 5 h has been reported [20]. However, they reported the beneficial effects of washing of spermatozoa with tris buffer by centrifugation without holding and subsequent preservation in tris extender at 5°C. The beneficial effect of washing on goat ejaculated spermatozoa was obtained due to the removal of the harmful egg yolk coagulating enzyme before their preservation in egg yolk based extender [22,20] which does not exist in ram cauda epididymal spermatozoa sample. Better quality during preservation of unwashed cauda epididymal ram spermatozoa in egg yolk citrate extender has also been reported [23]. Being the values in respect of all the parameters within the acceptable limits and the non-observance of any significant difference between the two processing methods, it could be concluded that epididymal spermatozoa could be cryopreserved with or without centrifugation depending on the need of the protocol or experimental study and washing of cauda epididymal spermatozoa has no significant adverse effect on the quality during cryopreservation. Therefore, this processing method can be applied wherever necessary before the extension of the recovered spermatozoa sample in different extenders.

Conclusion

From the above study, it can be concluded that centrifugation as method of washing cauda epididymal spermatozoa has no significant adverse effect on the quality during cryopreservation. Therefore, this processing method can be applied wherever necessary before the extension of the recovered spermatozoa sample in different extenders.

Authors' Contributions

This study is the part of M.V.Sc thesis work of TA, which was conducted under the guidance of RI. TA conducted the whole study and designed the manuscript under the supervision of RI. FAL and AAM revised the manuscript and helped in statistical analysis. All authors read and approved the final manuscript.

Acknowledgments

The authors are thankful to the Dean, FVSc & AH, SKUAST-K and authorities of Frozen Sperm Station, Srinagar, for providing the necessary facilities which paved the way for completion of this study.

Competing Interests

The authors declare that they have no competing interests.

References

1. Behera, S., Harshan, H.M., Bhai, K.L. and Ghosh, K.N.A. (2015) Effect of cholesterol supplementation on cryosurvival of goat spermatozoa. *Vet. World*, 8: 1386-1391.
2. Ali, A.T., Bomboi, G. and Floris, B. (2013) Replacing chicken yolk with yolks from other sources in ram semen diluents and their effects on fertility *in vitro*. *Small Rum. Res.*, 113: 405-410.
3. Naing, S.W., Haron, A.W., Goriman, M.A.K., Yusoff, R., Abu Bakar, M.Z., Sarsaifi, K., Bukar, M.M., Thein, M., Kyaw, T. and San, M.M. (2011) Effect of seminal plasma removal, washing solutions, and centrifugation regimes on boer goat semen cryopreservation. *Pertanika J. Trop. Agric. Sci.*, 34(2): 271-279.
4. Forouzanfar, M., Ershad, S.F., Hosseini, S.M., Hajian, M., Hosseini, S.O., Abid, A., Tavalaee, M., Shahverdi, A., Dizaji, A.V. and Esfahani, M.H.N. (2013) Can permeable super oxide dismutase mimetic agents improve the quality of frozen–thawed ram semen. *Cryobiology*, 66: 126-130.
5. Azeredo, G.A., Esper, C.R. and Resende, K.T. (2001) Evaluation of plasma membrane integrity of frozen-thawed goat spermatozoa with or without seminal plasma. *Small Rum. Res.*, 41(3): 257-263.
6. Peterson, K., Kappen, M.A.P., Ursem, P.J.F., Nothling, J.O., Colenbrander, B. and Gadella, B.M. (2007) Microscopic and flow cytometric semen assessment of Dutch AI-bucks: Effect of semen processing procedures and their correlation to fertility. *Theriogenology*, 67(4): 863-871.
7. Kozdrowski, R., Dubiel, A., Bielas, W. and Dzieciol, M. (2007) Two protocols of cryopreservation of goat semen with the use of computer-analysis system. *Acta Vet. Brno.*, 76: 601-604.
8. Sarıozkan, S., Bucak, M.N., Tuncer, P.B., Tasdemir, U., Kinet, H. and Ulutas, P.A. (2010) Effects of different extenders and centrifugation/washing on post thaw microscopic-oxidative stress parameters and fertilizing ability of Angora buck sperm. *Theriogenology*, 73: 316-323.
9. Carvajal, G., Cuello, C., Ruiz, M., Vazquez, J.M., Martinez, E.A. and Roca, J. (2004) Effect of centrifugation on Boar sperm. *J. Androl.*, 25: 389-396.
10. Webb, G.W. and Dean, M.M. (2009) Effect of centrifugation technique on post-storage characteristics of stallion spermatozoa. *J. Equine Vet. Sci.*, 29(9): 675-680.
11. Purdy, P.H. (2006) A review on goat sperm cryopreservation. *Small Rum. Res.*, 63(3): 215-225.
12. Lone, F.A., Islam, R., Khan, M.Z. and Sofi, K.A. (2011b) Effect of collection methods on the quality and quantity of spermatozoa recovered from the cauda epididymidis of slaughtered ram. *Indian Vet. J.*, 88(9): 46-48.
13. Lone, F.A., Islam, R., Khan, M.Z. and Sofi, K.A. (2012) Effect of different egg yolk-based extenders on the quality of ovine cauda epididymal spermatozoa during storage at 4°C. *Reprod. Domest. Anim.*, 47: 257-262.
14. Zemjanis, R. (1970) Diagnostic and Therapeutic Techniques in Animal Reproduction. 2nd ed. Williams and Willkins Co., Baltimore.
15. Foote, R.H. (1970) Influence of extender, extension rate and glycerolating technique on fertility of frozen bull semen. *J. Dairy Sci.*, 53: 1478-1482.
16. Blom, E. (1977) Sperm morphology with reference to bull infertility. In: Some Papers Contributed to the 1st All India Symposium on Animal Reproduction. Punjab Agricultural University, Ludhiana, India, p66-81.
17. Watson, P.F. (1975) Use of Giemsa stain to detect changes in acrosomes of frozen ram spermatozoa. *Microsc. Res. Tech.*, 61: 1-6.
18. Vasquez, J., Florentini, E.A., Camargo, L.A., Gonzales, J. and Valdivia, M. (2013) Hypo osmotic swelling test in epididymal ram (*Ovis aries*) spermatozoa. *Livest. Sci.*, 157: 618-622.
19. Hoogewijs, M., Rijsselaere, T., De Vliegher, S.,

Vanhaesebrouck, E., De Schauwer, C., Govaere, J., Thys, M., Hoflack, G., Soom, A.V. and de Kruif, A. (2010) Influence of different centrifugation protocols on equine semen preservation. *Theriogenology,* 74(1): 118-126.

20. Islam, R., Ahmed, K. and Deka, B.C. (2006) Effect of holding and washing on the quality of goat semen. *Small Rum. Res.,* 66: 51-57.

21. Jones, R.C. and Holt, W.V. (1974) The effect of washing on the ultra structure and cytochemistry of ram spermatozoa. *J. Reprod. Fertil.,* 41(1): 159-167.

22. Islam, R. and Ahmed, K. (2003) Effect of seminal plasma and of its removal on the quality of goat semen during preservation at 5°C. *Indian Vet. J.,* 80: 1302-1303.

23. Lone, F.A., Islam, R., Khan, M.Z. and Sofi, K.A. (2011a) Effect of transportation temperature on the quality of cauda epididymal spermatozoa of ram. *Anim. Reprod. Sci.,* 123: 54-59.

16

Phenotypic and genotypic detection of methicillin-resistant *Staphylococcus aureus* in hunting dogs in Maiduguri metropolitan, Borno State, Nigeria

Muhammad Mustapha, Yachilla Maryam Bukar-Kolo, Yaqub Ahmed Geidam and Isa Adamu Gulani

Department of Veterinary Medicine, Faculty of Veterinary Medicine, University of Maiduguri, PMB 1069 Maiduguri, Borno State, Nigeria.
Corresponding author: Muhammad Mustapha, e-mail: tanimuzimbos@yahoo.co.uk,
YMB: yachillabukar@yahoo.com, YAG: yageidam@unimaid.edu.ng, IAG: isagulani@gmail.com

Abstract

Aim: To determine the presence of MRSA in hunting dogs in Maiduguri metropolitan.

Materials and Methods: Phenotypic methods used includes microscopic technique, colony morphology study, catalase-coagulase tests, and the use of mannitol salt agar test, oxacillin resistance screening agar base, and antibiotic susceptibility testing methods. Genotypic approach was used for deoxyribonucleic acid extraction, and the presence of *nuc* and *mecA* gene was detected using polymerase chain reaction (PCR) techniques.

Results: Examination of 416 swab samples from nasal and perineal region of dogs revealed a total of 79.5% of *S. aureus*, where 62.5% of the isolates were MRSA. Molecular analysis revealed that 7*nuc* genes specific for *S. aureus* from 20 presumptive MRSA assay were all *mecA* PCR negative. The isolates were sensitive to gentamicin and ciprofloxacin but proved resistant to cefoxitin and oxacillin.

Conclusion: High isolation rate of MRSA was found in hunting dogs. Significant level (p<0.05) of MRSA was isolated in the nasal cavity of hunting dogs than its perineum. Only *nuc* genes were detected from the MRSA isolates.

Keywords: dogs, genotypic, methicillin, phenotypic, *Staphylococcus aureus*.

Introduction

Staphylococcal infections are of major importance in both Human and Veterinary Medicine. *Staphylococcus aureus* is a major resident or transient colonizer of the skin and the mucosa of humans and primates [1]. *S. aureus* is occasionally found on domestic animals, although other species of staphylococci predominate. *S. aureus* produces an extracellular thermostable nuclease, encoded by *nuc* gene [2].

S. aureus has characteristic ability to rapidly develop resistance to virtually any antibiotics coming into clinical use [3]. Resistance to methicillin that indicated resistance to all beta-lactam agents was first reported in 1961, which marked the appearance of methicillin-resistant *S. aureus* (MRSA) [4]. MRSA is becoming a major public health concern because companion animals often are in close physical contact (touching, petting, and licking) with their owners, exposing them to infection with pathogenic bacteria [5]. Dogs are usually colonized by MRSA strains from humans [6,7].

When *S. aureus* gains entry into the host, it is able to cause a variety of infections from mild skin infection to life-threatening invasive infections such as brain abscesses, endocarditis, pericarditis, pneumonia, arthritis, osteomyelitis, urinary tract infection, and toxic shock syndrome [1]. The report above therefore, indicates that hunting dogs could be colonized by MRSA. Colonization of MRSA in dogs has been extensively studied in Europe and most parts of the world. However, in Nigeria, there is very little documented information on (MRSA) colonization of dogs.

There is the presence of MRSA in hunting dogs in Maiduguri Borno State, which is evident as a result of the presence of *mecA* polymerase chain reaction (PCR) negative *S. aureus* in the isolate. Therefore, the objective of this research is to determine the presence of MRSA, antibiotic sensitivity pattern of MRSA isolates, and the presence of *nuc* and *mecA* gene from MRSA isolates using phenotypic and genotypic techniques.

Materials and Methods

Ethical approval

This research was approved by the Faculty of Veterinary Medicine Ethics and Research Committee, University of Maiduguri, Borno State, Nigeria.

Study area

Maiduguri is the capital and the largest urban center of Borno State, North Eastern Nigeria (Figure-1).

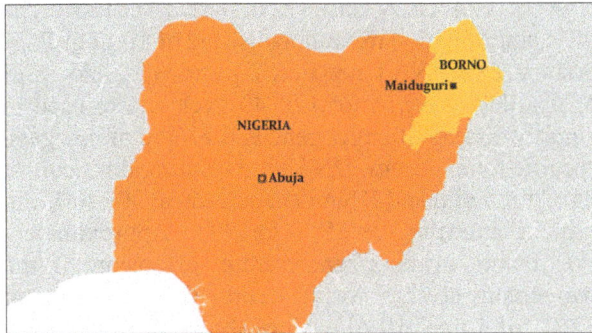

Figure-1: Map of Nigeria showing Maiduguri metropolitan in Borno State (study area).

The state lies between latitude 11°32′ North and 11°40′ North and latitude 13°20′ East and 13°25′ East between the Sudan Savanna and Sahel Savanna vegetation zones, characterized by short rainy season of 3-4 months (June-September) followed by a prolonged dry season of more than 8 months duration [8].

Sample collection

Total of 416 swab samples were collected from the four major hunting rendezvous in Maiduguri metropolitan. 211 and 205 swab samples from the nostril and perineum of the hunting dogs were analyzed. Cotton swab sticks were used to collect all the samples according to laboratory standard [9]. Each sample was labeled with an identification number and date of collection. The samples were kept on an ice pack and transported to the research laboratory, Department of Veterinary Medicine, Faculty of Veterinary Medicine, University of Maiduguri.

Hunting dogs

Dogs were sampled with owners consent. Cotton-tipped sterile swab (Everson Industries Limited, Nigeria) was inserted into one nostril of each dog where sample was taken from the nasal mucosa and immediately inserted into the aseptic tube. The tubes were labeled and dates of collection noted. Another sterile cotton-tipped swab is rolled on the perineal region and then immediately inserted back into its tube [9].

Isolation and identification

Enriched solid medium of 5% blood agar (Sigma® Switzerland) was prepared according to the manufacturer's instruction and inoculated with the swabs [10]. Sterile wire loop was used to streak the inoculums to get discrete colonies. The inoculated plates were incubated aerobically at 37°C for 24 h and observed for yellowish-white colonies with smooth slightly raised surfaces. Some positive colonies have complete zones of hemolysis while others were non-hemolytic.

Colony morphology

Gram-stain of the collected samples was performed to identify staphylococci by their gram reaction. Samples that were cocci arranged in grape-like clusters were subjected to catalase and coagulase tests.

The positive isolates were streaked on mannitol salt agar (MSA, Oxoid) which is a selective medium for *S. aureus,* and plates were incubated under an aerobic condition at 37°C for 24 h. The appearance of yellowish colonies on MSA was presumed to be *S. aureus.*

Oxacillin resistance screening agar base (ORSAB)

ORSAB is a medium for the screening of MRSA, the medium is nutritious, selective and contains peptones for the growth of microorganisms. The medium has high salt and lithium chloride concentration to suppress non-staphylococcal growth, with mannitol and aniline blue, for the detection of mannitol fermentation. The antibiotics contained in ORSAB selective supplement are oxacillin at 2 mg/L to inhibit methicillin-sensitive *S. aureus,* and polymyxin B for the suppression of other bacteria that are able to grow at such a high salt concentration,e.g. *Proteus* spp. typical colonies of MRSA are intense blue on a colorless background enabling the organism to be more easily identified in mixed culture than the pale yellow colonies seen on MSA.

Antibiotic susceptibility testing

The ATS of MRSA isolates was determined according to the method of Bauer-Kirby [11]. Using the commercially prepared disc (Oxoid, UK) with a known concentration of antibiotics, freshly sub-cultured MRSA and well-isolated colonies from ORSAB plates were emulsified in 3-4 ml of sterile normal saline. The turbidity of the suspension was adjusted to the turbidity of standard equivalent to 0.5 McFarland [12]. Mueller-Hinton agar medium was prepared, and a sterile cotton swab stick was dipped into the suspension. Excess fluid was removed by pressing and rotating the swab against the side of the tube above the suspension. The dried surface of the Mueller-Hinton agar was inoculated by streaking the swab evenly over the surface of the medium in three directions, rotating the plate approximately 60° to ensure even distribution [9]. Five antimicrobial discs were dispensed into each inoculated plates and incubated at 35°C for 24 h. Zone of inhibition were measured in millimeters (mm) using vernier caliper. The sizes of the zones of inhibition were interpreted according to CLSI [12] criteria. The following 10 antibiotics were tested FOX 30 ug, DA 2 ug, SXT 25 ug, CIP 5 ug, E 15 ug, KZ 30 ug, C 30 ug, CN 10 ug, TE 30 ug, and OX 1 g (Oxoid, UK). For the interpretation of susceptibility toward oxacillin disc, growth within the zone of inhibition was considered indicative of methicillin resistance. According to the classification criteria given by CLSI [12], a diameter of inhibition zones of ≤10, 11-12, and ≥13 by 1 ug of oxacillin is categorized as resistant (R), intermediate (I), or susceptible (S) to oxacillin accordingly. For cefoxitin disc, a diameter of inhibition zones of ≤24 and ≥25 mm correspond to the class of staphylococci considered as resistance or susceptible for oxacillin, accordingly. There is no intermediate category of classification for staphylococci using the cefoxitin disc diffusion test [12].

Genotypic characterization

A total of 80 phenotypically detected MRSA from hunting dogs, 20 samples from this number were randomly selected for the genotypic analysis using PCR for the detection of *S. aureus* specific gene (*nuc* gene), and the *mecA* gene encoding the resistance as described by Perez-Roth *et al.* [13].

Deoxyribonucleic acid (DNA) extraction

A loop full MRSA isolates were scooped into 1.5 ml tube that contained 400 µl of lysis buffer and 4 µl proteinase k and was vortexed (Fisher brand, Allied Fisher Scientific, USA), for 2 min to get a homogeneous mixture. This was followed by incubation at 55°C for 3 h in the thermocycler (Strata gene, USA). 400 µl of phenol/chloroform (PC) was added to the tube and mixed gently for 1min. It was then spun in a microcentrifuge for 10 min at maximum speed (10,000 rpm). The supernatant was transferred to another tube, and 400 µl of PC was added, vortexed, and then it was spun for 10 min at 10,000 rpm. The supernatant was transferred to a new tube, 300 µl of chloroform was added and vortexed, spun for 1 min at 10,000 rpm, and the supernatant was also transferred to another tube. 825 µl of 100% ethanol and 25 µl of sodium acetate were added and incubated in the freezer overnight.

The following day, the samples were centrifuged using high speed refrigerated centrifuge (Harvey Instruments Inc. USA) for 20 min and the supernatant was discarded. One (1 ml) of 70% ethanol was added to the samples, mixed and centrifuged for 20 min at 13500 rpm; the supernatant was discarded and dry spun for 1 min, and the residual ethanol was removed. The DNA pellets were allowed to dry at room temperature. The pellets were resuspended in 20 µl of water. After the DNA extraction, 10 µl of loading dye (bromophenol blue) was mixed with 5 µl of the DNA pellets and pipetted into the wells of the gel. Finally, electrophoresis was carried out to determine the presence of DNA.

PCR primers dilution

Primers that corresponded to *nuc* gene specific for *S. aureus* and *mecA* gene were obtained from Integrated DNA Technologies, USA. The primers were resuspended in sterile distilled water, and the diluted primers were stored at −20°C.

Detection of *nuc* and *mecA* gene by PCR

The PCR amplification was done according to Perez-Roth *et al.* [13]. Using the following primers that will detect the *nuc* gene in *S. aureus* and *mecA* gene with the amplicon size of 276 bp and 533 bp; The *nuc* primers were 5'-GCG ATT GAT GGT GAT ACG GTT-3' and 5'- AGC CAA GCC TTG ACG AAC TAA AGC-3', whereas the *mecA* primers were 5'-AAA ATC GAT GGT AAA GGT TGG C-3' and

5'-AGT TCT GCA GTA CCG GAT TTG C-3'. The PCR amplification mixture consisted of 10 µl of PCR premix, 2 µl DNA templates, 2 µl primers, and 16 µl of distilled water. A total of 40 cycles were used to amplify 533 bp of *mecA* gene and 276 bp of *nuc* gene specific for *S. aureus*. DNA pre-denaturation occurs at 94°C for 5 min and DNA denaturation at 30 s to 1 min primers annealing at 55°C for 30 s. Approximately 5°C below primers temperature, extension of the two strands at 72°C for 60 s and a final extension at 72°C for 4 min. 10 µl each of the PCR products for *mecA* and *nuc* gene were analyzed separately on 2% agarose gel (Biogene, UK). Electrophoresis was performed in TBE buffer at 180 V for 1 h, and the gel was subsequently stained with 3 µl of ethidium bromide (Sigma, UK). DNA bands were visualized using UV-light with the camera (Gel Doc 2000, Bio-Rad) and photographed.

Data analysis

Fisher's exact test (Graph pad®Software Inc.) was used to determine the probability and significance of MRSA detection from the skin, perineal region, and nasal cavity of hunting dogs. The values were considered significant (p< 0.05).

Results

Total of 416 swab samples from the nostril and perineal region of hunting dogs of *S. aureus* revealed 128 (79.5%) positive isolates. Microscopic examination of Gram-stained colonies showed Gram-positive cocci arranged in irregular grape-like clusters, some appearing in single, whereas others in pairs, short chain, or tetrads. Results of catalase and coagulase positive isolates are 141 (87.6) and 128 (79.5%), respectively. Table-1 shows results of Gram-staining, biochemical test and ORSAB screening of staphylococcal isolates in hunting dogs in Maiduguri metropolitan, Borno State. The values of *S. aureus* isolated from the nostril and perineum of hunting dogs were 78 (36.9%) and 50 (24.4%) respectively. The values of MRSA isolated from the nostril and perineum of hunting dogs were 50 (23.7%) and 30 (14.7%), respectively (Table-2). The result of antimicrobial susceptibility

Table-1: Gram-staining, biochemical test and ORSAB screening of *S. aureus* isolates in hunting dogs in Maiduguri metropolitan, Borno State.

Test	Result of positive isolates (%)	Result of negative isolates (%)	Total
Gram reaction	161 (38.7[a])	255 (61.3[b])	416
Catalase test	141 (87.6[c])	20 (12.4[d])	161
Coagulase test	128 (79.5)	33 (20.5)	161
ORSAB screening	80 (62.5[k])	48 (37.5[y])	128

Figures in brackets are percentage occurrence of staphylococcal isolate species. Values denoted by different superscripts for a given parameter are significantly different (p<0.05). ORSAB=Oxacillin resistance screening agar base, *S. aureus=Staphylococcus aureus*

Table-2: Percentage distribution of S. aureus and MRSA isolated from hunting dogs in Maiduguri metropolitan.

Source	Site	S. aureus (-ve)	S. aureus (+ve)	MRSA (+ve)	Number of samples
Dog	Nasal	133	78 (36.9)	50 (23.7)	211
	Perineum	155	50 (24.4)	30 (14.7)	205
	Total	288	128 (30.8)	80 (19.2)	416

MRSA=Methicillin-resistance Staphylococcus aureus, S. aureus=Staphylococcus aureus

Table-3: Antibiotic susceptibility pattern of MRSA isolated from hunting dogs in Maiduguri metropolitan, Borno State.

	Susceptibility pattern		
Antibiotics	Resistant number of isolates (%)	Intermediate number of isolates (%)	Susceptible number of isolates (%)
Cefoxitin	97 (99.0)	0 (0.0)	1 (1.0)
Cefazolin	69 (70.0)	6 (6.1)	23 (23.5)
Chloramphenicol	8 (8.2)	4 (4.1)	86 (87.8)
Ciprofloxacin	3 (3.1)	6 (6.1)	89 (90.8)
Clindamycin	15 (15.3)	5 (5.1)	78 (79.6)
Erythromycin	14 (14.3)	4 (4.1)	80 (81.6)
Gentamicin	1 (1.0)	1 (1.0)	96 (98.9)
Oxacillin	87 (88.8)	1 (1.0)	10 (10.2)
Tetracycline	72 (73.4)	4 (4.1)	22 (22.4)
Sulfa/Trimethoprim	7 (7.1)	5 (5.1)	86 (87.8)

MRSA=Methicillin-resistance Staphylococcus aureus

Table-4: Multidrug resistance profile of MRSA isolated from hunting dogs in Maiduguri metropolitan.

Number of drugs resisted (%)
0 (0.00)
1 (2.04)
2 (6.12)
3 (34.7)
4 (35.7)
≥5 (21.4)

MRSA=Methicillin-resistance Staphylococcus aureus

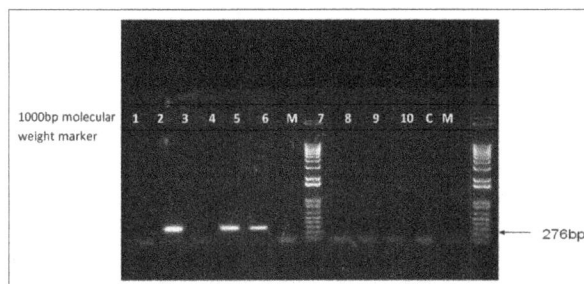

Figure-2: Agarose gel electrophoresis of polymerase chain reaction of methicillin-resistance Staphylococcus aureus isolate. Lanes 2, 4,and 5 are positive for nuc gene as indicated by 276 bp.Lane 1, 3, 6, 7, 8, 9, and 10 are negative samples. Lane M is the molecular weightmarker. Lane C is the negative control.

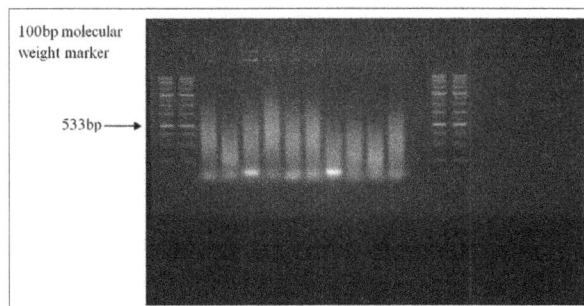

Figure-3: Agarose gel electrophoresis pattern of polymerase chain reaction of methicillin-resistance Staphylococcus aureus isolate. Lane M: Molecular weight marker. Lane 1-10: Negative for mecA. Lane C: Negative control.

test indicated that the isolates were highly resistant to FOX (99%), OX (88.7%), TE (73.4%), and KZ (70.0%), while they were highly susceptible to CN (98%), CIP (90.8%), C (87.6%), SXT (87.8%), E (81.6%), and DA(79.6%) as presented in Table-3. Multidrug Resistance (MDR) Profile of MRSA isolated from hunting dogs in Maiduguri Metropolitan is shown in Table-4. 20 presumptive MRSA isolates assayed 7 bands showed evidence expression of *nuc* gene specific for S. *aureus* with a molecular weight of 276 bp which is presented in Figure-2. This confirms the assumption based on the phenotypic detection that some of the strains were S. *aureus*. The result of PCR based on targeted *mecA* gene revealed that none of the isolates possessed *mecA* gene as represented in Figure-3.

Discussion

Investigations on phenotypic detection of MRSA in hunting dogs in Maiduguri Metropolitan revealed higher isolation rates (19.2%) of these pathogens in dogs compared to the findings of Loeffler *et al.* [14], Kottler *et al.* [15], and Chah *et al.* [16] who, respectively, recorded 9.0%, 3.3%, and 12.8% of MRSA in dogs in the UK, the US, and Nigeria.

This may probably be attributed to variation in the breeds of dogs used in this finding, indiscriminate antibiotic therapy, harsher environmental challenges commonly encountered during hunting and could also be associated to starvation which results in stress that affects dog's immunity. Kutdang *et al.*[17] supported the assertion above from his finding that hunting dogs are more exposed to the outside environment and hence stood the chance of contracting more infections than household dogs. Floras *et al.* [18] further augmented the findings of this study with a report of an increasingly higher detection rate of MRSA in dogs in Canada.

The distribution of *S. aureus* and MRSA recorded from the nasal cavity of hunting dogs was significantly different (higher) than the values recorded from the perineal region of dogs. These suggest that higher possibilities of contamination rate of dogs are through the nostril. Contaminations can also result through scavenging of death carcasses exposed to antibiotics from backyard poultry operations. These tallies, with the findings of Rich and Roberts [19] and Khanna *et al.* [20] who reported that MRSA colonization in animals, are better detected through nasal sampling. Rich and Roberts [19] further confirmed this through a record of a single case of MRSA detection from nasal swab samples of 255 dogs and not from the throat and skin of the same animals.

Antimicrobial susceptibility pattern of the MRSA isolates has also been investigated indicating a high level of resistance to FOX and OX . This finding, therefore, implies that FOX based assays are particularly important for low-level OX resistant MRSA detection [21]. Phenotypic antimicrobial susceptibility test needs particular care when using OX as a test substrate because of heterogeneous *in vitro* expression of Methicillin-resistance (hetero-resistance) in nearly all of currently disseminated MRSA clonal lineages. Heteroresistance can be either detected using high inocula as recommended by the Clinical Laboratory Standard Institutes, or by use of FOX disks since this antibiotic is less affected by heterogeneous expression [12].

The MRSA isolates were highly susceptible to CIP and CN. CIP, a member of the fluoroquinolones that are newer drugs with mode of action on DNA inhibition and are relatively expensive and less available for abuses [22]. In addition; CN, an aminoglycoside, also showed high activity against MRSA, which may be as a result of the complexity of the aminoglycoside and the route of administration [22].

It was concluded that 59 out of 80 isolates of MRSA were multidrug resistant (MDR) in this study. This finding was supported by Abeer *et al.* [23], who reported that 14 out of 51 MRSA isolates were MDR. Methicillin-resistant coagulase negative staphylococci (MRCoNS) from healthy dogs in Nsukka, Nigeria, isolated revealed that 13 out of 109 isolates of MRCoNS were MDR [16].

The PCR analysis did not reveal any *mecA* positive samples, and this might indicate the presence of *mecA* PCR negative MRSA isolates in Maiduguri. A previous study by Garcia-Alvarez *et al.* [24] had reported a novel allele of the *mecA* gene encoding an alternative penicillin binding protein that mediates methicillin resistance among bovine *S. aureus* isolates, and humans in the UK, Denmark, and Germany that were Methicillin-resistant but *mecA* PCR negative.

These novel alleles of the *mecA* gene ($mecA_{LGA251}$) have 70% nucleotide identity to the archetypal *mecA* gene. Moreover, the findings highlight the possibility that additional *mecA* allele is in circulation in the environment, and therefore, could be acquired by *S. aureus* and leads to the emergence of new MRSA strain. However, antimicrobial susceptibility testing and other routine culture will identify *S. aureus* isolates encoding $mecA_{LGA251}$ as methicillin-resistant [24]. Furthermore, Kriegeskorte *et al.* [25] also found MRSA isolates with novel genetic homolog among human in a study of human MRSA isolates in Germany.

The results of the PCR analysis in the current study which revealed *nuc* genes at 276 bp which tallied with the findings recorded by Merlino *et al.* [26], Saiful *et al.* [27], and Szczepanik *et al.* [28], who used modified PCR analysis (multiplex PCR) for the detection of *mecA* and *nuc* genes in multidrug resistance and non-multidrug resistance MRSA.

Conclusion

Conclusively, MRSA was phenotypically detected with significant (p<0.05) isolation rate in the hunting dogs. Microbiological and PCR results confirm the presence of MRSA in hunting dogs in Maiduguri Metropolitan, Borno State, Nigeria. Higher percentages (50.0%) of MRSA were detected from the nasal cavities of dogs than the perineal region (30.0%).

Author's Contributions

This study was conceived by MM, YMB, and YAG. MM collected the data during field work. The data were compiled by MM, analyzed by MM and IAG. Write up by MM. All authors read and approved the final manuscript.

Acknowledgments

My sincere appreciation goes to pet owners for permission to collect samples, DNA laboratory Kaduna, Nigeria, for molecular analysis and Dr. M.S. Auwal for objective criticism. The research is self-sponsored.

Competing Interests

The authors declare that they have no competing interests.

References

1.   Pantosti, A. (2012) Methicillin-resistant *Staphylococcus aureus* associated with animal and its relevance to human. *Microbiol*, 3: 137.

2.   Zhang, K., Sparkling, J., Chow, B.L., Elsayed, S., Hussain, Z. and Church, D.C. (2004) New quadriplex PCR assay for detection of methicillin and mupirocin resistance and simultaneous discrimination of *Staphylococcus aureus* from coagulase-negative *Staphylococci. J. Clin.Microbiol.*, 42(11): 4947-4955.

3. Pantosti, A., Sanchini, A. and Monaco, M. (2007) Mechanisms of antibiotic resistance in *Staphylococcusaureus*. *FutureMicrobiol.,* 2(3): 323-334.

4. Molton, J.S., Tambyan, P.A. and Ang, B.S.P. (2013) The global spread of healthcare associated multidrug-resistant bacteria: A perspective from Asia. *Clin. Infect. Dis.,* 56(3): 1310-1318.

5. Guardabassi, L., Loeber, M.E. and Jacobson, A. (2004) Transmission of multiple antimicrobial-resistant *Staphylococcus intermedius* between dogs affected by deep pyoderma and their owners.*Vet. Microbiol.,* 98:23-27.

6. Loeffler, A. and Lloyd, D.H. (2010) Companion animals: A reservoir for methicillin-resistant *Staphylococcus aureus* in the community? *Epidemiol. Infect.,*138(5):595-605.

7. Lin, Y., Barker, E., Kislow, J., Kaldhone, P., Stemper, M.E., Pantrangi, M., Moore, F.M., Hall, M., Fritsche, T.R., Novicki, T., Foley, S.L. and Shukla, S.K. (2011) Evidence of multiple virulence subtypes in nosocomial and community-associated MRSA genotypes in companion animals from the upper Midwestern and northeastern United States.*Clin. Med. Res.,* 9(1):7-16.

8. Borno State Ministry of Land and Survey, (BMLS). (2016) Annual Report 15-58.

9. Cheesbrough, M. (2010) District Laboratory Practice in Tropical Countries. 2nd ed. Cambridge University Press, Cambridge, UK. p45.

10. Vincze, A., Stamm, I., Kopp, P.A., Hermes, T., Adlhoh, C., Semmler, T., Wieler, LH., Lubke-Becker, A. and Walter, B. (2014) Alarming proportion on Methicillin-resistant *Staphylococcus aureus* (MRSA) in wound samples from companion animals, Germany 2010-2012. *PLoSOne,* 9(1): e85656.

11. Bauer, A.W., Kirby, W.M.M., Sherris, J.C. and Turck, M. (1966) Antibiotic susceptibility testing by standardized single disk method. *Am. J. Clin. Pathol.,* 45: 493-496.

12. CLSI. (2011) Performance Standards for Antimicrobial SusceptibilityTesting; Twenty- First Information Supplement. M100-S20.Vol.30. Clinical Laboratory Standard Institute, Wayne, PA, p157-165.

13. Perez-Roth, E., Claverie-Martin, F., Villar, J. and Mendez-Alvarez, S. (2001) Multiplex PCR for simultaneous identification of *Staphylococcus aureus* and detection of methicillin and mupirocin resistance.*J. Clin. Microbiol.,*39: 4037-4041.

14. Loeffler, A., Boag, A.K., Sung, J., Lindsay, J.A., Guardabassi, L., Dalsgaard, A., Smith, H., Stevens, K.B. and Lloyd, D.H. (2005) Prevalence of methicillin-resistant *Staphylococcus aureus* among staff and pets in a small animal referral hospital in the UK. *J. Antimicrob. Chemoth*er., 56(4): 692-697.

15. Kottler, S., Middleton, J.R., Perry, J., Weese, J.S. and Cohn, L.A. (2010) Prevalence of *Staphylococcusaureus* and methicillin-resistant *Staphylococcusaureus* carriage in three populations. *J. Vet. Int. Med.* 24(1):132-139.

16. Chah, K.F., Soaz, E.G., Nwanta, J.A., Asadu, B., Agbo, I.F., Lozano, C., Zarazaga, M. and Torres, C. (2014) Methicillin-resistant coagulase negative *Staphylococci* from healthy dogs in Nsukka, Nigeria. *Braz. J. Microbiol.,* 45(1): 215-220.

17. Kutdang, E.T., Bukbuk, D.N. and Ajayi, J.A.A. (2010) Theprevalence of intestinalhelminthes of dogs (Canisfamillaris) in Jos, Plateau State, Nigeria. *Researcher,* 2(8):51-56.

18. Floras, A., Lawn, K., Slavic, D., Golding, G.R., Mulvey, M.R. and Weese, J.S. (2010) Sequence type 398 meticillin-resistant *Staphylococcus aureus* infection and colonisation in dogs.*Vet. Rec.,* 166(26):826-827.

19. Rich, M. and Roberts, L. (2004) Methicillin-resistant *Staphylococcus aureus*isolates from companion animals. *Vet. Rec.,* 154(10):310.

20. Khanna, T., Friendship, R., Dewey, C. and Weese, J.S. (2008) Methicillin resistant *Staphylococcus aureus* colonization in pigs and pig farmers. *Vet.Microbiol.,* 128(3-4):298-303.

21. Witte, W., Pasemann, B. and Cuny, C. (2007) Detection of low-level oxacillin resistance in *mecA* positive *Staphylococcus aureus*.*Clin. Microbiol. Infect.,* 13(4): 408-412.

22. Onanuga, A., Oyi, A.R. and Onaolapa, A.J. (2005) Prevalence and susceptibility pattern of Methicillin resistant *Staphylococcus aureus* isolates amongst healthy women in Zaria,Nigeria. *Afr. J. Biotechnol.,* 4(11):1321-1324.

23. Abeer, A.R., Mohamed, S.S. and Amal, S.O. (2007) Detection of methicillin/oxacillin resistant *Staphylococcus aureus* isolated from clinical Hospital in Cairo using mecA/nuc gene and antibiotic susceptibility profile. *Int.J. Agric. Biol., 9(6):800-806*:

24. Garcia-Alvarez, L., Holden, M.T., Lindsay, H., Webb, C.R., Brown, D.F. and Curran, M.D. (2011) Methicillin-resistant *Staphylococcus aureus* with a novel mecA homologue in human and bovine population in the UK and Denmark: A descriptive study. *Lancet Infect.Dis.,* 11:595-603.

25. Kriegeskorte, A., Ballhausen, B., Idelevich, E.A., Kock, R., Friedrich, A.W. and Karch, H. (2012) Human methicillin-resistant *Staphylococcus aureus* isolates with novel genetic homolog, Germany. *Emerg.Infect. Dis.,* 18(6):1016-1018.

26. Merlino, J., Watson, J., Rose, B., Beard-Pegler, M., Gottlieb, T., Bradbury, R. and Harbour, C. (2002) Detection and expression of methicillin/oxacillin resistance in multidrug-resistant and non-multidrug-resistant *Staphylococcus aureus* in Central Sydney, Australia. *J. Antimicrob. Chemother.,* 49: 793-801.

27. Saiful, A.J., Mastura, M., Zarizal, S., Mazurah, M.I., Shuhaimi, M. and Ali, A.M. (2006) Detection of methicillin-resistant *Staphylococcus aureus* using *mecA/nuc* genes and antibiotic susceptibility profile of Malaysian clinical isolates.*World J. Microbiol. Biotechnol.,* 22:1289-1294.

28. Szczepanik, A., Koziol-Montewka, M., Al-Doori, Z., Morrison, D. and Kaczor, D. (2007) Spread of a single multi-resistant methicillin-resistant *Staphylococcus aureus* clone carring a variant of staphylococcal cassette chromosome mecType III isolated in a university hospital. *Eur. J. Clin. Microbiol. Infect. Dis.,* 26: 29-35.

17

Ultrastructural changes in the sublingual salivary gland of prenatal buffalo (*Bubalus bubalis*)

A. D. Singh and Opinder Singh

Department of Veterinary Anatomy, Guru Angad Dev Veterinary and Animal Sciences University, Ludhiana - 141 004, Punjab, India.
Corresponding author: Opinder Singh, e-mail: singhopinder68@gmail.com,
ADS: dramandeep287@gmail.com

Abstract

Aim: The present study was aimed to elucidate ultrastructural changes in the development of sublingual salivary gland of buffalo during prenatal life.

Materials and Methods: The study was carried out on sublingual salivary gland of 36 buffalo fetuses ranging from 13.2 cm curved crown-rump length (CVRL) (88th day) to full term. The fetuses were categorized into three groups based on their CVRL.

Results: The cells lining the terminal tubules were undifferentiated with poorly developed cytoplasmic organelles but lacked secretory granules (SGs) at 13.2 cm CVRL (88th day). The SGs appeared first in the form of membrane-bound secretory vesicles with homogeneous electron-dense as well as electron-lucent contents at 21.2 cm CVRL (122nd day); however, mucous acinar cells contained electron-lucent granules, while serous secretory cells as well as serous demilunes showed electron-dense granules at 34 cm CVRL (150th day) of prenatal life. At 53.5 cm CVRL (194th day), both mucous and serous acini were differentiated by the density of SGs.

Conclusion: The cytoplasm of acinar cells was filled with mitochondria, rough endoplasmic reticulum, and Golgi profiles in mid and late fetal age groups. The SGs were increased in number during the late fetal age group. The myoepithelial cells (MECs) were located at the base of the acinar cells as well as intercalated and striated ducts and were stellate in shape. The ultrastructure of MEC revealed a parallel stream of myofilaments in the cytoplasm and its processes. The mucous cells were predominantly present in the sublingual salivary gland and were pyramidal in shape.

Keywords: buffalo, prenatal, sublingual salivary gland, transmission electron microscopy.

Introduction

The sublingual salivary gland contributes to the secretion of saliva which plays a key role in maintaining ruminants healthy by facilitating mastication and deglutition, helping in the restoration of normal ruminal pH. Ruminant saliva is an isotonic, bicarbonate-phosphate buffer with high pH. It has an important role in providing lubrication for eating and vocalization, aid digestion, and supply saliva for pH buffering [1]. This well-buffered solution is necessary for neutralizing acids formed by fermentation in the rumen to maintain the acid-base equilibrium of the ruminal contents. Salivary glands are composed of specialized epithelial cells, and the basic secretory units of salivary glands are clusters of cells called acini. These cells can be classified as serous cells as well as mucous cells [2]. The distribution of these types varies from species to species [3]. The salivary glands also secrete immunoglobulin A, potassium, and sodium [4].

This paucity and the precious role of the sublingual salivary gland in digestion prompted to study the histogenesis which may be serving as a tool for future research on stem cell analysis of primordia of the salivary gland. The study of prenatal development is prerequisite to understand the normal developmental biology of an organ. The documentation of normal fetal growth can serve as a guide for understanding the consequence of harmful influences at various stages of gestation [5].

Various prenatal as well as postnatal studies have been done on salivary glands of rat [6], Japanese quail [7], birds [8], and buffalo [9,10]; however, there is no detailed information about the ultrastructural studies of buffalo sublingual salivary gland during prenatal development; therefore, the present work was aimed to observe the ultrastructural changes in the sublingual salivary gland of prenatal buffalo.

Materials and Methods

Ethical approval

This study was conducted after approval by the Research Committee and Institutional Animal Ethics Committee.

Collection of samples

The present study was conducted on sublingual salivary gland of 36 buffalo fetuses, during different stages of prenatal development. Immediately after collection, the fetuses were measured for their curved crown-rump length (CVRL) in centimeters with a calibrated inelastic thread. The approximate age of fetuses was calculated using the following formula in buffalo [11].

$Y = 28.66 + 4.496X$ (CVRL <20 cm)

$Y = 73.544 + 2.256X$ (CVRL ≥20 cm)

Where, Y is age in day(s) and X is curved crown-rump length (CVRL) in cm(s). Depending on CVRL, fetuses were divided into three groups with a minimum of 12 samples in each group:

Group I: CVRL between 0 and 20 cm

Group II: CVRL >20-40 cm

Group III: CVRL >40 cm

Fixation and processing of samples

Immediately after measuring CVRL, the tissue samples, collected from the sublingual salivary gland of buffalo fetuses, were thoroughly washed in phosphate buffer saline solution (pH 7.4) and trimmed to 1 mm³ size. These samples were fixed in Karnovsky's fixative (2.5% glutaraldehyde and 2% paraformaldehyde in 0.1 M phosphate buffer solution) for 8-12 h, and their secondary fixation was done in 2% osmium tetroxide for 2 h. Subsequently, tissue samples were dehydrated, cleared, infiltrated, embedded, and polymerized. The ultrathin sections of 70-90 nm were cut and stained with uranyl acetate for 15 min followed by lead citrate for 10 min [12]. The grids with sections were examined under transmission electron microscope for detailed study.

Results and Discussion

Group I

The cells lining the terminal tubules were undifferentiated with poorly developed cytoplasmic organelles but lacked secretory granules (SGs) at 13.2 cm CVRL (88th day). However, the apical ends of cells showed electron-lucent and some electron-dense granules. In sublingual salivary gland of rat, at 19 days of intrauterine life, more cells of the terminal buds contained granules, and larger numbers of granules were present in the cells. Cells containing electron-lucent mucous granules and cells containing electron-dense serous granules were present around a common lumen. The mucous granules usually had fine fibrillar content; their membranes were indistinct, and adjacent granules often were fused. The size and density of serous granules varied from granule to granule, although the content of individual granules was generally of uniform density [6].

Group II

Accumulations of SGs were seen in the acinar cells at 21.1 cm CVRL (121st day). Flattened myoepithelial cells (MECs) with long cytoplasmic processes containing homogeneous cytoplasm were observed around the developing acinar cells (Figure-1). These cells contained myofilaments in the cytoplasmic processes during late age groups.

In sublingual salivary gland of Japanese quail, two cell types were clearly distinguished within tubules: A great majority of secretory cells with a lot of granules, and a few intercalated non-secretory cells with a high content of mitochondria. Both secretory and mitochondria-rich cells surround a lumen where secretory products are exocyted [7]. The SGs appeared in the form of membrane-bound secretory vesicles with homogeneous electron-dense as well as electron-lucent contents.

At 34 cm CVRL (150th day), mucous acinar cells contained electron-lucent granules, while serous cells as well as serous demilunes showed electron-dense granules. The Golgi complex, mitochondria, and rough endoplasmic reticulum (ER) were markedly developed in the cells of acini (Figure-2). The

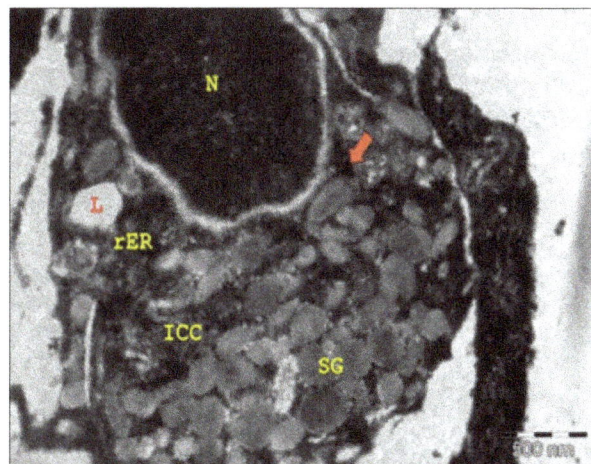

Figure-1: Transmission electron micrograph of sublingual salivary gland of 21.1 cm curved crown-rump length (121st day) buffalo fetus showing electron-lucent secretory granules (SGs) in developing mucous acinar cells (L - Lipofuscin pigment, N - Nucleus, rER - Rough endoplasmic reticulum, ICC - Intercellular canaliculi, Arrow - Mitochondria) (×8000).

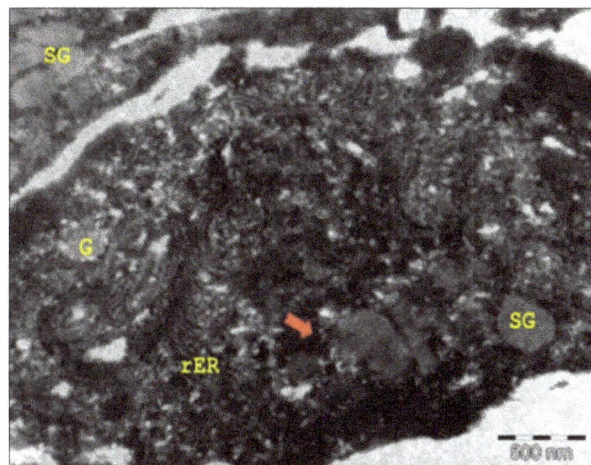

Figure-2: Transmission electron micrograph of the sublingual salivary gland of 34 cm curved crown-rump length (150th day) buffalo fetus showing electron-lucent granules (SGs), Golgi complex (G), rough endoplasmic reticulum (rER), and mitochondria (arrow) (×8000).

proportion of serous cells located at the periphery of the terminal buds increased from mid to late intrauterine life in the sublingual salivary gland of rat. The mixed granules had a variable density, and some contained a dense core located either peripherally or centrally within the granule [6]. The SGs might represent of storage of secretory products that are located to the heterogeneous and complex ultrastructural patterns of granules in the mucous and seromucous cells in the sublingual salivary gland of some bird species [8]. Electron-lucent granules with a delimiting membrane were observed in the trans-surface of the Golgi saccules. These observations were in accordance with the findings in buffalo [9].

Group III

The ultrastructure of sublingual salivary gland revealed both mixed acini, mucous, and serous at 53.5 cm CVRL (194th day) and was differentiated by the density of SGs. The mucous cells were predominantly present in the sublingual salivary gland and were pyramidal in shape, as reported at the 141st day of prenatal life in buffalo [10]. The mucous cells had a flattened nucleus occupying the basal region of the cytoplasm and a well-organized cisternal rough ER arranged in parallel arrays. The Golgi complex was prominent and contained a significant number of smooth transport vesicles budding from the transitional ER, as well as coated vesicles formed from membranes of the Golgi saccules. In the late prenatal life of rat, the sublingual glands showed all of the epithelial structures, i.e. mucous acini, serous demilunes, intercalated ducts, striated ducts, and excretory ducts. The gland increased markedly in size, mainly through an increase in the number of acinar and demilune cells [13].

Stellate shaped MECs with cytoplasmic processes were observed around the base of mucous acinar cells and ducts (Figure-3). These observations were in total agreement with the findings in buffalo at the 141st day of prenatal life [10]. The ultrastructure of MECs revealed the parallel stream of myofilaments in the cytoplasm and its processes. These MECs were found to be attached to the glandular cells by desmosomes (Figure-4). Fat cells were observed in between the acinar cells. The size of the mucous cells and the number of granules increased during the late fetal and early postnatal period in rat. Cells containing mixed granules were present in decreasing numbers through 5 days of age [6]. There was a gradual decrease in the stromal spaces accompanied by intense collagen deposition in the intra and interlobular connective tissue. Occasionally, an electron-dense band formed by non-collagen fibrils was observed in sublingual gland close to the basement membrane of the excretory ducts. During the late intrauterine life of rat, elongated MECs were frequently seen around the acini and intercalated ducts. In contrast to the abundance of myofilaments in cell prolongation, the perinuclear

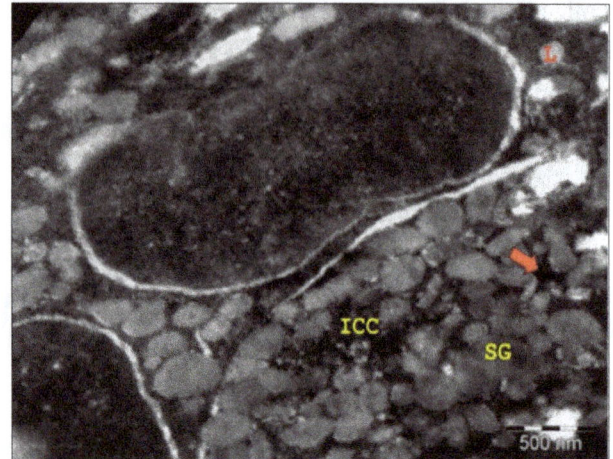

Figure-3: Transmission electron micrograph of sublingual salivary gland of 53.5 cm curved crown-rump length (194st day) buffalo fetus showing electron-lucent secretory granules (SGs), lipofuscin pigment (L), intercellular canaliculi (ICC), and mitochondria (arrow) (×8000).

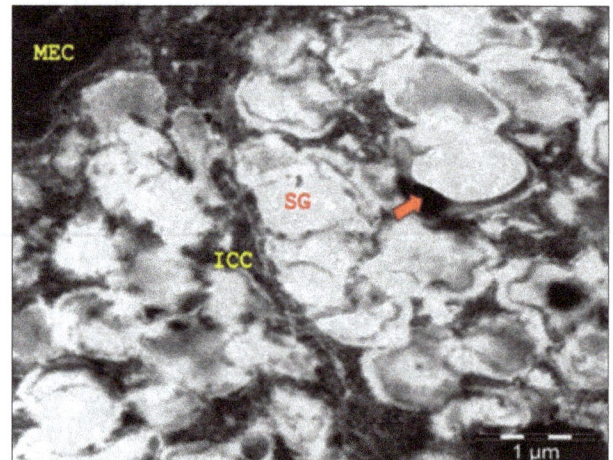

Figure-4: Transmission electron micrograph of sublingual salivary gland of 53.5 cm curved crown-rump length (194th day) buffalo fetus showing presence of myoepithelial cell (MEC) around the basement membrane of mucous cells having electron-lucent secretory granules (SGs) (ICC - Intercellular canaliculi, Arrow - Mitochondria) (×5000).

cytoplasm contained a well-developed rough ER consisting of flattened and dilated cisternae, a large amount of polyribosomes and a conspicuous Golgi complex always facing the acinar or intercalated duct cells [14].

The ultrastructure of intercalated duct cells contained few electron-dense granules. The cells appeared cuboidal to low columnar with the broader base. The apical cytoplasm of the epithelial cells lining the intercalated ducts contained SGs. The basal and lateral plasma membranes of intercalated duct cells were fairly smooth with few plications, microvilli, and extensive junctional complexes. Flattened MECs with long cytoplasmic processes were observed between the epithelial cells and basement membrane of intercalated ducts. The ultrastructure of the secretory cells of rabbit sublingual gland, during last prenatal stage, was not morphologically different from that at earlier ages, except for an increase in the area of the Golgi complex in acinar cells. The larger excretory ducts were multilayered with high prismatic and basal cuboidal cells as found in adult rabbit [15].

Conclusion

It may be concluded that the cytoplasm of acinar cells was filled with mitochondria, rough ER, and Golgi profiles in mid and late fetal age groups. The SGs appeared first in the form of membrane-bound secretory vesicles with homogeneous electron-dense as well as electron-lucent contents at 21.2 cm CVRL (122nd day); however, mucous acinar cells contained electron-lucent granules, while serous secretory cells as well as serous demilunes showed electron-dense granules at 34 cm CVRL (150th day) of prenatal life. The SGs were increased in number during the late fetal age group. The MECs were located at the base of the acinar cells as well as intercalated and striated ducts and were stellate in shape. The ultrastructure of MEC revealed the parallel stream of myofilaments in the cytoplasm and its processes.

Authors' Contributions

ADS has planned and designed the study. OS analyzed the data and provided technical support. The manuscript was prepared under the guidance of OS. All authors read and approved the final manuscript.

Acknowledgments

The authors are thankful to Guru Angad Dev Veterinary and Animal Sciences University, Ludhiana for providing all type of facilities to carry out the study. The funding was provided by the Department of Science and Technology (DST), New Delhi, Government of India for research under INSPIRE program (DST-INSPIRE Fellowship, IF 120277).

Competing Interests

The authors declare that they have no competing interests.

References

1. Moghaddam, Y.F., Darvish, J., Mahdavi, S.N., Abdulamir, A.S., Mousavi, M. and Daud, S.K. (2009) Comparative histological and histochemical inter-species investigation of mammalian submandibular salivary glands. *Res. J. Appl. Sci.*, 4: 50-56.

2. Pfaffe, T., White, J.C., Beyerlein, P., Kostner, K. and Punyadeera, C. (2011) Diagnostic potential of saliva: Current state and future applications. *Clin. Chem.*, 57(5): 675-687.

3. Konig, H.E. and Liebich, H.G. (2004) Veterinary Anatomy of Domestic Animals: Textbook and Colour Atlas. 1st ed. Schattauer Co., Stuttgart, Germany, p284-286.

4. Aspinall, V. and Reilly, M.O. (2004) Introduction to Veterinary Anatomy and Physiology. An Imprint of Elsevier Ltd., London, p110-111.

5. Heinrich, I. and Johannes, Z. (2014) Salivary gland diseases in children. *GMS Curr. Topics Otorhinolaryngol. Head Neck Surg.*, 13: 1-30.

6. Wolff, M.S., Mirels, L., Lagner, J. and Hand, A.R. (2002) Development of the rat sublingual gland: A light and electron microscopic immunocytochemical study. *Anat. Rec.*, 266: 30-42.

7. Capacchietti, M., Sabbieti, M.G., Agas, D., Materazzi, S., Menghi, G. and Marchetti, L. (2009) Ultrastructure and lectin cytochemistry of secretory cells in lingual glands of the Japanese quail (*Coturnix coturnix japonica*). *Histol. Histopathol.*, 24: 1087-1096.

8. Bakry, A.M. and Iwasaki, S. (2014) Ultrastructure and histochemical study of the lingual salivary glands of some bird species. *Pak. J. Zool.*, 46: 553-559.

9. Singh, A.D. and Singh, O. (2014) Histoenzymatic studies on prenatal development of submandibular salivary gland in buffalo (*Bubalus bubalis*). *Vet. World*, 7(12): 1032-1036.

10. Raja, K., Santhi Lakshmi, M., Raghavender, K.B.P. and Purushotham, G. (2015) Prenatal development of sublingual salivary glands in the buffalo (*Bubalus bubalis*). *Indian Vet. J.*, 92(8): 31-33.

11. Soliman, M.K. (1975) Studies on the physiological chemistry of the allantoic and amniotic fluids of buffalo at various periods of pregnancy. *Indian Vet. J.*, 52: 106-111.

12. Bozolla, J.J. and Russell, L.D. (1992) Electron Microscopy: Principles and Techniques for Biologists. 2nd ed. Jones and Bartlett Publishers International, London, UK.

13. Taga, R. and Sesso, A. (2002) Ultrastructure of the rat sublingual gland during period of high proliferative activity in postnatal development. *Braz. J. Morphol. Sci.*, 19(2): 55-62.

14. Amal, A.E.B. (2013) Histological and ultrastructural evaluation of the protective effect of ginseng on gamma-irradiated rats' salivary glands. *Nat. Sci.*, 11(8): 114-121.

15. Al-Saffar, F.J. and Simawy, M.S.H. (2014) Histomorphological and histochemical study of the major salivary glands of adult local rabbits. *Int. J. Adv. Res.*, 2(11): 378-402.

18

Characterization of promoter sequence of toll-like receptor genes in Vechur cattle

R. Lakshmi[1], K. K. Jayavardhanan[1] and T. V. Aravindakshan[2]

1. Department of Veterinary Biochemistry, College of Veterinary and Animal Sciences, Thrissur, Kerala, India;
2. Centre for Advanced Studies in Animal Genetics and Breeding, College of Veterinary and Animal Sciences, Thrissur, Kerala, India.
Corresponding author: R. Lakshmi, e-mail: lakshmivetbio@gmail.com,
KKJ: jayavardhanan@kvasu.ac.in, TVA: aravindakshantv@kvasu.ac.in

Abstract

Aim: To analyze the promoter sequence of toll-like receptor (TLR) genes in Vechur cattle, an indigenous breed of Kerala with the sequence of *Bos taurus* and access the differences that could be attributed to innate immune responses against bovine mastitis.

Materials and Methods: Blood samples were collected from Jugular vein of Vechur cattle, maintained at Vechur cattle conservation center of Kerala Veterinary and Animal Sciences University, using an acid-citrate-dextrose anticoagulant. The genomic DNA was extracted, and polymerase chain reaction was carried out to amplify the promoter region of TLRs. The amplified product of TLR2, 4, and 9 promoter regions was sequenced by Sanger enzymatic DNA sequencing technique.

Results: The sequence of promoter region of TLR2 of Vechur cattle with the *B. taurus* sequence present in GenBank showed 98% similarity and revealed variants for four sequence motifs. The sequence of the promoter region of TLR4 of Vechur cattle revealed 99% similarity with that of *B. taurus* sequence but not reveals significant variant in motifregions. However, two heterozygous loci were observed from the chromatogram. Promoter sequence of TLR9 gene also showed 99% similarity to *B. taurus* sequence and revealed variants for four sequence motifs.

Conclusion: The results of this study indicate that significant variation in the promoter of TLR2 and 9 genes in Vechur cattle breed and may potentially link the influence the innate immunity response against mastitis diseases.

Keywords: mastitis, promoter, sequence, toll-like receptor, Vechur breed.

Introduction

Toll-like receptors (TLRs) are critical sensors of microbial attack and effectors of the TLR dependent innate defense mechanism, enabling the host to eliminate pathogens that otherwise would cause disease or mortality [1]. TLRs recognize a wide variety of pathogen-associated molecular patterns (PAMPs) from bacteria, viruses, and fungi as well as some of the host molecules which in turn trigger intracellular signal transduction cascades that result in the expression of pro-inflammatory cytokines, chemokines, and antiviral molecules [2]. So far, 13 TLRs have been identified in mammals of which 10 TLRs are known to occur in cattle, and the expression of TLR transcripts varies among different mammalian species. Among the members of TLR family, TLR2, 4, and 9 play an essential role in both innate immunity and adaptive immune response by ligand recognition and signal transduction. TLR2 is essential for the recognition of a variety of PAMPs from Gram-positive bacteria, including bacterial lipoproteins, lipomannans, and lipoteichoic acids, whereas TLR4 is predominantly activated by lipopolysaccharides [3]. TLR9 is a pattern recognition receptor that plays a key role in cell survival through recognition of various bacterial components including unmethylated CpG-DNA [4]. The expression of TLR 2, 4, and 9 are critical sensors of innate defense against bacterial infection.

Vechur cattle, a rare breed of *Bos indicus*, are an indigenous breed of Kerala, and it is the smallest cattle breed in the world. They are well adapted for the hot, humid tropical climate of Kerala and are high disease resistant. In dairy industry, mastitis is considered to be one of the expensive diseases and a major economic issue for dairy farmers [5]. In India, the economic loss due to mastitis is about 2500 million per annum. Vechur breeds are not prone to mastitis. Characterization of factors involved in the innate immune system of this breed might provide an insight into the mechanisms involved in the disease resistance.

The promoter region of a gene, through binding of a specific transcription factor, is directly involved in gene transcription initiation. Therefore, sequence variation in this region may alter transcription factor binding sites, which in turn can affect gene expression and exert biological impacts [6]. Given their key role as sentinels of the innate immune defense, TLR structure, and function are tightly regulated. Numerous attempts have been made to identify variation affecting TLR structural genes, but studies on genetic variation in the promoter region of TLRs gene are relatively rare, and their contribution to disease remains unclear. In this study, promoter sequence of TLR2, 4, and 9 genes in Vechur cattle breed was examined and accessed the differences that could be attributed to innate immune responses against bovine mastitis.

Materials and Methods

Ethical approval

The study was approved by the committee framed for the research by the university authority. Adequate measures were taken to minimize pain or discomfort in accordance with the International Animal Ethics Committee.

Experimental animals and DNA extraction

Blood samples were collected using acid-citrate-dextrose anticoagulant from Jugular vein of Vechur cattle, maintained at Vechur cattle conservation center of Kerala Veterinary and Animal Sciences University. The genomic DNA was extracted by phenol-chloroform method. The DNA concentration was assessed by NanoDrop (Thermo Scientific, USA) spectrophotometer, and the purity was confirmed by measuring absorbance at 260 nm and 280 nm, followed by quality of the DNA was also assessed by agarose gel (1%) electrophoresis.

Primer designing and polymerase chain reaction (PCR) amplifications

Primers used to amplify the promoter region of TLR2 (AC_000174), TLR4 (AC_000165), and TLR9 (AC_000179) genes in Vechur cattle were designed from *Bos taurus* sequences available in National Centre for Biotechnology Information (NCBI) database. Primers were designed using an online tool from NCBI, Primer-BLAST. The designed forward and reverse primers were custom synthesized at Sigma-Aldrich India (Table-1). The primers were reconstituted in nuclease-free water to a concentration of 10 p M/µl.

The promoter regions of TLRs were amplified through PCR. 20 µL of PCR were carried out in 0.2 mL PCR tube and each tube contained 2 µL of genomic DNA (50 ng) as template, 1 µl of each forward primer and reverse primer (10 pM/µl), ×2 concentration of 10 µl of PCR reaction mix (contain dNTPs- 0.4 mM each, Taq polymerase-0.05 U/µl, magnesium chloride-4 mM), and 6 µL of nuclease-free water. PCR conditions followed for amplification of promoter region of TLR2, 4, and 9 genes are presented in Table-2. Amplified PCR products were separated by agarose gel electrophoresis (1.5%) and visualized by ethidium bromide staining.

Sequencing and analysis

The purified PCR products of the promoter regions of TLR2, 4, and 9 genes were commercially sequenced by Sanger's enzymatic DNA sequencing

Table-1: Primers designed for TLR promoter regions from NCBI databank sequences.

Target	Primer sequence (5′→3′)	Size
Promoter region of TLR2	Forward TGTGGCATCTCTCGTTTCCT	934 bp
	Reverse CTGGTTACTCTGCTCCCTGA	
Promoter region of TLR4	Forward GTCCCTTGCTCTATCAGGCA	898 bp
	Reverse ATGCTGTCCCCTTGGCTTAT	
Promoter region of TLR9	Forward CTGGGGTAGGGGCTTTATAAGA	1005 bp
	Reverse CCATCTGTCACATCCCACGT	

TLR=Toll-like receptor

Table-2: PCR program for amplification of TLR promoter region in Vechur cattle.

Steps	Temperature and time
Initial denaturation	95°C for 3 min
Denaturation	95°C for 30 s
Annealing	53.2°C for 30 s for TLR2
	56.0°C for 30 s for TLR4
	53.0°C for 30 s for TLR9
Extension	72°C for 1 min
	Step 2 to 4 set for 35 cycles
Final extension	72°C for 5 min

TLR=Toll-like receptor, PCR=Polymerase chain reaction

technique. The nucleotide sequences for the promoter of TLR2, 4, and 9 genes were submitted to GenBank. Sequence alignment of Vechur breed promoter regions of TLR2, 4, and 9 genes with *B. taurus* sequences was performed using CLUSTALW.

Results and Discussion

Bovine mastitis, defined as an inflammation of the mammary gland, is generally considered the most economically imposing diseases of dairy cattle. Financial losses due to mastitis occur for animals experiencing both subclinical and clinical disease. Subclinical mastitis is the most economically important form of mastitis because of long-term reductions in milk yield. Vechur cattle breed found in Kerala state are known for less susceptible to mastitis than any other cattle breeds. The marked differences in susceptibility to mastitis predict that there is substantial variation in the efficiency of the antimicrobial defense within the cattle breeds. Yet, the mechanisms underlying exaggerated or attenuated response of Vechur breed to mastitis remain unclear. As TLRs are essential for innate immunity, understanding the genetic basis of varied TLRs receptor expression and function is of great importance for the many biological end points that depend on TLRs signaling. The promoter region of TLRs plays a key role in the transcription of genes. Promoter region consists of various consensus sequences, capable of regulating the rate of transcription by inducing or suppressing the respective genes. TLR2, 4, and 9 are reported as critical sensors of innate defense against bovine mastitis [3]. In this study, sequence variation of these TLRs promoter region in Vechur breed was examined for the important regulatory motifs that might influence the expression of TLR genes and innate immune response dynamics against bovine mastitis.

The promoter region of TLR2, 4, and 9 of Vechur cattle was successfully amplified using specific primer pairs. The sizes of amplified products were verified using agarose gel electrophoresis (Figure-1). Nucleotide sequences for promoter regions of these TLRs genes were deposited in GenBank and assigned with the following accession numbers: TLR2 promoter, KR559022.1; TLR4 promoter, KR559023.1; TLR4 promoter, KR559024.1.

TLR2 is essential for the recognition of a variety of PAMPs from Gram-positive bacteria. TLR2 forms heterodimers with TLR1 or TLR6, each dimer having different ligand specificity thus increasing its binding receptors. TLR2 mRNA expression was strongly increased in mammary tissue in cattle. The promoter sequences of TLRs genes in Vechur cattle were assessed with *B. taurus* for the important sequence motifs, consensus sequence, and their functions. The sequence of promoter region of TLR2 of Vechur cattle with the *B. taurus* sequence present in GenBank showed 98% similarity and revealed variants for four sequence motifs. All of these motifs were located in sequences with a high degree of homology

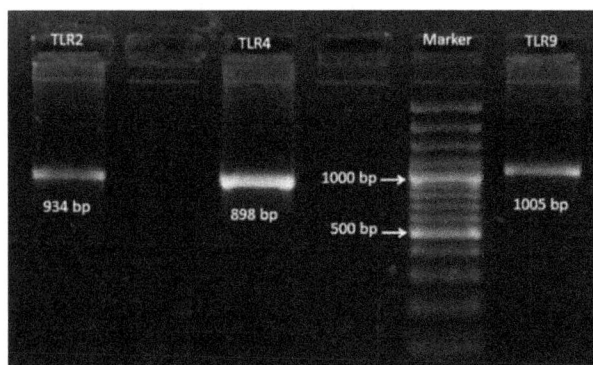

Figure-1: Polymerase chain reaction product size of toll-like receptor 2, 4, and 9 promoter region.

to possible transcription factor binding site. The important sequence motif and variations observed in Vechur cattle with that of *B. taurus* sequence are listed in Table-3 and also highlighted in Figure-2.

A consensus TATA boxwas observed in the promoter sequence of TLR2 gene of Vechur, which might consider as the core promoter for transcription initiation [7], to which RNA polymerase II binds is found to be present in the region between −726 and −723 bp. In addition, TATA-like sequences such as TATAA also present in the region of −85 to −81 bp and −752 to −748 bp with one single nucleotide polymorphism (SNP) at bp −751 in Vechur cattle. The AT-rich region of TATA box can facilitate easy unwinding of DNA due to weak interaction between the bases than GC during initiation of transcription.

Cyclic adenosine monophosphate (cAMP) responsive elements (CRE) are ubiquitous regulator of inflammatory and immunological reactions [8]. CRE is expressed in a wide variety of cell types. It has been established that cAMP induces phosphorylation of CRE, which then activates cAMP-responsive genes, leading to increased cell proliferation, differentiation, or modulation of various cell functions [9]. TLR2 found to be mediated by cAMP production [8]. CRE-like sequence (TGACGTCA) is detected at two positions in both *B. taurus* and Vechur sequence. First, CRE is positioned at −379 to −372 bp with one SNP at bp −375 in both Vechur cattle and *B. taurus,* and second, CRE is positioned at −470 to −463 bp is observed with three mismatch base pair in Vechur and two mismatch base pair in *B. taurus.*

Nuclear factor-kappa B (NF-kB) transcription factor was observed at position −440 to −431 bp with two mismatch base pairs in both Vechur and *B. taurus* sequence with reference consensus sequence. NF-kB consists of a family of transcription factor that play critical roles in inflammation, immunity, cell proliferation, differentiation, and survival [10]. This NF-kB plays an important role in the regulation of TLR2 gene expression [11]. The special protein binding sites (Sp site), which enhance the expression of TLR2 gene [12] is also present in the region between −571

Table-3: Important sequence motifs and variants observed in the TLR2 promoter region of *B. taurus* and Vechur cattle breed.

Motif	Consensus sequence	Region	*B.taurus* sequence	Vechur sequence
TATA sequence	TATA	−726 to−723	TATA	TATA
		−85 to 81	TATAA	TATAA
		−752 to−748	TATAA	T**C**TAA
CRE	TGACGTCA	−379 to−372	TGAC**T**TCA	TGAC**T**TCA
		−470 to−463	TGA**AT**TCA	TG**GAT**TCA
E-box	CANNTTG	−200 to−195	CATATG	CATATG
EC	GTGG (A/T)(A/T)(A/T)	−645 to−639	GTGGAAA	GTGGAAA
CAAT	CAAT	−11 to−8	CAAT	CAAT
NF-kB	GGGRNNYYCC, R-purine, Y-pyrimidine	-440 to -431	GGGAAAT**AT**C	GGGAAAT**AT**C
IRF	GAAANNGAAAGG	−73 to−62	GAAAGAGAAA**AA**	GAAAGAGAAA**AA**
Sp-1 site	GGGCGG	−571 to−567	**A**GGCG	**G**GGCG

EC=Enhancer core, TLR=Toll-like receptor, CRE=Cyclic adenosine monophosphate responsive elements, NF-kB=Nuclear factor-kappa B, IRF=Interferon regulatory factor 3, *B. taurus=Bos taurus*

and −567 bp in Vechur, whereas *B. taurus* reveals one mismatch at −571 bp.

In the present study, the sequence of the promoter region of TLR4 of Vechur cattle revealed 99% similarity with that of *B. taurus* sequence and had important motifs such as TATA, CAAT, E-box, NF-kB, CRE, and CpG regions required for regulation of transcription but not reveals significant variant in motif regions. The important sequence motif for TLR4 observed in Vechur cattle with that of *B. taurus* sequence are

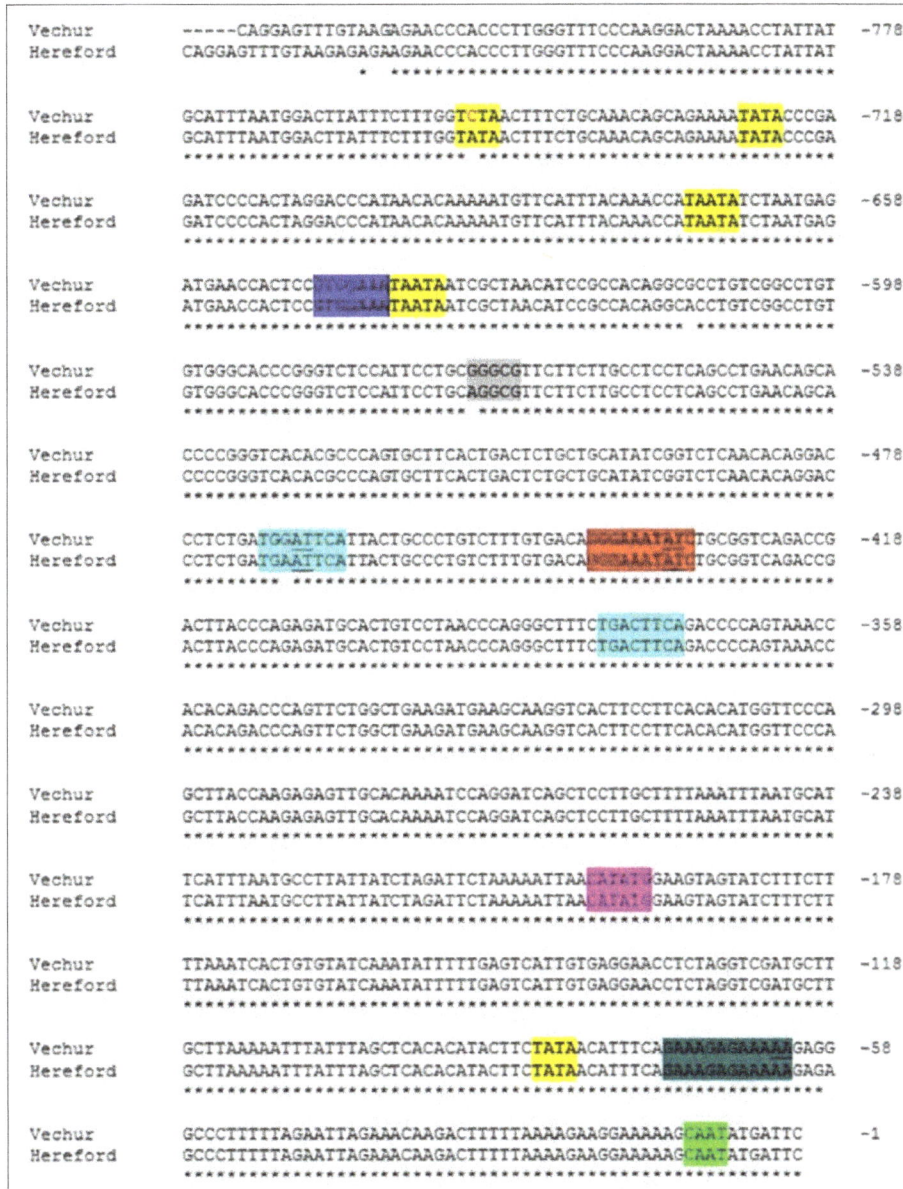

Figure-2: Sequence alignment of toll-like receptor 2 promoter region of Vechur cattle breed and *Bos taurus* (Hereford) highlighted with important motifs.

Table-4: Important sequence motifs and variants observed in the TLR4 promoter region of *B. taurus* and Vechur cattle breed.

Motif	Consensus sequence	Region	*Bos taurus* sequence	Vechur sequence
TATA	TATA	−513 to−510 −101 to−98	TATA	TATA
E-box	CANNTTG	−823 to−818	CATGTG	CATGTG
CRE	TGACGTCA	−17 to−10	TGACGT<u>G</u>A	TGACGT<u>G</u>A
CAAT	CAAT	−732 to−729 −229 to−226	CAAT	CAAT
NF-kB	GGGRNNYYCC, R-purine, Y-pyrimidine	−92 to−81	GGGTGGC<u>TCT</u>	GGGTGGC<u>TCT</u>
Sp-1 site	GGGCGG	−284 to−278	GGGCGG	GGGCGG

EC=Enhancer core, TLR=Toll-like receptor, CRE=Cyclic adenosine monophosphate responsive elements, NF-kB=Nuclear factor-kappa B, *B. taurus=Bos taurus*

listed in Table-4 and highlighted in Figure-3. TLR4 plays an important role in the induction of the inflammatory response by recognizing exogenous PAMPs and endogenous ligands [13]. TLR4 is linked to the activation of NF-κB factor in several cell types [14]. Increased NF-κB activity was found in the milk and intra-mammary epithelial cells of mastitis-affected cows. Although Vechur promoter sequence of TLR4 did not show any polymorphism with *B. taurus* sequence, however, chromatograph reveals two heterozygous conditions in Vechur breed (Figure-4).

Promoter sequence of TLR9 gene also showed 99% similarity to *B. taurus* sequence and revealed variants for four sequence motifs. The sequence variation in TLR9 promoter region for the important motifis presented in Table-5 and Figure-5. TLR9, which is localized intracellularly, is involved in the recognition

of specific unmethylated CpG-oligodeoxynucleotides (ODN) sequences that distinguish bacterial DNA from mammalian DNA. Bacterial DNA can stimulate immune cells mainly because of the unmethylated CpG motifs, which are rarely detected in vertebrate DNA, and if present, are highly methylated. Species difference in TLR9 expression during mastitis exists as CpG-ODN has been shown to promote the expression of its specific receptor (TLR9 mRNA) in goat mammary tissue [15].

The promoter sequence of TLR9 in Vechur and *B. taurus* shows variation for enhancer core (EC) region, CAAT box, nuclear factor-kappa binding protein, and Sp-1 binding site. EC region is expressed in a variety of tissues, and transgenic animal studies have demonstrated that EC region plays a critical role in thymocyte and macrophage development [16]. Three EC regions were observed in the sequence of Vechur

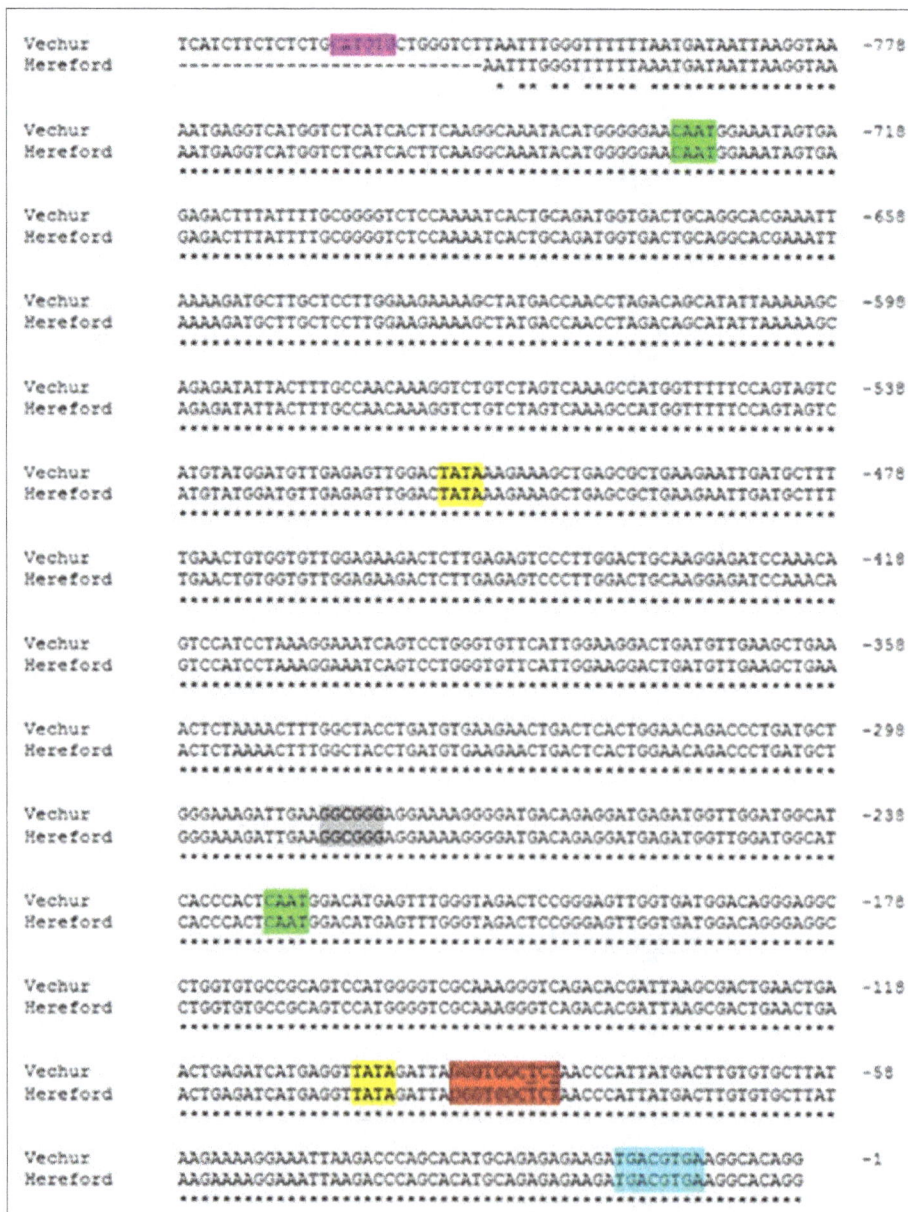

Figure-3: Sequence alignment of toll-like receptor 4 promoter region of Vechur cattle breed and *Bos taurus* (Hereford) highlighted with important motifs.

cattle. CAAT box region also found in Vechur, however, *B. taurus* sequence reveals variation for this box at −307 bp. ECs, CAAT enhancer binding protein might physically and functionally interact with each other, leading to maximal transcription of the TLR9 gene [17].

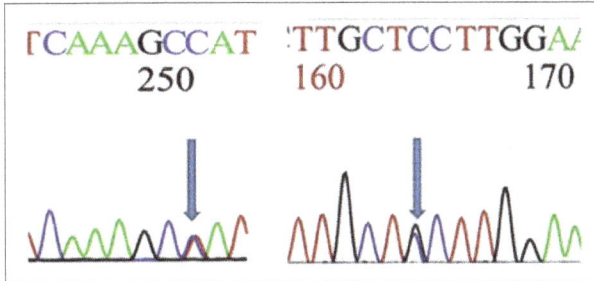

Figure-4: Sequence chromatographs reveal heterozygous peaks in the promoter region of toll-like receptor 4 gene.

NF-kB was observed at three positions; one SNP was observed in both Vechur and *B. taurus* at −307 bp, respectively. Vechur sequence also reveals another SNP in the NF-kB region of −61 bp. Sp1 binding sites were noticed at two regions, no variation was observed between Vechur and consensus sequence for this binding sites, however, *B. taurus* reveals an SNP at −403 bp.

Conclusion

The TLR2 and TLR9 promoter regions are considerably more variable than TLR4 in Vechur breed to that of *B. taurus* as revealed by four different important motifs which further identified with SNPs. TATA and CAT boxes and multiple putative binding sites present in the TLR2 and TLR9 promoter sequences may influence the transcription. This study is, therefore, the first to propose that genetic variation in the

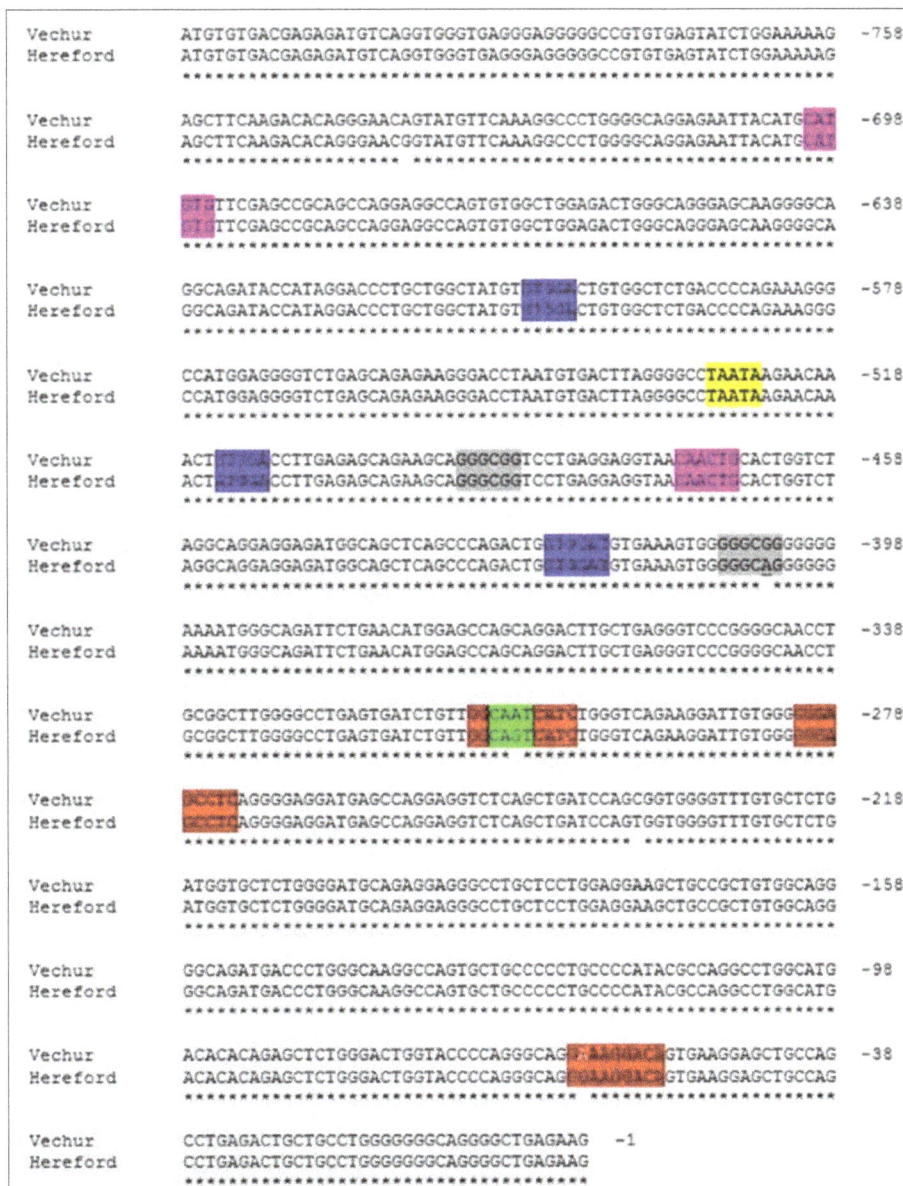

Figure-5: Sequence alignment of toll-like receptor 9 promoter region of Vechur cattle breed and *Bos taurus* (Hereford) highlighted with important motifs.

Table-5: Important sequence motifs and variants observed in the TLR9 promoter region of *B. taurus* and Vechur cattle breed.

Motif	Consensus sequence	Region	*B. taurus* sequence	Vechur sequence
TATA sequence	TATA	−529 to−525	T**A**ATA	T**A**ATA
E-box	CANNTTG	−700 to−695	CATGTG	CATGTG
		−72 to−467	CAACTG	CAACTG
EC	GTGG (A/T) (A/T) (A/T)	−606 to−602	GTGGA	GTGGA
		−514 to−510	GTGGA	GTGGA
		−424 to−419	GTGGAT	GTGGAT
CAAT	CAAT	−309 to−306	CA**G**T	CAAT
NF-kB	GGGRNNYYCC, R-purine, Y-pyrimidine	−281 to−271	GGGAGCCTC	GGGAGCCTC
		−311 to−302	GGCA**G**TCATC	GGCA**A**TCATC
		−62 to−54	GGAAGGACA	G**A**AAGGACA
Sp-1 site	GGGCGG	−492 to−487	GGGCG**G**	GGGCGG
		−408 to−402	GGGGC**A**G	GGGGCGG

EC=Enhancer core, TLR=Toll-like receptor, NF-kB=Nuclear factor-kappa B, *B. taurus=Bos taurus*

TLRs promoter might influence the TLRs expression. A significant finding is the identification of SNPs in the promoter of TLR2 and 9 genes in Vechur cattle breed. The variation in TLR promoter sequence of Vechur breed might potentially influence the innate immunity response against mastitis.

Authors' Contributions

RL - The research work mentioned in this article is a part of the Ph.D. research work of the first author and first author carried out all the work mentioned in this article. KKJ - The entire work mentioned in this article was carried out under the guidance and supervision of the second author. TVA- Member of research advisory committee reviewed the manuscript. All authors read and approved the final manuscript.

Acknowledgments

The first author acknowledging the INSPIRE Fellowship program of Department of Science and Technology, Ministry of Science and Technology, Government of India, for providing fellowship for the Ph.D. program. The authors are thankful to the Dean, College of Veterinary and Animal Science, for providing facilities to conduct this experiment.

Competing Interests

The authors declare that they have no competing interests.

References

1. Uematsu, S. and Akira, S. (2006) Toll-like receptors and innate immunity. *J. Mol. Med.*, 84: 712-725.
2. Akira, S. and Hemmi, H. (2003) Recognition of pathogen associated molecular patterns by TLR family. *Immonol. Lett.*, 85: 85-95.
3. Fernando, N., Eduardo, M.R.S., Marcos, B.H., Magnus, A.G., Luiza, C.R., Maiara, G.B. and Alice, M.M. (2012) The innate immunity in ovine mastitis: The role of pattern-recognition receptors. *Am. J. Immunol.*, 8: 166-178.
4. Tanaka, J., Sugimoto, K., Shiraki, K., Tameda, M., Kusagawa, S., Nojiri, K., Beppu, T., Yoneda, K., Yamamoto, N., Uchida, K., Kojima, T. and Takei, Y. (2010)

Functional cell surface expression of toll-like receptor 9 promotes cell proliferation and survival in human hepatocellular carcinomas. *Int. J. Oncol.*, 37: 805-814.
5. Hogeveen, H., Huijps, K. and Lam, T.J.G. (2011) Economic aspects of mastitis: New developments. *N. Z. Vet. J.*, 59: 16-23.
6. Muhaghegh-Dolatabady, H. and Habibizad, J. (2014) Sequence characterization of promoter region at the melanocortin-1 receptor (MC1R) gene in karakul sheep breed. *J. Agric. Sci. Technol.*, 16: 551-560.
7. Viola, H., Lucia, S., Matthew, J.F. and Michal, R. (2002) Transcription regulation of the human toll-like receptor 2 gene in monocytes and macrophages. *J. Immunol.*, 168: 5629-5637.
8. Eun, Y.M., Yu, S.L., Wahn, S.C. and Mi, H.L. (2011) Toll-like receptor 4 mediated cAMP production upregulates B-cell activating factor expression in raw264.7 macrophages. *Sci. Direct*, 317: 2447-2455.
9. Blobel, G.A. (2000) CREB-binding protein and p300: Molecular integrators of hematopoietic transcription. *Blood*, 95: 745.
10. Oeckinghaus, A. and Ghosh, S. (2009) The NF-kB family of transcription factors and its regulation. *Cold Spring Harb. Perspect. Biol.*, 1: 1-14.
11. Musikacharoen, T., Matsuguchi, T., Kikuchi, T. and Yoshikai, Y. (2001) NF-kB and STAT5 play important roles in the regulation of mouse toll-like receptor 2 gene expression. *J. Immunol.*, 166: 4516-4524.
12. Haehnel, V., Schwarzfischer, L., Fenton, M.J. and Rehli, M. (2002) Transcription regulation of the human toll-like receptor 2 gene in monocytes and macrophages. *J. Immunol.*, 168: 5629-5637.
13. Miyake, K. (2007) Innate immune sensing of pathogens and danger signals by cell surface toll-like receptors. *Semin. Immunol.*, 19: 3-10.
14. Kuhn, H., Petzold, K., Hammerschmidt, S. and Wirtz, H. (2014) Interaction of cyclic mechanical stretch and toll-like receptor 4-mediated innate immunity in rat alveolar Type II cells. *Respirology*, 19: 67-73.
15. Zhu, Y.M., Miao, J.F., Zhang, Y.S., Li, Z., Zou, S.X. and Deng, Y.E. (2007) CpG ODN enhances mammary gland defense during mastitis induced by *Escherichia coli* infection in goats. *Vet. Immunol. Immunopathol.*, 120: 168-176.
16. Zaldumbide, A., Carlotti, F., Pognonec, P. and Boulukos, K.E. (2002) The role of the Ets2 transcription factor in the proliferation, maturation, and survival of mouse thymocytes. *J. Immunol.*, 169: 4873.
17. Takeshita, F., Leifer, C.A., Gursel, I., Iashii, K.L., Takeshita, S., Gursel, M. and Klinman, D.M. (2001) Transcriptional regulation of the human TLR9 gene. *J. Immunol.*, 173: 2552-2561.

19

Effect of *in ovo* supplementation of nano forms of zinc, copper, and selenium on post-hatch performance of broiler chicken

P. Patric Joshua[1], C. Valli[2] and V. Balakrishnan[3]

1. Department of Pharmacology, Sri Muthukumaran Medical College Hospital and Research Institute, Dr. M.G.R. Medical University, Chennai, Tamil Nadu, India; 2. Department of Animal Nutrition, Institute of Animal Nutrition, Tamil Nadu Veterinary and Animal Sciences University, Chennai, Tamil Nadu, India; 3. Department of Animal Nutrition, Madras Veterinary College, Tamil Nadu Veterinary and Animal Sciences University, Chennai, Tamil Nadu, India.
Corresponding author: P. Patric Joshua, e-mail: patricvet@gmail.com, CV: valliviba@yahoo.co.in, VB: drbalakrishnanphd@yahoo.co.in

Abstract

Background and Aim: Nanoparticles can bypass conventional physiological ways of nutrient distribution and transport across tissue and cell membranes, as well as protect compounds against destruction prior to reaching their targets. *In ovo* administration of nanoparticles, may be seen as a new method of nano-nutrition, providing embryos with an additional quantity of nutrients. The aim of the study is to examine the effect of *in ovo* supplementation of nano forms of zinc, copper and selenium on the hatchability and post hatch performance of broiler chicken.

Materials and Methods: Nano form of zinc at 20, 40, 60 and 80 μg/egg, nano form of copper at 4, 8, 12 and 16 μg/egg and nano form of selenium at 0.075, 0.15, 0.225 and 0.3 μg/egg were *in ovo* supplemented (18th day incubation, amniotic route) in fertile broiler eggs. Control group *in ovo* fed with normal saline alone was also maintained. Each treatment had thirty replicates. Parameters such as hatchability, hatch weight and post hatch performance were studied.

Results: *In ovo* feeding of nano minerals were not harmful to the developing embryo and did not influence the hatchability. Significantly ($p < 0.05$) best feed efficiency for nano forms of zinc (2.16), copper (2.46) and selenium (2.51) were observed, when 40, 4 and 0.225 μg/egg respectively were *in ovo* supplemented. Except in nano form of copper at 12 μg per egg which had significantly ($p < 0.05$) highest breast muscle percentage there was no distinct trend to indicate that dressing percentage or breast muscle yield was influenced in other treatments.

Conclusion: Nano forms of zinc, copper and selenium can be prepared at laboratory conditions. *In ovo* feeding of nano forms of zinc, copper and selenium at 18th day of incubation through amniotic route does not harm the developing embryo, does not affect hatchability.

Keywords: hatchability, hatch weight, *in ovo* feeding, nanoparticles, and post hatch performance.

Introduction

Indian poultry sector has been growing at around 8-10% annually over the last decade with broiler meat volumes growing at more than 10%, and table egg growing at 5-6% [1]. The growth of the industry can be attributed to the production performance of commercial poultry which has grown linearly every year, and the trend is likely to continue in future with the advent of development in the field of genetics, nutrition, biotechnology, developmental biology, etc. Early nutritional strategies offer the promise of sustaining progress in production efficiency and welfare of commercial poultry [2].

One-way to give hatchlings a nutritional jump start before they start eating feed is to feed them before they hatch (*In ovo* feeding). *In ovo* injection technology developed and patented by Uni and Ferket [3] provides a method to safely introduce external nutrients into developing embryos. During late embryogenesis, solutions injected into the amniotic fluid are subsequently swallowed, digested, and absorbed by the embryo before piping [4]. Rapid growth coupled with a high nutrient requirement, especially during late embryogenesis, may make *in ovo* feeding of supplemental nutrients beneficial to poultry. Supplementing the amnion with appropriate nutrients is a novel way to feed critical dietary nutrients to embryos. Mineral reserves in yolk decrease significantly from the day of setting; this leaves the embryo with low mineral reserves for the last period of incubation and probably leads to a mineral deficiency status of the embryo [5]. *In ovo* feeding of minerals has also gained importance as the high-metabolism, fast-growing broiler embryos may reach levels of mineral deficiency that can lead to metabolic disorders [6].

In ovo feeding could lead to improved digestive capacity, increased growth rate and feed efficiency, reduced post-hatch mortality and morbidity, improved immune response to enteric antigens, reduced incidence of developmental skeletal disorders, and increased muscle development and breast meat yield [7].

The *in ovo* injection of L-carnitine has shown many beneficial effects in post-hatch performance [8,9]. The protection level against *Salmonella enteritidis* was evaluated in chickens after *in ovo* treatment with different species of *Lactobacillus* spp. inoculated into the air cell or by immersion in broth culture [10]. *In ovo* fed birds exhibited higher glycogen reserves, body weight, pectoral muscle weight and body weight gain than control birds [11]. The *in ovo* administration of manan oligosaccharides (MOS) showed a short-term effect resulting in a hatching chick with more mature enterocytes in the small intestine and enhanced digestive capacity and epithelial barrier, which can, in turn, improve development and growth in the 1st days after hatch. The beneficial effects of MOS began 72 h after *in ovo* administration and lasted at least until date of hatch [12].

Zinc plays a role in the development of the immune system of the broiler embryo [13,14]. In a large number of studies, additional zinc used in the diet of broilers has improved antibody production [15]. Zinc is crucial for normal development and function of cells mediating non-specific immunity such as neutrophils and natural killer cells [16]. Effects of dietary copper-loaded chitosan nanoparticle (CNP-Cu) supplementation on growth performance, hematological and immunological characteristics and the cecal microbiota in broilers were investigated. Results indicated that supplemental CNP-Cu could improve growth performance; affect the immune system [17]. Selenium supplementation in experimental animals has been shown to be associated with increases in natural killer cell activity, T-cell proliferation, lymphokine-activated killer cell activity, delayed-type hypersensitivity skin responses, and vaccine-induced immunity [18]. Examination of the effect of *in ovo* enrichment of phosphorus (P), calcium (Ca), iron (Fe), zinc (Zn), copper (Cu), and manganese (Mn) along with vitamins, amino acids and carbohydrates showed that the enrichment resulted in increased iron, zinc, copper, and manganese levels in the yolk even though the minerals are supplemented in the amniotic fluid [19]. This research study is the first of its kind in exploring the significant beneficial effects of nano forms of zinc, copper, and selenium when fed *in ovo*.

Nanoparticles have different physical and chemical characteristics compared to their larger equivalents because of a very high surface to volume ratio, physical activity, and chemical stability. The small size of nanoparticles allows for penetration inside tissues and even enables them to cross cell membranes. Nanoparticles can bypass conventional physiological ways of nutrient distribution and transport across tissue and cell membranes, as well as protect compounds against destruction before reaching their targets.

In ovo administration of nanoparticles, acting as bioactive agents and as carriers of nutrients may be seen as a new method of nano-nutrition, providing embryos with bioactive compounds and/or with an additional quantity of nutrients or energy. Nutrient supplementation through *in ovo* was reported to be a more efficient when a compound was attached to nanoparticles (silver or gold), which delivered it inside the body tissues and cells [20]. It is with this background a research was carried out wherein the post-hatch performance of broiler chicken *in ovo* supplemented with nano forms of zinc, copper, and selenium was studied. Thus, the aim of this research study is to examine the effect of *in ovo* supplementation of nano forms of zinc, copper and selenium on the hatchability and post-hatch performance of broiler chicken.

Materials and Methods

Ethical approval

No Ethical Committee approval was necessary for this study as we conducted experiment on broiler chicken with a lifespan of about 5-6 weeks. However, we conducted experiment under very fine confinement without giving any undue stress to the birds.

Experimental design

In an earlier study, Bakyaraj *et al.* [21] recommended *in ovo* feeding levels for zinc, copper and selenium as 80, 16 and 0.3 µg, respectively/egg. For this study, these levels were considered as 100% of the requirement of the respective minerals. The efficacy of the respective nano minerals *viz.* zinc, copper and selenium at four graded levels (25%, 50%, 75% and 100%) were tested. A control group wherein only normal saline was *in ovo* fed was maintained. Each egg was weighed and randomly distributed into respective treatment groups (Table-1) maintaining similar average weight across treatment groups. In each treatment, 30 eggs were set in the incubator in three separate groups so that the hatch record could be maintained for three replicates per treatment. Thus, each nano mineral had five treatments (four graded levels and one control).

Production of nano forms of zinc, copper, and selenium and their characterization

Nano form of zinc, copper, and selenium was produced in triplicate adopting the procedure as explained in this section. Nano form of zinc was produced by a chemical method using starch as a stabilizing agent. Starch solution (0.5%) was prepared and 20-50 ml of 0.2 M zinc acetate dihydrate was added with few drops of 0.2 M of sodium hydroxide. The pH was adjusted to 8.5 using 0.2 M NaOH. The contents were stirred continuously at 100°C. A milky white colloid was obtained; the colloid was stirred for 2 h and centrifuged at 9000 rpm for 15 min. The sediment was filtered and washed using initially acetone, followed by ethanol and water. After which the sediment was dried in hot air oven at 80°C for 3 h. Thus, produced

Table-1: Treatment groups experimented to assess optimum level of nano forms of zinc, copper and selenium required to be fed *in ovo* to fertile broiler eggs.

Treatment	Normal saline ml/egg	Percent inclusion of nano form of minerals	Nano form of minerals µg/egg
Control	0.5 ml	0	0
Nano form of zinc	0.5 ml	25	20
	0.5 ml	50	40
	0.5 ml	75	60
	0.5 ml	100	80
Control	0.5 ml	0	0
Nano form of copper	0.5 ml	25	4
	0.5 ml	50	8
	0.5 ml	75	12
	0.5 ml	100	16
Control	0.5 ml	0	0
Nano form of selenium	0.5 ml	25	0.075
	0.5 ml	50	0.15
	0.5 ml	75	0.225
	0.5 ml	100	0.3

nano form of zinc's yield was determined and characterized [22].

Nano form of copper was produced by electrochemical method. An indigenous laboratory electrolysis unit was fabricated and feed grade copper sulfate solution was subjected to electrolysis using copper rods as anode and cathode. The flow of a steady current into the electrolytic cell caused the ionization and disassociation of copper sulfate solution which removed the copper from the anode and deposited it in the cathode. Such deposited copper, was collected dried, yield determined, and characterized [23].

Nano form of selenium was prepared by adopting the procedure of Razi *et al.* [24]. Selenium powder 0.1 g was mixed with 2.4 g sodium hydroxide in 40 ml of distilled water. The contents were maintained at a temperature of 140°C for 1 h. The contents were then cooled to room temperature, filtered and washed using water and ethanol. The residue was dried yield determined and characterized.

The size and zeta potential of the nano zinc, copper, and selenium produced was determined using particle size analyzer (Malvern make Model No. 2000). The zinc, copper and selenium content of the respective samples from each of the method were determined using Atomic Absorption Spectrophotometer (Perkin-Elmer, Model 3110, 1994) as per the procedure outlined in the reference manual.

Fumigation and incubation

A total of 390 fertile broiler eggs (Vencobb 400) were procured, fumigation of all the eggs was carried out in a fumigation hood. Fumigation was done using 57 g of potassium permanganate (×1 concentration) and 85 ml of formalin (×1.5 concentration). The eggs were set in an incubator with setter temperature of 100°F and relative humidity of 85%. Eggs were candled on 7th and 14th day to remove infertile eggs.

***In ovo* feeding procedure**

On 18th day of incubation, candling of eggs were carried out and amniotic route was marked and a small pinpoint hole was made in the broad end of the egg to remove the egg shell by using Topaz Engraver as egg driller and *in ovo* supplementation was done according to the treatments through the amniotic route using a 24G hypodermic needle (25 mm long) and the pinpoint hole was sealed using wax [25]. The eggs were placed back in incubator with hatcher temperature of 100°F and relative humidity of 90%.

Parameters studied

Parameters studied included hatchability, hatch weight of chicks, chick weight is to egg weight ratio, post-hatch performance relating to weight gain, feed efficiency, and slaughter studies. The percent hatchability was determined using the following formulae:

$$\text{Percent hatchability} = \frac{\text{Number of chicks hatched on 21 days}}{\text{Number of eggs that were } in~ovo \text{ fed}} \times 100$$

The hatch weight of chicks was determined by weighing the chicks in an electronic weighing balance and expressed in grams. The chick weight is to egg weight ratio was determined using the following formula:

$$\text{Chick weight is to egg weight ratio} = \frac{\text{Chick weight (g)}}{\text{Egg weight (g)}} \times 100$$

To study the post-hatch performance 20 chicks from each treatment were weighed, wings banded, maintained in their same respective groups and were reared for a period of 5 weeks. The experimental birds were housed in five-tiered, well-ventilated battery cages provided with artificial lighting.

The standard managemental practices were adopted, and they were uniform for all the treatment groups. All the chicks in the various treatments were fed *ad libitum* quantity of a common experimental ration. The chicks were fed with broiler starter ration from 0 to 3 weeks and broiler finisher ration from 4 to 5 weeks. Clean drinking water was provided *ad libitum.* The ingredient and nutrient composition of the experimental ration are presented in Table-2.

Every day the left over feed and wastage that spilled outside the feed trough was collected and weighed so as to record the accurate feed intake in grams. The chicks were sex corrected to calculate

Table-2: Ingredient and nutrient composition of the experimental rations.

Ingredients	Broiler starter	Broiler finisher
Ingredient composition (%)		
Maize	50	45
Bajra	-	18
Soyabean meal	32	23
De-oiled rice bran	1	-
Fish meal	10	8
Oil	4.5	4
Mineral mixture	2	1.6
L-lysine	0.1	0.05
DL-methionine	0.15	0.10
Salt	0.25	0.25
Total	100.00	100.00
Nutrient composition		
Crude protein (%)	21.73	19.78
Metabolizable energy (kcal/kg)	3160	3252
Crude fiber (%)	3.00	2.85
Calcium (%)	1.31	1.22
Availablephosphorus (%)	0.49	0.46
Lysine (%)	1.21	0.94
Methionine (%)	0.50	0.31

Additives added per 100 kg feed - Vitamin AB_2D_3K - 0.01 g, Ultracil - 0.05 g, Unicox - 0.02 g, Tefroli - 0.05 g, Ultra B_{12}-0.01 g, Perivac - 0.02 g, Spectra - 0.01 g, Larvadex - 0.05 g

weight gain and feed efficiency. The birds were weighed individually every week in a calibrated balance to document their weight gain which was expressed in grams. The feed efficiency per kilogram weight gain was calculated using the following formulae:

$$\text{Feed efficiency} = \frac{\text{Feed consumed per bird in kg}}{\text{Weight of bird in kg}} \times 100$$

At the end of the trial (5 weeks of age), six birds from each treatment were selected randomly and slaughtered by decapitation to record the live weight, carcass weight, and giblets weight. The dressing percentage and giblet percentage were calculated. Breast muscle was separated, and breast muscle yield was recorded and expressed in terms of percent dressed weight.

Statistical analysis

The design of all the experiments in this study was completely randomized design. Data were analyzed with analysis of variance as per procedure of statistical analysis system (SAS/SPPSS, 1999, version 10.0 for windows). When a significant difference ($p<0.05$) were detected, the multiple range test was used to separate the mean value.

Results and Discussion

The product yield, particle size, zeta potential, mineral content in nano forms of zinc, copper, and selenium are presented in Table-3.

The particle size of nano form of zinc, copper and selenium were below 100 nm confirming their

Table-3: Product yield, particle size, zeta potential and mineral content in nano forms of zinc, copper and selenium, respectively.

Parameters	Nano form minerals		
	Zinc	Copper	Selenium
Mean product yield (g/h)	1.0	1.0	0.1
Size (assessed through particle size analyser) nm*	78.3±0.35	72.3±0.27	74.9±0.28
Zeta potential (mV)*	−24.7±0.45	−27.2±0.27	−26.1±0.28
Mineral content (ppm)*	92.06±0.12	88.10±0.15	94.56±0.38

*Mean of three samples

nano size. Yadav et al. [26] reported a lower size (50 nm) for zinc oxide nanoparticles. Similar to this study Ramyadevi et al. [27] also reported 35-80 nm sized copper nano particles produced by polyol process. Zhang et al. [28] also had reported the size of nano red elemental selenium (Nano-Se) in the range from 20 to 60 nm.

The stability of the nano form of zinc, copper and selenium ascertained by their zeta potential, lies well within the stable limits viz. > +25 mV or < −25 mV [29]. The respective mineral content in nano forms of zinc, copper, and selenium were indicative of a high level of purity. The yield of the products produced was low. Earlier studies in the laboratory also evinced that production of nano forms of minerals by wet chemical method or electrochemical method was 160-200 times lower than that produced by physical method using ball mill [30]. However, the quantity produced through wet chemical (zinc and selenium), or electrochemical (copper) methods was sufficient to meet the *in ovo* feeding, and hence these methods were adopted. Nanoparticles can bypass conventional physiological ways of nutrient distribution and transport across tissue and cell membranes, as well as protect compounds against destruction prior to reaching their targets. In which case *in ovo* administration of nano particles, acting as bioactive agents and as carries of nutrients may be seen as a new method of nano-nutrition [20].

The effect of *in ovo* feeding of broiler eggs with nano form of zinc, copper and selenium at graded levels on egg weight, hatch weight of chicks and their ratio, hatchability percent is presented in Table-4.

No significant variation ($p>0.05$) existed in the egg weight, hatch weight of the chicks or their ratio and hatchability percent between the treatment groups (control and graded levels of nano form of zinc/copper/selenium) studied.

The hatchability percentage obtained in this study for nano forms of zinc, copper and selenium at graded levels were higher than that previous study reported by Bakyaraj et al. [21], who reported hatchability of 81.3% on *in ovo* feeding of selenium 0.3 µg, zinc 80 µg, copper 16 µg and manganese 120 mg/egg. They also reported a hatchability of 61.3% on *in ovo* feeding of selenium 0.3 µg, zinc 80 µg, iron 160 µg and iodine 0.7 µg/egg. The chick weights on hatch in this study for nano forms of zinc, copper and selenium at graded levels were similar to that reported by Bakyaraj *et al.* [21]. However, the chick weight to egg weight ratio was higher in the present study. More than minerals, *in ovo* feeding of energy sources or protein sources is likely to improve hatch weight of chicks as they would supplement the crucial needs of these nutrients during the vital period of hatching [31]. The degree of response to *in ovo* feeding may depend on genetics, breeder hen age, egg size, and incubation conditions [32]. Salmanzadeh [33] reported a reduced hatchability on *in ovo* injection of glucose and attributed it to the development of allergic reactions under air sac that stopped the respiration of the embryo causing its death. Whether such type

of change occurred with regard to *in ovo* feeding of coarse form of minerals when particle size was larger is uncertain. However, nano form of minerals owing to its particle size, have an ability to remain in colloidal state and might have not caused harm to the embryo.

The effect of *in ovo* feeding of broiler eggs with nano form of zinc, copper and selenium at graded levels on overall weight gain, feed efficiency and mortality of broilers at 0-5 weeks is presented in Table-5.

No significant variation (p>0.05) existed in the chick weight or mortality percentage between control and graded levels of nano form of zinc studied. Significantly (p<0.05) highest final weight and weight gain was observed in 50% inclusion of nano form of zinc. This inclusion level also resulted in significantly (p<0.05) the best feed efficiency.

No significant variation (p>0.05) existed in the chick weight or mortality percentage between control

Table-4: Effect of *in ovo* feeding of broiler eggs with nano form of zinc, copper and selenium at graded levels on egg weight, hatch weight of chicks and their ratio and hatchability percent*.

Treatments	Level of inclusion (%)	Level of inclusion (µg/egg)	Egg weight (g)[NS]	Hatch weight of Chicks (g)[NS]	Ratio of chick weight to egg weight[NS]	Hatchability percent[NS]
Control	0	0	60.73±0.68	47.52±0.72	78.24±0.37	96.66±3.33
Nano form zinc	25	20	60.31±1.05	47.30±0.86	78.81±1.84	96.29±3.70
	50	40	61.90±1.99	46.56±0.93	75.54±1.69	96.29±3.70
	75	60	60.93±0.88	46.29±0.68	76.01±0.62	92.96±3.53
	100	80	61.50±0.79	47.62±0.69	77.40±0.36	88.42±0.46
Nano form of copper	25	4	61.14±0.94	47.53±0.73	77.79±0.62	92.96±3.53
	50	8	60.76±0.68	47.17±0.68	77.62±0.58	92.96±3.53
	75	12	62.41±0.82	47.46±0.64	76.07±0.50	92.12±3.95
	100	16	59.82±0.95	46.14±0.77	77.39±1.55	92.96±3.53
Nano form of selenium	25	0.075	61.44±0.99	46.96±0.72	76.47±0.47	83.33±11.02
	50	0.15	62.10±0.90	47.04±0.81	76.03±1.72	83.33±11.02
	75	0.225	60.69±1.06	48.02±0.76	79.41±1.55	92.59±3.70
	100	0.3	60.78±0.73	47.69±0.63	78.56±1.00	88.88±6.41

*Mean of 25 observations. NS=Non-significant difference between treatments

Table-5: Effect of *in ovo* feeding of broiler eggs with nano form of zinc, copper and selenium at graded levels on overall weight gain, feed efficiency and mortality of broilers (0-5 weeks)*.

Treatments	Level of inclusion	Level of inclusion (µg/egg)	Chick weight (g)[NS]	Final weight (g)	Weight gain (g)	Feed efficiency	Mortality percent[NS]
Control	0	0	47.52±0.72	1374.0[a]±22.82	1326.63[a]±22.63	2.30[b]±0.04	0
Nano form of zinc	25	20	47.28±0.78	1360.93[a]±26.15	1313.26[a]±25.84	2.33[b]±0.04	4.5
	50	40	47.01±0.90	1419.29[b]±17.28	1372.05[b]±17.64	2.16[a]±0.03	4.5
	75	60	46.43±0.69	1300.92[a]±8.69	1254.55[a]±8.86	2.42[bc]±0.01	0
	100	80	47.44±0.65	1348.62[a]±23.01	1301.09[a]±22.93	2.89[c]±0.06	0
Control	0	0	47.52±0.72	1374.0[b]±22.82	1326.63[b]±22.63	2.30[a]±0.04	0
Nano form of copper	25	4	47.68±0.67	1315.91[a]±14.23	1268.12[a]±14.01	2.46[a]±0.02	0
	50	8	47.07±0.64	1388.94[b]±22.53	1341.76[b]±22.34	2.55[a]±0.04	0
	75	12	47.17±0.63	1377.94[b]±21.46	1330.47[b]±21.49	2.68[b]±0.04	0
	100	16	46.08±0.70	1336.67[ab]±14.75	1289.88[ab]±14.96	2.46[a]±0.03	4.5
Control	0	0	47.52±0.72	1374.0[a]±22.82	1326.63[a]±22.63	2.30[a]±0.04	0
Nano form of selenium	25	0.075	46.56±0.72	1453.97[b]±22.54	1406.86[b]±22.38	2.90[c]±0.04	0
	50	0.15	46.92±0.74	1470.90[b]±15.59	1423.56[b]±15.82	2.85[c]±0.02	0
	75	0.225	47.85±0.70	1355.57[a]±16.96	1307.55[a]±16.92	2.51[a]±0.03	4.5
	100	0.3	47.94±0.72	1386.10[a]±19.49	1338.41[a]±19.44	2.66[b]±0.03	4.5

*Mean of 25 observations. Means bearing different superscripts within columns differ significantly (p<0.05). NS=Non significant difference between treatments

Table-6: Effect of *in ovo* feeding of broiler eggs with nano form of zinc, copper and selenium at graded levels on dressing, giblet and breast muscle percentage of broilers (0-5 weeks)*.

Treatments	Level of inclusion	Level of inclusion (µg/egg)	Dressing percentage	Giblet percentage	Breast muscle percentage[NS]
Control	0	0	66.26[bc]±0.82	4.84[a]±0.12	27.25±0.66
Nano form of zinc	25	20	59.84[a]±1.92	5.07[ab]±0.18	30.32±0.96
	50	40	66.33[bc]±1.38	5.66[c]±0.17	30.24±1.52
	75	60	62.44[ab]±1.23	5.16[ab]±0.15	30.33±2.46
	100	80	68.39[c]±1.85	5.45[bc]±0.17	26.72±0.93
Control	0	0	66.26±0.82	4.84±0.12	27.25[a]±0.66
Nano form of copper	25	4	65.28±2.09	5.51±0.09	26.74[a]±0.48
	50	8	62.84±0.96	4.98±0.39	26.73[a]±0.82
	75	12	63.94±0.95	5.17±0.07	29.31[b]±0.63
	100	16	65.45±0.74	5.14±0.17	26.12[a]±0.64
Control	0	0	66.26[b]±0.82	4.84[a]±0.12	27.25±0.60
Nano form of selenium	25	0.075	64.70[ab]±0.33	5.65[c]±0.25	27.34±0.3
	50	0.15	66.31[b]±0.77	5.43[bc]±0.16	27.11±0.28
	75	0.225	63.17[a]±0.51	5.06[ab]±0.05	27.06±0.28
	100	0.3	64.14[a]±0.53	5.10[ab]±0.16	26.30±0.39

*Mean of six observations. Means bearing different superscripts within columns differ significantly (p<0.05).
NS=Non-significant variation between treatments

and graded levels of nano form of copper studied. Significantly (p<0.05) lowest final weight and weight gain was observed in 25% (4 µg/egg) and 100% (16 µg/egg). The feed efficiency was comparable between control, 25% (4 µg/egg), 50% (8 µg/egg), and 100% (16 µg/egg) inclusion level of nano form of copper. The inclusion level of nano form of copper at 75% (12 µg/egg) revealed a significantly (p<0.05) highest feed efficiency value. Among the various graded level of inclusion of nano form of copper, 25% (4 µg/egg) inclusion proved to be the best in terms of feed efficiency.

No significant variation (p>0.05) existed in the chick weight or mortality percentage between control and graded levels of nano form of selenium studied. The final weight and weight gain were significantly (p<0.05) highest in 25% (0.075 µg/egg) and 50% (0.15 µg/egg) inclusion level of nano form of selenium. However, the feed efficiency value was significantly (p<0.05) lower, and therefore, the best in control and 75% (0.225 µg/egg) inclusion level of nano form of selenium. Nano form of selenium included at 75% (0.225 µg/egg) level lead to a significantly (p<0.05) lowest feed efficiency. Among the various graded level of inclusion of nano form of selenium, 75% inclusion (0.225 µg/egg) proved to be the best in terms of feed efficiency.

Similar to the results obtained in this study wherein the feed efficiency on *in ovo* feeding of nano form of copper and selenium showed no improvement over that of control, Bakyaraj *et al.* [21] also reported that there was no significant (p<0.05) difference observed in feed conversion ratio of *in ovo* trace elements injected chicks.

The effect of *in ovo* feeding of broiler eggs with nano form of zinc, copper and selenium at graded levels on dressing, giblet and breast muscle percentage of broilers at 0-5 weeks is presented in Table-6.

The effect of *in ovo* feeding of broiler eggs with nano form of zinc revealed that dressing percentage was significantly (p<0.05) higher in 100% inclusion (80 µg/egg) level of nano form of zinc. However, significantly (p<0.05) highest giblet percentage was in 50% inclusion (40 µg/egg) level of nano form of zinc. No significant variation (p>0.05) existed in breast muscle percentage among the treatment groups (control and graded levels of nano form of zinc) studied.

The effect of *in ovo* feeding of broiler eggs with nano form of copper revealed that no significant variation (p>0.05) existed in dressing percentage and giblet percentage between control and graded levels of nano form of copper studied. However, significantly (p<0.05) higher breast muscle percentage was in 75% inclusion (12 µg/egg) level of nano form of copper.

The effect of *in ovo* feeding of broiler eggs with nano form of selenium at graded levels revealed significantly highest (p<0.05) dressing percentage in control and 50% inclusion (0.15 µg/egg) level of nano form of selenium. However, significantly highest (p<0.05) giblet percentage was observed in 25% inclusion level (0.075 µg/egg) of nano form of selenium. No significant variation (p>0.05) existed in breast muscle percentage between control and graded levels of nano form of selenium studied. Increasing protein above requirement enhanced the activation of components related to translation initiation in the neonate chick muscle but the role of trace elements is not clear [34].

Conclusion

Stable forms of nano sized zinc and selenium with high purity can be produced by wet chemical method and stable nano sized copper with high purity can be produced by electrochemical method. *In ovo* feeding of nano forms of zinc, copper and selenium at the 18th day of incubation through amniotic route does not harm the developing embryo and does not affect hatchability. Nano forms of zinc, copper and selenium gave best feed efficiency at certain inclusion levels. There existed no trend to indicate that the dressing percentage was influenced by different levels of nano forms of minerals. The breast muscle percentage was higher for nano form of copper at certain inclusion level. The research clearly shows that nano minerals are not harmful to the embryo and can be used to improve the post-hatch performance of broiler chicken. However, further many advanced researches are required to explore further beneficial effects and safety of nano forms of minerals.

Authors' Contributions

The present study was a part of original research work by PPJ during his M.V.Sc., thesis program under the eminent guidance of CV. CV and VB conceptualized the aim of the study, designed, planned and supervised the experiment. Collection of samples, execution of experimental study was done by PPJ. Analysis of data, interpretation of the results and drafting of the manuscript was done by PPJ, CV, and VB. All authors read and approved the final manuscript.

Acknowledgments

The authors are thankful to Tamil Nadu Veterinary and Animal Sciences University for allocation of funds to carry out this research work and also we extend our gratitude to all the Teaching Faculty, Staffs, and Post-Graduate students of Department of Animal Nutrition, Poultry Science and Poultry Research Station of Tamil Nadu Veterinary and Animal Sciences University for their untiring help to carry out this study.

Competing Interests

The authors declare that they have no competing interests.

References

1. ICRA. (2013) Indian Poultry Industry – Broiler Meat and Table Egg, Corporate Ratings. Available from: http://www.icra.in/files/ticker.

2. Noy, Y. and Uni, Z. (2010) Early nutritional strategies. *World Poult. Sci. J.*, 66: 639-646.

3. Uni, Z. and Ferket, P.R. (2003) Enhancement of development of oviparous species by *in ovo* feeding. US Patent Number 6, 592, 878.

4. Uni, Z., Ferket, P., Tako, E. and Kedar, O. (2005) *In ovo* feeding improves energy status of late term chicken embryos. *Poult. Sci.*, 84: 764-770.

5. Yair, R. and Uni, Z. (2011) Content and uptake of minerals in the yolk of broiler embryos during incubation and effect of nutrient enrichment. *Poult. Sci.*, 90: 1523-1531.

6. Angel, R. (2007) Metabolic disorders: Limitations to growth of and mineral deposition into the broiler skeleton after hatch and potential implications for leg problems. *J. Appl. Poult. Res.*, 16: 138-149.

7. Ferket, P.R. (2011) *In ovo* feeding and the promise of perinatal nutrition. In: Proceedings of Alltech International Nutrition Symposium, Lexington, Kentucky, United States of America.

8. Zhai, W., Neuman, S., Latour, M.A. and Hester, P.Y. (2008) The effect of *in ovo* injection of L-carnitine on hatchability

9. Keralapurath, M.M., Corzo, A., Pulikanti, R., Zhai, W. and Peebles, E.D. (2010) Effects of *in ovo* injection of L-carnitine on hatchability and subsequent broiler performance and slaughter yield. *Poult. Sci.*, 89: 1497-1501.

10. Yamawaki, R.A., Milbradt, E.L., Coppola, M.P., Rodrigues, J.C., Andreattifilho, R.L., Padovani, C.R. and Okamoto, A.S. (2013) Effect of immersion and inoculation *in ovo* of *Lactobacillus* spp. in embryonated chicken eggs in the prevention of *Salmonella enteritidis* after hatch. *Poult. Sci.*, 92(6): 1560-1563.

11. Kornasio, R., Halevy, O., Kedar, O. and Uni, Z. (2011) Effect of *in ovo* feeding and its interaction with timing of first feed on glycogen reserves, muscle growth, and body weight. *Poult. Sci.*, 90(7): 1467-77.

12. Cheled-Shoval, S., Amit-Romach, E., Barbakov, M. and Uni, Z. (2011) The effect of *in ovo* administration of mannan oligosaccharide on small intestine development during the pre-and post-hatch periods in chickens. *Poult. Sci.*, 90(10): 2301-2310.

13. Kidd, M.T., Anthony, N.B. and Lee, S.R. (1992) Progeny performance when dams and chicks are fed supplemental zinc. *Poult. Sci.*, 71: 1201-1206.

14. Kidd, M.T. (2003) A treatise on chicken dam nutrition that impacts progeny. *World Poult. Sci. J.*, 59: 475-494.

15. Cardoso, A., Albuquerque, R. and Tessari, E. (2007) Humoral immunological response in broilers vaccinated against Newcastle disease and supplemented with dietary zinc and vitamin E. *Rev. Bras. Cien. Avic.*, 8(2): 2501-2509.

16. Shankar, A.H. and Prasad, A.S. (1998) Zinc and immune function: The biological basis of altered resistance to infection. *Am. J. Clin. Nutr.*, 68: 447-463.

17. Wang, C., Wang, M.Q., Ye, S.S., Tao, W.J. and Du, Y.J. (2011) Effects of copper-loaded chitosan nanoparticles on growth and immunity in broilers. *Poult. Sci.*, 90(10): 2223-2228.

18. McKenzie, R.C., Rafferty, T.S. and Beckett, G.J. (1998) Selenium: An essential element for immune function. *Immunol. Today*, 19: 342-345.

19. Yair, R., Uni, Z. and Shahar, R. (2012) Bone characteristics of late term embryonic and hatchling broilers: Bone development under extreme growth rate. *Poult. Sci.*, 91(10): 2614-2620.

20. Sawosz, F., Pineda, L., Hotowy, A., Hyttel, P., Sawosz, E., Szmidt, M., Niemiec, T. and Chwalibog, A. (2012) Nano-nutrition of chicken embryos. Effect of silver nanoparticles and glutamine on molecular responses and morphology of pectoral muscle. *Balt. J. Comp. Clin. Syst. Bio.*, 2: 29-45.

21. Bakyaraj, S., Bhanja, S.K., Majumdar, S. and Dash, B. (2012) Modulation of post-hatch growth and immunity through *in ovo* supplemented nutrients in broiler chickens. *J. Sci. Food Agric.*, 92: 313-320.

22. Yadav, A., Prasad, V., Kathe, A.A., Raj, S., Yadav, D., Sundaramoorthy, C. and Vigneshwaran, N. (2006) Functional finishing in cotton fabrics using zinc oxide nanoparticles. *B. Mater. Sci.*, 29: 641-645.

23. Theivasanthi, T. and Alagar, M. (2011) Nano sized copper particles by electrolytic synthesis and characterizations. *Int. J. Phys. Sci.*, 6(15): 3662-3671.

24. Razi, K.M., Maamoury, R.S. and Banihashemi, S. (2011) Preparation of nano selenium particles by water solution phase method from industrial dust. *Int. J. Nano Dimens.*, 1(4): 261-267.

25. Bhanja, S.K., Mandal, A.B. and Johri, T.S. (2004) Standardisation of injection sites, needle length, embryonic age and concentration of amino acids for *in ovo* injected in broiler breeder eggs. *Indian J. Poult. Sci.*, 39: 105-111.

26. Yadav, B.C., Srivastava, R., Yadav, A. and Srivastava, V. (2008) LPG sensing of nanostructured zinc oxide and zinc niobate. *Sensors Lett.*, 6: 1-5.

27. Ramyadevi, J., Jeyasubramanian, K., Marikani, A., Rajakumar, G. and Rahuman, A. (2012) Synthesis and

antimicrobial activity of copper nanoparticles. *Mater. Lett.*, 71: 114-116.

28. Zhang, J., Wang, H., Bao, Y. and Zhang, L. (2004) Nano red elemental selenium has no size effect in the induction of seleno-enzymes in both cultured cells and mice. *Life Sci.*, 75(2): 237-244.

29. Nanocomposix. (2012) Zeta potential analysis of nanoparticles. V1.1.

30. Ramesh, J.R. (2014) Effect of nano mineral supplementation in TANUVAS – SMART mineral mixture on performance of the lambs. Ph.D., Thesis Submitted to Tamil Nadu Veterinary and Animal Sciences University, Chennai, Tamil Nadu, India.

31. Shafey, T.M., Alodan, M.A., Al-Ruqaie, I.M. and Abouheif, M.A. (2012) *In ovo* feeding of carbohydrates and incubated at a high incubation temperature on hatchability and glycogen status of chicks. *S. Afr. J. Anim. Sci.*, 42(3): 211-220.

32. Uni, Z. and Ferket, P.R. (2004) Methods for early feeding and their potential. *World Poult. Sci. J.*, 60: 101-111.

33. Salmanzadeh, M. (2012) The effects of *in-ovo* injection of glucose on hatchability, hatching weight and subsequent performance of newly-hatched chicks. *Rev. Bras. Cien. Avic.,* 14(2). Available from: http://www.dx.doi.org/10.1590/S1516635X20100008.

34. Everaert, N., Swennen, Q., Metayer, C.S., Willemsem, H., Careghi, C., Buyse, J., Bruggeman, V., Decuypere, E. and Tesseraud, S. (2010) The effect of the protein level in a pre-starter diet on the post-hatch performance and activation of S6K1 in muscle of neonatal broilers. *Br. J. Nutr.,* 103: 206-211.

20

Awareness, knowledge, and risks of zoonotic diseases among livestock farmers in Punjab

Jaspal Singh Hundal[1], Simrinder Singh Sodhi[1], Aparna Gupta[2], Jaswinder Singh[1] and Udeybir Singh Chahal[1]

1. Department of Veterinary and Animal Husbandry Extension Education, Guru Angad Dev Veterinary and Animal Sciences University, Ludhiana, Punjab, India; 2. Krishi Vigyan Kendra, Ropar, Punjab Agricultural University, Ludhiana, Punjab, India.
Corresponding author: Jaspal Singh Hundal, e-mail: drjshundal@yahoo.com,
SSS: simrindersodhi@gmail.com, AG: aparnapau@gmail.com, JS: jaswindervet@rediffmail.com,
USC: udeybirchahal@gmail.com

Abstract

Aim: The present study was conducted to assess the awareness, knowledge, and risks of zoonotic diseases among livestock farmers in Punjab.

Materials and Methods: 250 livestock farmers were selected randomly and interviewed with a pretested questionnaire, which contained both open and close ended questions on different aspects of zoonotic diseases, i.e., awareness, knowledge, risks, etc. Knowledge scorecard was developed, and each correct answer was awarded one mark, and each incorrect answer was given zero mark. Respondents were categorized into low (mean − ½ standard deviation [SD]), moderate (mean ± ½ SD), and high knowledge (Mean + ½ SD) category based on the mean and SD. The information about independent variables *viz.*, age, education, and herd size were collected with the help of structured schedule and scales. The data were analyzed by ANOVA, and results were prepared to assess awareness, knowledge, and risks of zoonotic diseases and its relation with independent variables.

Results: Majority of the respondents had age up to 40 years (70%), had their qualification from primary to higher secondary level (77.6%), and had their herd size up to 10 animals (79.6%). About 51.2% and 54.0% respondents had the history of abortion and retained placenta, respectively, at their farms. The respondents not only disposed off the infected placenta (35.6%), aborted fetus (39.6%), or feces (56.4%) from a diarrheic animal but also gave intrauterine medication (23.2%) bare-handedly. About 3.6-69.6% respondents consumed uncooked or unpasteurized animal products. About 84.8%, 46.0%, 32.8%, 4.61%, and 92.4% of livestock farmers were aware of zoonotic nature of rabies, brucellosis, tuberculosis, anthrax, and bird flu, respectively. The 55.6%, 67.2%, 52.0%, 64.0%, and 51.2% respondents were aware of the transmission of zoonotic diseases to human being through contaminated milk, meat, air, feed, or through contact with infected animals, respectively. The transmission of rabies through dog bite (98.4%), need of post-exposure vaccination (96.8%), and annual vaccination of dogs (78%) were well-known facts but only 47.2% livestock owners were aware of the occurrence of abortion due to brucellosis and availability of prophylactic vaccine (67.6%) against it as a preventive measure. About 69.2% respondents belonged to low to medium knowledge level categories, whereas 30.8% respondents had high knowledge (p<0.05) regarding different aspects of zoonotic diseases. Age, education, and herd size had no significant effect on the knowledge level and awareness of farmers toward zoonotic diseases.

Conclusion: Therefore, from the present study, it may be concluded that there is a need to create awareness and improve knowledge of livestock farmers toward zoonotic diseases for its effective containment in Punjab.

Keywords: awareness, knowledge level, livestock farmers, risk factors, zoonotic diseases.

Introduction

Zoonoses, diseases and infections that are naturally transmissible between vertebrate animals and humans [1], are among the most frequent and dreaded risks to which mankind are exposed. The emergence and re-emergence of zoonoses and its potentially disastrous impact on human health are a growing concern around the globe [2]. Brucellosis, rabies, human African trypanosomiasis, bovine tuberculosis, cysticercosis, echinococcosis, and anthrax are listed as seven endemic zoonoses of concern [3]. In developing countries, they constitute an important threat to human health [4] especially for societies that domesticate and breed animals for food and clothing.

The Indian subcontinent has been identified as one of the four global hot-spots at increased risk for emergence of new infectious diseases (Public Health Foundation of India). The latest high-resolution climate change scenarios and projections for India (based on a regional climate modeling system known as Providing Regional Climates for Impact Studies, forecasts the likely increase in annual mean surface temperature by the end of the century from 2.5°C to 5°C and with warming more pronounced in the northern parts of India and a more than 20% rise in summer monsoon rainfall is projected which indicates a pronounced impact of zoonoses in future [5]. Hence, Veterinary Public Health has become a much more active field of enquiry in India and is involved with human health than that it was before.

The zoonotic diseases may be transmitted to livestock farmers through contamination during production, processing, and handling of food products of animal origin. About 68% of workforce in India is in close contact with domestic animals [6] and their activities, such as working with animals and in their sheds, improper disposal of waste from animal sheds, skinning of infected animals, slaughtering of diseased animals, disposal of infective material from the diseased animals, and poor personal hygiene practices, have been reported to be important risk factors. Lack of awareness about the occurrence of zoonotic diseases and their impact on public health have acted as a major hurdle in commencing adequate and effective control measures [7]. In our perspective dairy farming management, culture and eating habits and perception of farmers about zoonotic diseases and their prevention needs to be assessed as an understanding about awareness and practices of farmers can be a useful tool in developing and improving existing control measures [8]. Thus, the present study aimed at investigating risks of zoonotic diseases among livestock farmers and to assess their awareness and knowledge level toward zoonotic diseases.

Materials and Methods

Ethical approval

No ethical approval was required as it is a survey based study; however, after obtaining consent from all the participants involved in the study, the data were collected.

Study site

Guru Angad Dev Veterinary and Animal Sciences University, Ludhiana act as a knowledge hub to the farmers of Punjab. The livestock farmers regularly visit the university for trainings, cattle fairs, learning new technologies, solution of livestock problems, treatment of diseased animals, purchasing of university publications, mineral mixture, bypass fat, uromin lick, etc., from all over the state. The present study was conducted based on data collected from livestock farmers who visited the University from different districts of Punjab between January 1st, 2015 and August 31st, 2015.

Sampling size

250 farmers were selected randomly who visited the university and interviewed with a questionnaire.

Data collection

The respondents were interviewed with a questionnaire contained both open and close ended questions on different aspects of zoonotic diseases, i.e., awareness, knowledge, risks, etc. The

questionnaire had 14 questions to assess potential sources of infection to the farmers and 20 questions to test their awareness and knowledge level. The questionnaire was pre-tested on a few selected farmers, and the easiness of completion of the questionnaire and ambiguity of questions were noted and subsequently revised before a large-scale interview of the farmers. The information about independent variables *viz.,* age, education, and herd size were collected with the help of structured schedule and scales.

Statistical analysis

Knowledge scorecard was developed, and each correct answer was awarded one mark, and each incorrect answer was given zero mark. Respondents were categorized into three groups [9] based on the mean (9.53 ± 0.19) and standard deviation (3.12) as a measure of check.

Total score on knowledge	Knowledge category
Less than (mean − ½ SD)	Low
Between (mean ± ½ SD)	Moderate
More than (mean + ½ SD)	High

SD=Standard deviation

The data were analyzed by ANOVA [10] using the software package SPSS version 16 [11], and results were prepared to assess awareness, knowledge, and risks of zoonotic diseases and its relation with independent variables.

Results

The study revealed that 28% of farmers belonged to up to 25 year age category, and 42% belonged to 26-40 years age group, and rest 30% were of higher age groups (Figure-1) indicated that higher number of younger farmers were involved in the occupation of dairy farming. The education level of most of the farmers (77.6%) was up to matriculation or higher secondary, whereas merely 13.6% farmers were having a higher qualification (Figure-2). This is probably due to the fact that up to higher secondary level education is easier to be acquired at the local level. It was observed that 79.6% farmers in the selected population were small farmers with herd size up to 10 (Figure-3).

Risk factors associated with conventional management and eating habits

The critical analysis of data revealed that around 51.2% and 54.0% respondents had the history of

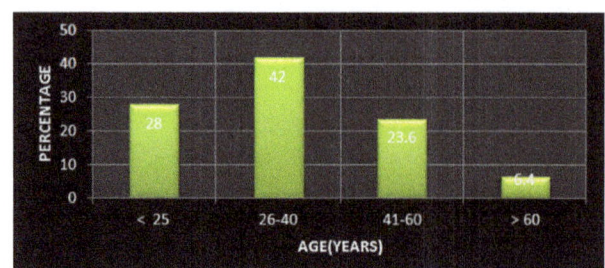

Figure-1: Distribution of respondents according to age.

abortion and retained placenta, respectively, at their farm and the respondents not only disposed off the infected placenta (35.6%), aborted fetus (39.6%), or feces (56.4%) from diarrheic animal but also gave intrauterine medication (23.2%) bare handedly (Table-1). The majority of respondents assisted calving (80.4%) and did milking (93.6%) which could be a source of infection to them. As for as consumption of raw milk, egg, and meat is concerned, about 3.6 to 69.6% respondents not only consumed uncooked or unpasteurized animal products but also applied cream from raw milk on their skin cracks. Even sleeping in animal shed may be one of the risk factor associated with the occurrence of zoonotic diseases and about 30% respondents were following this practice. Newly purchased animal if suffered from diseases such as brucellosis or tuberculosis may act as a potential source of infection to farmers as well as to other animals, but merely 14% respondents got their animals tested for brucellosis and tuberculosis before making purchase.

Awareness and knowledge of livestock farmers toward zoonotic diseases

On the basis of knowledge score, respondents were divided into low, medium, and high-level knowledge groups (Table-2). About 69.2% respondents belonged to low and medium knowledge level categories, whereas only 30.8% respondents had high knowledge regarding different aspects of zoonotic diseases. The differences were statistically significant ($p<0.05$) among all the groups.

As for as the awareness toward zoonotic diseases is concerned (Table-3), about 84.8%, 46.0%, 32.8%, 4.61%, and 92.4% of livestock farmers were aware of zoonotic nature of rabies, brucellosis, tuberculosis, anthrax, and bird flu, respectively, whereas as they had never heard about cysticercosis and echinococcosis. Even 92.8% of farmers listed swine fever among zoonotic diseases which may be due to the fact that media presented H_1N_1 as swine fever or swine flu in most of their reports. The zoonotic diseases may be transmitted to the human being through contaminated milk, meat, air, feed, or through contact with infected animals but this fact was known to 55.6%, 67.2%, 52.0%, 64.0%, and 51.2% respondents, respectively. Avian influenza virus may stick to the egg shell and may be enteredinto the food chain, but its transmission through raw egg was a lesser known fact (29.6%).

Rabies and brucellosis are the two most common diseases of zoonotic importance. The awareness level of farmers about rabies (Table-3) indicated that its transmission through dog bite was a well-known fact (98.4%) while it can also be transmitted through saliva (24.8%) and contact (6.8%) of infected dog were known to a lesser extent. About 69.2% respondents were aware of the use of soap to wash the wound immediately after dog bite but still 30.8% farmers opined to apply chili powder on it which is a mere misconception, and there is need to educate the people

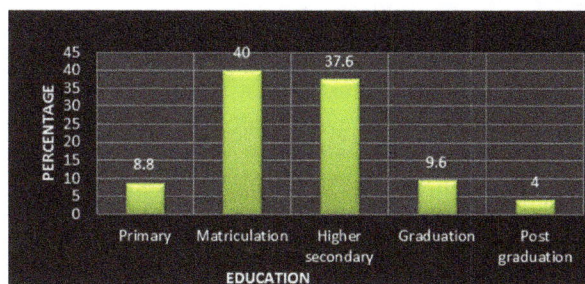

Figure-2: Distribution of respondents according to education.

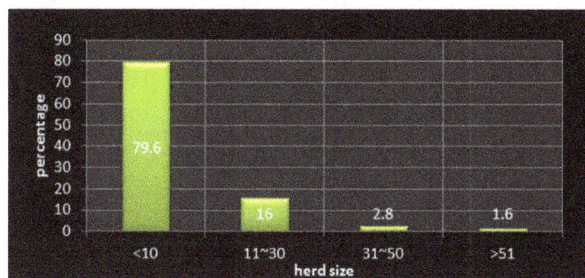

Figure-3: Distribution of respondents according to herd size.

Table-1: Exposure of livestock farmers to risk factors associated with various types of farm activities and eating habits.

Risk factors	Exposure	
	Frequency (n=250)	Percent
Eating habits		
Drinking raw milk	174	69.6
Eating raw meat	9	3.6
Eating raw eggs	65	26.0
Farm activities		
Milking	201	80.4
Sleeping in animal shed	75	30.0
Dealing with diarrheic animals	141	56.4
Assisting cow during calving	234	93.6
History of animal abortion at the farm	128	51.2
Disposed off aborted fetus with naked hands	99	39.6
Incidence of retained placenta	135	54.0
Disposed off placenta without bearing gloves	89	35.6
Intrauterine medication after abortion	58	23.2
Apply milk cream (raw milk) on cracks of lips	92	36.8
Testing of animal for brucellosis and tuberculosis before purchasing	35	14.0

Table-2: Knowledge level of livestock farmers toward zoonotic diseases.

Knowledge level	Frequency (n=250)	Percent
Low (upto 7.97 score)	71[a]	28.4
Moderate (7.98-11.09 score)	102[c]	40.8
High (≥11.10 score)	77[b]	30.8

Figures with different superscript in column differ significantly, $p<0.05$

on this aspect. 96.8% respondents were aware of need of post-exposure vaccination in human, but 55.2% of them were still thinking that intra peritoneal was the only route of administration. Remarkably, 78% respondents were aware of annual vaccination of dogs for prevention of rabies. Brucellosis is another common disease of dairy animals which is zoonotic in nature and can cause economic loss as well as a health hazard to the farmers. However, only 47.2% livestock farmers were aware of the fact that animals may abort in the third trimester of their pregnancy due to brucellosis. Now-a-days, prophylactic vaccine is available for female dairy animals as a preventive measure, and about 67.6% of respondents were aware of it. When farmers asked about the disease/s that they acquired from their animals, about 6% respondents said yes, and it was a skin infection.

Table-3: Awareness of livestock farmers toward zoonotic diseases and their possible means of transmission.

Parameter	Frequency (n=250)	Percentage
Diseases transmit from animals to human being		
Rabies	212	84.8
Brucellosis	115	46.0
Bovine tuberculosis	82	32.8
Anthrax	12	4.61
Bird flu	231	92.4
Cysticercosis	0	0
Echinococcosis	0	0
Swine fever	232	92.8
Possible means of transmission of diseases from animals to human being		
Contaminating milk	139	55.6
Contaminating meat	168	67.2
Contaminating egg	74	29.6
Aerosol	130	52.0
Infected contaminating water or feed	160	64.0
Contact with infected animal	128	51.2
Awareness about rabies and brucellosis		
Rabies may result from		
Bite of rabid dog	246	98.4
Contact with rabid dog	17	6.8
From saliva of rabid dog	62	24.8
Rabid dog bite wound		
Wash with soap	173	69.2
Apply chili powder	77	30.8
Do we need vaccination after rabid dog bite	242	96.8
Vaccination of rabies in human		
Intra muscular	112	44.8
Intra peritoneal	138	55.2
Is annual vaccination of dog against rabies is necessary?	197	78.8
Brucellosis can cause abortion in dairy animals during which trimester of gestation period?	118	47.2
Is vaccination available against brucellosis?	169	67.6
Have you ever got disease transmitted to you from your animal	15	6.0

Independent variables and knowledge level of farmers toward zoonotic diseases

The effect of age, education, and herd size on knowledge level and awareness of farmers toward zoonotic diseases was given in Table-4. The data revealed that age, education, and herd size didn't affect the knowledge level and awareness of farmers toward zoonotic diseases as mean correct responses difference among different age, education, and herd size groups remained non-significant.

Discussion

Risk factors associated with conventional management and eating habits

Incidence of abortions, retained placenta, consumption of raw animal products, bare-handed handling of animal excreta and milking are the prime sources of infection [12]. The findings are in agreement with earlier results [13], who also reported similar practices of consumption of raw animal products. Researcher [14] observed that majority of the dairy farmers practiced hand milking. Ingestion of infected raw unpasteurized milk was cited as the most possible way of contracting milk-borne zoonoses [15]. The unpasteurized or un-boiled milk have been reported to be associated with brucellosis and bovine tuberculosis [16-18]. Newly purchased animal if suffered from diseases such as brucellosis or tuberculosis may act as a potential source of infection to farmers as well as to other animals. Many of the respondents under study also followed these practices which may be due to the lack of awareness about the transmission of zoonotic diseases. The facts clearly indicated that the farmers were at high-risk end to get zoonotic diseases, and

Table-4: Effect of age, education and herd size on knowledge level of livestock farmers toward zoonotic diseases.

Parameter	Mean correct responses	Significance
Effect of age (years) on knowledge level of livestock farmers		
≤25	9.56±0.40	NS
26-40	9.63±0.27	NS
41-60	9.17±0.43	NS
>60	10.12±0.87	NS
Effect of education on knowledge level of livestock farmers		
Primary	9.77±0.53	NS
Matriculation	8.93±0.30	NS
Higher secondary	9.85±0.31	NS
Graduation	10.96±0.77	NS
Post-graduation	8.60±1.27	NS
Effect of herd size on knowledge level of livestock farmers		
≤10	9.39±022	NS
11-30	10.45±0.51	NS
21-50	8.57±1.28	NS
>50	9.0±1.58	NS

NS=Non-significant, i.e., $p>0.05$

there is need to educate them about scientific management methods, safe disposal of infected material, and handling of livestock products for effective containment of zoonoses.

Awareness and knowledge of livestock farmers toward zoonotic diseases

Healthy herd and health of livestock farmers both are equally important. However, the study indicated that knowledge level of livestock farmer was low to medium. This stressed on the need for providing better knowledge to them for effective control of zoonosis. As for as the awareness toward zoonotic diseases is concerned, awareness about rabies was high and findings are in agreement with another researcher [19], but awareness toward brucellosis, tuberculosis, and anthrax was low and even they had never heard the name of cysticercosis and echinococcosis diseases. Most of the farmers listed swine fever among zoonotic diseases which may be due to lack of awareness and printing of misinformation in a section of media. It not only creates a fear psychosis among pork consumers but also have huge economic impact on pig farmers as well as the nation. The zoonotic diseases may be transmitted to the human being through contaminated milk, meat, air, feed, or through contact with infected animals but this fact is not known to all of the farmers. Similar levels of knowledge were also reported by others [13] regarding the transmission of zoonotic diseases.

Like rabies, brucellosis is another disease of zoonotic importance which the livestock farmers may get from animals and clinically it may manifest as an acute or chronic form [20]. Awareness about rabies was good among livestock farmers, which may be due to the fact that dog bite is common in India due to a huge population of stray dogs and we always go for post-exposure vaccination. However, still the misconception like the application of chili powder on dog bite wound was there, which is need to be stressed. However, on other hand, farmers were not well aware of brucellosis as less than half of the respondents knew that *Brucella* can cause abortions in dairy animals. Now-a-days, prophylactic vaccine is available for female dairy animals as a preventive measure, but only two third farmers were aware of it. When farmers asked about the disease/s that they acquired from their animals, about 6% respondents said yes and it was the skin infection. It may be due to the reason that skin infection is visible easily, and other diseases cannot be diagnosed at farmer level. Some [21] also reported a low level of knowledge in respondents regarding zoonotic diseases. However, knowledge on rabies was found to be higher than other zoonotic diseases and this fact also conjoins with this study. Similar results were also reported by a researcher [22] where they concluded that 87% small scale holders had low to fair level of knowledge regarding zoonosis. This low and medium level of awareness could be due to remoteness, lack of health facilities, poor extension services, low training status on rearing and handling of animals, and low literacy rate which have been reported as major contributors to the low level of awareness among dairy farmers [23]. Now-a-days, improvement in the zoonotic diseases research should also be based newer basic science techniques and areas of genetic algorithms and ant colony optimization to combinatorial optimization problems [24-26].

Independent variables and knowledge level of farmers toward zoonotic diseases

Age, education, and herd size didn't affect the knowledge level and awareness of farmers toward zoonotic diseases significantly. It may be due to the reason that exposure to disease, training, and extension contacts might have played their role [23].

Conclusion

Livestock farmers were well aware of rabies, but the knowledge toward other zoonotic diseases was low to medium. Even the farmers did not hear the name of cysticercosis and echinococcosis. Livestock holders were mostly not aware of the risk of contracting zoonotic pathogens from consuming contaminated raw milk, meat, and eggs. In addition, proper disposal of infected milk or dairy products, aborted materials, and use of hygienic procedures during milking and milk storage are extremely important steps in successful control of zoonotic pathogens [27]. These zoonotic diseases have a direct effect on human and animal health and production, but this may influence the economy of the country by being barriers to trade, increased cost of marketing the product to ensure it is safe for human consumption and the loss of market because of decreased consumer confidence. Inspite of its utmost importance, awareness to livestock farmers regarding their needs to be stressed on because due to lack of awareness most of them go undiagnosed and uncontrolled. Even though the government is practicing most disease control schemes including vaccination, organization of animal health camps but preponderance over the issue of improving awareness among the livestock owners could become a milepost in prevention and control of zoonotic diseases.

Authors' Contributions

JSH: Prepared, pretested and revised questionnaire for collection of data by personal interview and statistical analysis; SSS & AG: Provided valuable suggestions regarding the design of the study and analysis of the collected data; JS & USC: Provided guidance throughout the study period as well as helped in academic/legislative aspects. All authors read and approved the final manuscript.

Acknowledgments

The authors are highly thankful to Head, Department of Veterinary and Animal Husbandry Extension Education, GADVASU, Ludhiana for allowing us to carry out this survey work.

Competing Interests

The authors declare that they have no competing interests.

References

1. World Health Organisation. (2015) Zoonoses. Available from: http://www.who.int/topics/zoonoses/en/. Retrieved on 18-10-2015.

2. Woolhouse, M.E.J. and Sequeria, S. (2005) Host range and emerging and re-emerging pathogens. *Emerg. Infect. Dis.,* 11: 1842-1847.

3. World Health Organisation. (2006) The Control of Neglected Zoonotic Diseases: A Route to Poverty Alleviation. Geneva Report of a Joint WHO/DFID-AHP Meeting with the participation of FAO and OIE, Geneva, 20-21, September, 2005.

4. Wastling, J.M., Akanmori, B.D. and Williams, D.J.L. (1999) Zoonoses in West Africa: Impact and control. *Parasitol. Today,* 15: 309-311.

5. Singh, B.B., Sharma, R., Gill, J.P.S., Aulakh, R.S. and Banga, H.S. (2011) Climate change, zoonoses and India. *Rev. Sci. Tech. Off. Int. Epiz.,* 30: 779-788.

6. Pavani, G. (2014) Zoonotic diseases with special reference to India. *Int. J. Basic Appl. Med. Sci.,* 4: 73-87.

7. Asokan, G.V., Vanitha, A. and Prathap, T. (2011) One Health National Programme across species on zoonoses: A call to the developing world. *Infect. Ecol. Epidemiol.,* 1: 8293.

8. Swai, E.S. and Schoonman, L. (2010) The use of Rose Bengal plate test to assess cattle exposure to *Brucella* infection in traditional and smallholder dairy production systems of Tanga Region of Tanzania. *Vet. Med. Int.,* Article ID: 837950. Available from: http://www.dx.doi. org/10.4061/2010/837950.

9. Chandrashekar, B.R., Lakshminnarayan, M.T., Krishnamurthy, B. and Shivaramu, K. (1998) Rabies: Factors influencing the knowledge of veterinarians. *Mysore J. Agric. Sci.,* 32: 225-228.

10. Snedecor, G.W. and Cochran, W.G. (1994) Statistical Methods. 8th ed. Oxford and IBH Publications, New Delhi.

11. SPSS. (2007) Statistical Packages for Social Sciences. Ver. 126, SPSS Inc., Illinois, USA.

12. Madkour, M.M, editor. (2001) Brucellosis: Overview. In: Madkour Medical Microbiology. 2nd ed. Springer-Verlag Press, Berlin. p1-14.

13. Tebug, S.F., Njunga, G.R., Chagunda, M.G.G., Mapemba, J.P., Awah-Ndukum, J. and Wiedemann, S. (2014) Risk, knowledge and preventive measures of smallholder dairy farmers in northern Malawi with regard to zoonotic brucellosis and bovine tuberculosis, *Onderstepoort J. Vet. Res.,* 81:1-6. Available from: http://www.dx.doi. org/10.4102/ojvr.v81i1.594.

14. Milligo, V., Ouedraogo, G.A., Agenas, S. and Svennersten-Sjaunja, K. (2008) Survey on dairy cattle milk production and milk quality problems in Peri-urban areas in Burkina Faso. *Afr. J. Agric. Res.,* 3: 215-224.

15. Chahota, R., Sharma, M., Katoch, R.C., Verma, S.,

16. Singh, M.M., Kapoor, V. and Asrani, R.K. (2003) Brucellosis outbreak in an organized dairy farm involving cows and in contact human beings in Himachal Pradesh. *Vet. Arch.,* 73:95-102.

16. Fetene, T., Kebede, N. and Alem, G. (2011) Tuberculosis infection in animal and human populations in three districts of Western Gojam, Ethiopia. *Zoonoses Public Health,* 58: 47-53. Available from: http://www.dx.doi.org/10.1111/j.1863-2378.2009.01265.

17. Kochar, D.K., Gupta, B.K., Gupta, A., Kalla, A., Nayak, K.C. and Purohit, S.K. (2007) Hospital-based case series of 175 cases of serologically confirmed brucellosis inBikaner. *J. Assoc. Phys. India,* 55: 271-275.

18. Makita, K., Fèvre, E.M., Waiswa, C., Kaboyo, W., De Clare Bronsvoort, B.M., Eisler, M.C. and Welburn, S.C. (2008) Human brucellosis in urban and peri-urban areas of Kampala,Uganda. *Ann. NY. Acad. Sci.,* 1149: 309-311.

19. Emmanuel, J., Awosanya, H.O. and Akande, H.O. (2015) Animal health care seeking behavior of pets or livestock owners and knowledge and awareness on zoonoses in a university community. *Vet.World,* 8(7): 841-847.

20. Ananthnarayan, R. and Paniker, J. (2013) *Brucella.* In: Arti, K., editor. Textbook of Microbiology. 9th ed. University Press, Hyderabad. p340-343.

21. Babu, A.J., Ramya, P., Rao, L.V., Swetha, C.S., Sudhanthiramani and Venkateswara R. (2015) A study on the awareness and knowledge of zoonotic diseases among the public in and around Proddatur -YSR Kadapa district, Andhra Pradesh, India. *Int. J. Rec. Sci. Res.,* 67: 5131-5138.

22. Mosalagae, D., Pfukenyi, D.M. and Matope, G. (2011) Milk producers' awareness of milk-borne zoonoses in selected smallholder and commercial dairy farms of Zimbabwe. *Trop. Anim. Health Prod.,* 43:733-739.

23. Munyeme, M., Muma, J.B., Munangandu, H.M., Kankya, C., Skjerve, E. and Tryland, M. (2010) Cattle owners' awareness of bovine tuberculosis in high and low prevalence settings of the wildlife-livestock interface areas in Zambia. *BMC Vet. Res.,* 6:21.

24. Markand, S., Tawfik, A., Ha, Y., Gnana-Prakasam, J., Sonne, S., Ganapathy, V. and Smith, S.B. (2013) Cystathionine beta synthase expression in mouse retina. *Curr. Eye Res.,* 38:597-604.

25. Markand, S., Saul, A., Roon, P., Prasad, P., Martin, P., Rozen, R., Ganapathy, G. and Smith, S.B. (2015) Retinal ganglion cell loss and mild vasculopathy in methylene tetrahydrofolate reductase deficient mice: A model of mild hyperhomocysteinemia. *Invest. Ophthalmol. Vis. Sci.,* 56:2684-2695.

26. Rajappa, G.P. (2012) Solving combinatorial optimization problems using genetic algorithms and ant colony optimization. PhD Dissertation, University of Tennessee; 2012. Available from: http://www.trace.tennessee.edu/utk_ graddiss/1478. Retrieved on 26-9-2015.

27. Al-Majali, A.M., Talafha, A.Q., Ababneh, M.M. and Ababneh, M.M. (2009) Seroprevalence and risk factors for bovine brucellosis in Jordan. *J. Vet. Sci.,* 10: 61-65.

21

In vitro larvicidal effects of ethanolic extract of *Curcuma longa* Linn. on *Haemonchus* larval stage

Norisal Binti Nasai[1], Yusuf Abba[2], Faez Firdaus Jesse Abdullah[1,3], Murugaiyah Marimuthu[1,2], Abdulnasir Tijjani[2], Muhammad Abubakar Sadiq[2], Konto Mohammed[1], Eric Lim Teik Chung[1] and Mohammed Ariff Bin Omar[1,3]

1. Department of Veterinary Clinical Studies, Faculty of Veterinary Medicine, Universiti Putra Malaysia, 43400 UPM Serdang, Selangor, Malaysia; 2. Department of Veterinary Pathology and Microbiology, Faculty of Veterinary Medicine, Universiti Putra Malaysia, 43400 UPM Serdang, Selangor, Malaysia; 3. Research Centre for Ruminant Disease, Faculty of Veterinary Medicine, Universiti Putra Malaysia, 43400 UPM Serdang, Selangor, Malaysia.
Corresponding author: Faez Firdaus Jesse Abdullah, e-mail: jesseariasamy@gmail.com,
NBN: usuba5050@live.com, YA: yabbavet@gmail.com, MM: researchofficer2002@yahoo.com,
AT: nasirvet69@gmail.com, MAS: masadiqvet@gmail.com, KM: kontomohammed@gmail.com,
ELTC: ericlim88@gmail.com, MAO: mo_ariff@upm.edu.my

Abstract

Aim: Gastrointestinal helminthosis is a global problem in small ruminant production. Most parasites have developed resistance to commonly available anthelminthic compounds, and there is currently an increasing need for new compounds with more efficacies. This study evaluated the *in vitro* effects of ethanolic extract of *Curcuma longa* (EECL) as a biological nematicide against third stage *Haemonchus* larvae (L3) isolated from sheep.

Materials and Methods: *Haemonchus* L3 were cultured and harvested from the feces of naturally infected sheep. EECL was prepared and three concentrations; 50, 100, and 200 mg/mL were tested for their efficacies on *Haemonchus* L3. Levamisole at concentration 1.5 and 3 mg/mL were used as positive controls.

Results: EECL showed anthelmintic activity in a dose-dependent manner with 78% worm mortality within 24 h of exposure at the highest dose rate of 200 mg/mL. There was a 100% worm mortality rate after 2 h of levamisole (3 mg/mL) admisntration. However, there was a comparable larvicidal effect between when levamisole (1.5 mg/mL) and EECL (200 mg) were administered.

Conclusion: The study shows that EECL does exhibit good anthelmintic properties at 200 mg/mL which is comparable with levamisole at 1.5 mg/mL.

Keywords: *Curcuma longa*, ethanolic extract, *Haemonchus*, larvae 3, levamisole, strongyle.

Introduction

Gastrointestinal helminths are among the most significant factors causing retarded growth in ruminants. Helminthosis is also one of the growing threats to the livestock production worldwide [1]. Treatment of helminthosis has become worrisome over the years due to the development of resistance by the parasites to chemical drugs available commercially in the market. Thus, there is an increasing need for alternative natural compounds that are safe and effective in combating this menace. Turmeric has been investigated widely and is said to exhibit different properties such as anti-inflammatory, hypercholesterolemic, choleretic, antimicrobial, insect repellent, antirheumtaic, antifibrotic, antivenomous, antiviral, antidiabetic, and antihepatotoxic as well as anticancerous properties [2,3].

The antiparasitic effect of curcumin, which is one of the active compounds in *Curcuma longa* has been observed to be dose-dependent, with higher concentrations of the compounds exhibiting the greatest effects. However, the exact mechanism of its action is still poorly understood and need to be studied in more detail [4]. Curcumin extract has been found to be effective against *Shistosoma mansoni* and earthworm muscle cells in a dose-dependent manner [5,6]. Its efficacy in *Ascaridia galli* in chicken has also been evaluated both *in vitro* and *in vivo* with success [7].

This study was designed to evaluate the effect of ethanolic extract of *C. longa* (EECL) as a treatment alternative for gastrointestinal heminths (strongyles) of sheep. The study will also evaluate the comparable efficacies of *C. longa* and levamisole on the survival rate of *Haemonchus* third stage larvae (L3) *in vitro*.

Materials and Methods

Ethical approval

Ethical approval was not required for this study as only fecal samples were collected from naturally infected sheep.

Preparation of plant materials

C. longa (turmeric) tubers were collected from the field in Serdang area. These tubers were thoroughly washed in water, cut into smaller pieces and left to dry at room temperature for 4 days. The dried turmeric was ground to powder form with a mortar and pestle and stored at room temperature in sealed plastic bags until it was used.

Preparation of EECL (turmeric)

Ethanolic extract of curcuma was prepared as previously described by Salama *et al.* [8]. Briefly, the fresh curcuma rhizomes were washed, dried, ground into powder, and weighed. 100 g of the powder was dissolved in 1 L of 95% ethanol at a ratio of 1:10 and left for 3 days at 25°C. The mixture was shaken at 4-6 h intervals. Filtration was done, and the liquid was evaporated to form a concentrated extract. This was kept in an incubator for a further 72 h to evaporate the residual. The sediment was then diluted with distilled water at a ratio of 200:1 to prepare the extract stock solution (200 mg/mL). Concentrations ranging from 100, 50, and 25 mg/mL were prepared by dilution of the stock solution with distilled water.

Preparation of levamisole concentrations

The initial concentration of levamisole was 32 mg/mL (Nilverm® Oral Drench, India) and was diluted with distilled water to get concentrations of 1.5 and 3.0 mg/mL.

Fecal culture and harvesting of third larval stage (L3) *Haemonchus*

Fecal samples were collected from naturally infected sheep (containing <250 epg), crushed and placed in a clean glass jar. The moisture of the feces in glass jar was maintained everyday by putting a few drops of distilled water for 7 days. A few scoops of charcoal were mixed with fecal material collected from diarrhoeric animals to prevent excessive moisture. After 7 days, the L3 stages were harvested from the culture by filling the glass jar with warm distilled and inverting the glass jar on a petri dish for 30 min. The L3 was observed under a dissecting microscope and harvested into a clean glass bottle and stored in the refrigerator at 4°C. Identification of the worm larvae was done by putting them on a glass slide with one drop of Lugol's iodine added before putting a cover slip onto it and examining under light microscopy.

Treatment and motility assessment

About 50 active L3 were put in a petri dish and maintained with 8.0 mL distilled water. The L3 were then treated with 1.0 mL *C. longa* extract at 200, 100, and 50 mg/mL. 1.0 mL levamisole at concentration 1.5 and 3 mg/mL was used as positive control and 1.0 mL distilled water was used as negative control. The petri dishes were shaken manually for 1 min and were kept at room temperature. Each Petri dish was examined every 2, 4, 6, and 24 h post-treatment. 4 replicates were done for each treatment. For every 2 h, the motility of the L3 was checked and recorded for each motile and non-motile or dead L3. The dead L3 were confirmed by observing the absence of motility for up to 10 s. The mortality index formula was used to determine the rate of L3 mortality.

$$\text{Mortality Index} = \frac{\text{No of dead L3}}{\substack{\text{Total number of} \\ \text{L3 in petri dish}}} \times 100\%$$

Statistical analysis

Statistical analysis was performed using SPSS version 20.0 statistical software. Results were assessed for its normality. One-way ANOVA was used for normally distributed data and $p<0.05$ was considered to be significant. Independent sample t-test was used for data in two independent or unrelated groups that have different means.

Results

Parasite larvae identification

Before the experiment was conducted, identifications were done on 100 strongyles that were harvested from the fecal culture by microscopic examination as previously described [9]. Based on the examination, the harvested strongyles comprised 97% *Haemonchus contortus* and 3% *Oesophagostomum* sp.

Effects of turmeric on *Haemonchus* L3 Viability

The different effects exhibited by different concentration of turmeric on the *Haemonchus* larvae mortality are shown in Figure-1. There was an increase in the number of dead larvae over time as turmeric concentrations exhibited the highest antihelmintic activity in a dose-dependent way with the maximum effect observed at the highest dose of turmeric extract; 200 mg/mL, where 78% of the worms died 24 h post-exposure. The mean mortality of larvae showed that it increased as turmeric concentration increased (Figure-2). The LC_{50} for MECL was estimated to be 128.2 mg, while the LC_{90} was 231 mg. The mortality of larvae was compared to the levamisole as the reference drugs or positive control at concentration of 1.5 mg/mL at 24 h and 3.0 mg/mL at 2 h post-exposure. At 1.5 mg/mL of levamisole, 72% larvae mortality was observed at 24 h post-exposure, while at 3.0 mg/mL, 100% larvae died at 2 h post-exposure. There was no mortality of larvae observed in distilled water (negative control) at 24 h post-exposure.

Comparative effects of turmeric at 200 mg/mL against levamisole at 1.5 mg/mL

The effect of turmeric extract was compared at 200 mg/mL with levamisole at 1.5 mg/mL. The result showed that there is no significance difference ($p<0.05$) between the two concentrations over a course of 24 h post-exposure (Figure-3).

Discussion

Tumeric has been long shown to exhibit different properties [2]. Turmeric hydroalcoholic extracts

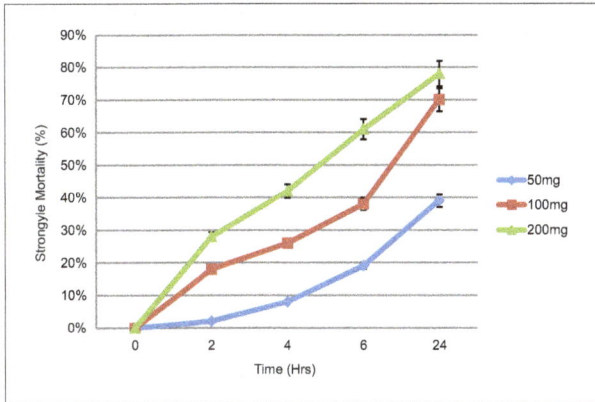

Figure-1: Percentage of larvae mortality at different hours following treatment with different concentrations of ethanolic extract of tumeric.

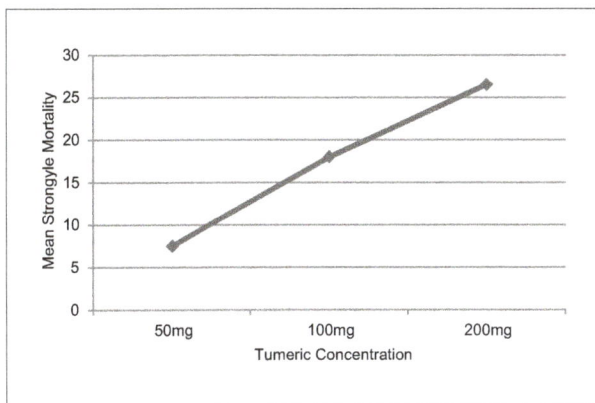

Figure-2: Mean non-motile strrongyle L3 following treatment with different concentrations of ethanolic extract of tumeric.

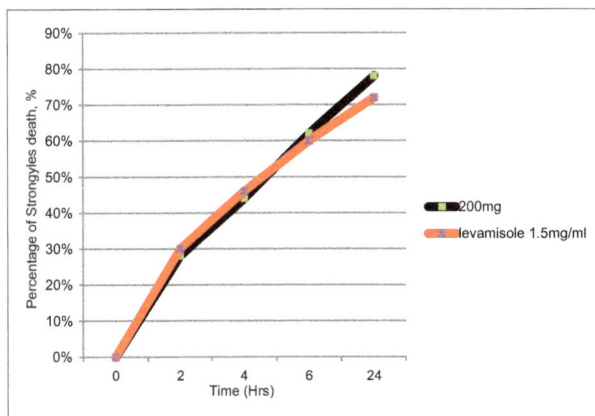

Figure-3: Comparison of larvae mortality at different hours following treatment with 200 mg/mL of ethanolic extract of tumeric and 1.5 mg/mL of levamisole.

have shown a remarkable anthelmintic potential against intestinal parasitism [10]. According to Kulkarni *et al.* [11], a maximum concentration of curcuminoids was obtained in methanol extract in the form of a dark black orange color compared to other extraction solvent such as acetone, chloroform, and ethyl acetate. This shows that methanol is a good solvent to be used to extract a high

concentration of curcumin content compared to any other solvent.

In this study, we observed that the efficacy of ethanolic extract of tumeric increased in a time and dose-dependent manner, as the number of larvae mortality increased with increasing dose and time. This could be due to the presence of more cucurminoid content in the extract as the concentration increased from 50 to 200 mg. Effects of *C. longa* as an anthelmintic revealed that some parts of cucurbits possess anthelmintic properties due to secondary metabolites such as cucurbitacin [1]. Previous studies reported that worms exposed to turmeric extract were paralyzed and died in a time and dose-dependent manner. The effect of turmeric extract on earthworm muscle cells was also found to be dosage dependent [5]. Similarly, Magalhães *et al.* [6] observed that curcumin at 50 and 100 μM caused 100% mortality in adult *S. mansoni* and at 5 and 20 μM decreased worm viability in comparison to negative control. The authors also reported that 5 and 10 μM reduced egg production by 50%, which was recently associated with transcriptional repression observed in Notch and transforming growth factor-β pathways [12].

With an increasing problem of anthelmintic resistance in small ruminants, especially sheep, there is an increasing demand to find alternative treatment for the helminthosis. According to Mohammed *et al.* [13], *H. contortus* is the major cause of small ruminant internal parasitism in warm and moist climatic regions. This is true as we observed 97 out of 100 isolated strongyles larvae to be *H. contortus* and only 3 were *Trichostrongylus* sp.

There was no significance difference between the effects of levamisole at 1.5 mg/mL and turmeric extract at 200 mg/mL on the mortality rate of larvae after 24 h of treatment. Levamisole kills worms by depolarizing nicotinic acetylcholine receptors in muscular junction and cause paralysis and death of worms [14,15]. While for turmeric, the curcuminoid is believed to be the main component that causes mortality of the worms, perhaps in a similar manner to that of levamisole. As stated earlier, a study by Vidya *et al.* [5] showed turmeric extract to have good growth suppression on earthworm muscle cells. Since nematodes or helminthes are only one level lower than earthworms, it may be considered that turmeric extract has similar effects on nematodes as it did on earthworms. Curcumin is a natural polyphenol that is responsible for antiproliferative activity on dividing cells; this activity may have caused the muscle growth suppression in earthworm. Although the antiparasitic effect of curcumin is more obvious at a higher concentration, the exact mechanism of action is not yet fully understood and may vary depending on the helminth parasite [4].

Conclusion

Turmeric extract at 200 mg/ml showed the highest anthelmintic properties with 78% mortality in L3 within 24 h. Similarly, it also showed a comparable effect at this dose with 1.5 mg/mL of levamisole. It can thus be concluded that the EECL exhibits good anthelmintic activity against *Haemonchus* larvae and can serve as a potential substitute for levamisole.

Authors' Contributions

MM, FFJA, and MAO designed and conceptualized the work. YA, AT, MAS, NBM, KM, and ELTC conducted the work and drafted the manuscript. All authors have read and approved the final manuscript.

Acknowledgments

The authors wish to acknowledge technical assistance rendered by staff of the Veterinary Pharmacology and Veterinary Pharmacology. Funds for this study were provided by Universiti Putra Malaysia.

Competing Interests

The authors declare that they have no competing interests.

References

1. Ullah, S., Khan, M.N., Sajid, M.S. and Muhammad, G. (2013) Comparative anthelmintic efficacy of *Curcuma longa, Citrullus colocynthis* and *Peganum harmala. Glob. Vet.,* 11(5): 560-567.

2. Akram, M., Shahab-Uddin, A.A., Usmanghani, K., Hannan, A., Mohiuddin, E. and Asif, M. (2010) *Curcuma longa* and Curcumin: A review article. *Rom. J. Plant Biol.,* 55(2): 65-70.

3. Velayudhan, K.C., Dikshi, N. and Nizar, M.A. (2012) Ethnobotany of turmeric (*Curcuma longa* L.). *Indian J. Tradit. Knowl.,* 11(4): 607-614.

4. Shahiduzzaman, M. and Daugschies, A. (2011) Curcumin: A natural herb extract with antiparasitic properties. In: Nature Helps. Springer, Berlin Heidelberg. p141-152.

5. Vidya, J., Kale, R.D. and Nair, P. (2012) Earthworm muscle cells as models to study anthelminitic properties of plant extracts. *Int. J. Res. Pharm. Biomed. Sci.,* 3(2): 489-496.

6. Magalhães, L.G., Machado, C.B., Morais, E.R., De Carvalho, M.É.B., Soares, C.S., Da Silva, S.H. and Rodrigues, V. (2009) *In vitro* schistosomicidal activity of curcumin against *Schistosoma mansoni* adult worms. *Parasitol. Res.,* 104(5): 1197-1201.

7. Bazh, E.K. and El-Bahy, N.M. (2013) *In vitro* and *in vivo* screening of anthelmintic activity of ginger and curcumin on *Ascaridia galli. Parasitol. Res.,* 112(11): 3679-3686.

8. Salama, S.M., Abdulla, M.A., AlRashdi, A.S., Ismail, S., Alkiyumi, S.S. and Golbabapour, S. (2013) Hepatoprotective effect of ethanolic extract of *Curcuma longa* on thioacetamide induced liver cirrhosis in rats. *BMC Compl. Altern. Med.,* 13(1): 56.

9. Hansen, J.W. and Perry, B.D. (1994) Techniques for parasite assays and identification in faecal samples. The Epidemiology, Diagnosis and Control of Helminth Parasites of Ruminants. International Laboratory for Research on Animal Diseases, Nairobi, Kenya.

10. Singh, R., Mehta, A. and Shukla, K. (2011) Anthelmintic activity of rhizome extracts of *Curcuma longa* and *Zingiber officinale* (Zingiberaceae). *Int. J. Pharm. Pharm. Sci.,* 3(2): 236-237.

11. Kulkarni, S.J., Maske, K.N., Budre, M.P. and Mahajan, R.P. (2012) Extraction and purification of curcuminoids from turmeric (*Curcuma longa* L.). *Int. J. Pharmacol. Pharm. Technol.,* 1(2): 29-34.

12. Morais, E.R., Oliveira, K.C., Magalhães, L.G., Moreira, É.B., Verjovski-Almeida, S. and Rodrigues, V. (2013) Effects of curcumin on the parasite *Schistosoma mansoni*: A transcriptomic approach. *Mol. Biochem. Parasitol.,* 187(2): 91-97.

13. Mohammed, K., Abba, Y., Ramli, N.S.B., Marimuthu, M., Omar, M.A., Abdullah, F.F.J., Sadiq, M.A., Tijjani, A., Chung, E.L.T. and Lila, M.A.M. (2016) The use of FAMACHA in estimation of gastrointestinal nematodes and total worm burden in Damara and Barbados Blackbelly cross sheep. *Trop. Anim. Health Prod.,* 1-8.

14. Martin, R.J. (1997) Review: Modes of action of anthelmintic drugs. *Vet. J.,* 154: 11-34.

15. Martin, R.J. and Robertson, A.P. (2007) Mode of action of levamisole and pyrantel, anthelmintic resistance, E153 and Q57. *Parasitology,* 134: 1093-1104.

22

Comparison of rapid immunodiagnosis assay kit with molecular and immunopathological approaches for diagnosis of rabies in cattle

Ajaz Ahmad and C. K. Singh

Department of Veterinary Pathology, College of Veterinary Science, Guru Angad Dev Veterinary and Animal Sciences University, Ludhiana - 141 004, Punjab, India.
Corresponding author: Ajaz Ahmad, e-mail: ajazpatho786@gmail.com,
CKS: rabiesck@gmail.com

Abstract

Aim: Presently, diagnosis of rabies is primarily based on, conventional fluorescent antibody technique (FAT), immunopathological and molecular techniques. Recently, rapid immunodiagnostic assay (RIDA) - A monoclonal antibody-based technique has been introduced for rapid diagnosis of rabies. The present investigation is envisaged to study the efficacy of RIDA kit for the diagnosis of rabies in cattle.

Materials and Methods: About 11 brain samples from cattle, clinically suspected for rabies, were screened by the FAT, Heminested reverse transcriptase polymerase chain reaction (HnRT-PCR), Immunohistochemistry (IHC), and RIDA.

Results: The sensitivity for detection of rabies from brain tissue by RIDA was 85.7% as compared to 100% by IHC as well as HnRT-PCR. The accuracy of detection of rabies by RIDA was 91.6% as compared to 100% that of IHC and HnRT-PCR, whereas specificity of RIDA was 100% like that of the IHC and HnRT-PCR.

Conclusion: Despite a comparatively low-sensitivity and accuracy of RIDA, latter can still be useful in screening a large number of field samples promptly. However, it is recommended that negative results with RIDA in cattle need to be authenticated by suitable alternative diagnostic approaches.

Keywords: cattle, diagnosis, fluorescent antibody technique, heminested reverse transcriptase, immunohistochemistry, rabies.

Introduction

Rabies is the most important zoonotic disease of animals that has a significant impact on human beings. Authentic diagnostic approaches, therefore, have to be employed to distinguish this disease from other encephalitic conditions.

A rapid immunodiagnostic assay (RIDA) using a specific monoclonal antibody against rabies virus (RABV) is commercially available (Bio note, Korea). RIDA kit is rapid and simple and does not require any special equipment or technical expertise [1]. The efficacy of the diagnostic kits might vary with different species.

Immunohistochemistry (IHC) is a sensitive diagnostic technique which can demonstrate rabies antigen in fixed paraffin embedded tissue sections. In cattle, the distribution of viral antigen was revealed either in granular form or as inclusion bodies in the cerebellum, brain stem, hippocampus, and cerebrum [2-4].

Heminested reverse transcriptase polymerase chain reaction (HnRT-PCR) has been used to diagnose RABV worldwide due to its sensitivity and immense versatility and can even be useful for examining paraffin-fixed archived and decomposed samples [5]. The nucleoprotein (N) gene of RABV is targeted for diagnosing and analyzing hereditary characteristics and antigenic properties since this gene is highly conserved and combined with encapsidation of genomic RNA [6,7]. Recently, RIDA - A monoclonal antibody-based technique has been introduced for rapid diagnosis of rabies. The efficacy of the assay might vary in different species.

The present study was, therefore, envisaged to study the efficacy of RIDA in cattle where in comparison of its sensitivity, specificity and accuracy of detection of RABV in clinically suspected cattle with molecular technique *viz.* HnRT-PCR and an immunopathological technique *viz.* IHC.

Materials and Methods

Ethical approval

The study was approved by Institutional Animal Ethics Committee under memo no. IAEC/2014/241-70, Dated 04/12/14.

Sample collection

Brain tissue samples of cattle (n=11) suspected for rabies were collected from post-mortem hall, Department of Veterinary Pathology, Guru Angad

Dev Veterinary and Animal Sciences University (GADVASU), Ludhiana, Punjab and different dairy farms of Punjab, India, between January 2014 and January 2015. All brain samples were stored at −20°C in the laboratory for further processing. Diagnostic tests like fluorescent antibody technique (FAT), HnRT-PCR and RIDA were carried out to detect the RABV infection. Direct FAT is a gold standard [8], thus, the sensitivity of RIDA kit was analyzed in comparison to FAT in brain tissue samples. For histopathology and IHC, brain tissue samples were fixed and stored in 10% neutral buffered formalin for further analysis.

Fluorescent antibody test

FAT was carried out on fresh brain sample following the standard protocol [9]. Briefly, glass slides with impression smears of brain tissue were placed in coplin jar containing acetone and fixed at −4°C for 1 h. Positive slides from a known rabies positive case and negative slide from a normal and uninfected animal were used as a positive and negative control, respectively. The slides were air-dried, incubated with lyophilized anti-rabies nucleocapsid conjugate (Bio-Rad, France) for 35 min at 37°C in a humid chamber and washed with phosphate buffered saline (PBS) in three successive washes for 5-10 min. The slides were rinsed with distilled water, air-dried and a cover slip was mounted by adding buffered glycerol on the smear. The slides were visualized under an immuno-fluorescent microscope (Zeiss) for bright apple-green, round to oval bodies. Positive and negative controls were run together with the test specimens.

Histopathology

Brian tissues samples including cerebellum, cerebrum, and hippocampus were collected and fixed in 10% neutral buffered formalin solution and given overnight washings under tap water. Dehydration of samples was done through ascending grades of alcohol (70%, 80%, 90%, and absolute alcohol) followed by clearing with acetone. Tissues were embedded in paraffin wax (Leica Microsystem) for further processing. Approximately, 4-5 μ thick sections were cut, stained with routine hematoxylin and eosin (H and E) staining technique [10] and examined by BX61 Research Photomicrograph Microscope System (Olympus Corporation, USA), the facility provided by the department.

IHC

Anti-rabbit polyclonal antisera raised in Rabies Research-cum-Diagnostic Laboratory of the Department of Veterinary Pathology, GADVASU, Ludhiana was used as primary antibody in IHC. Advanced SS™ One step polymer horseradish peroxidase (HRPO) IHC detection system (BioGenex Laboratories Inc., San Ramon, California, USA) counterstained with Gill's hematoxylin was used. IHC was done as recommended by the manufacturer with minor modifications. Formalin-fixed brain samples were thoroughly washed in running water; dehydrated

in ascending grades of alcohol and acetone; cleared in benzene and embedded in paraffin at 58°C [11,12]. Paraffin-embedded tissues were cut into 5 μm thick sections, and sister sections were taken on Superfrost/Plus, positively charged, microscopic slides (Fisher Scientific, USA). The sections were deparaffinized and rehydrated by immersing in 250 ml EZ-AR common solution at 70°C for 10 min in EZ-Retriever R System V.2.1. Subsequent antigen retrieval was done in citrate buffer (0.01 M, pH 6.0-6.2) at 95°C for 10 min and at 98°C for 5 min in EZ-Retriever R System V.2.1. Three washing were given in PBS buffer for 3 min each. The endogenous tissue peroxidases were inactivated by immersing slides in 3% hydrogen peroxide solution in methanol for 15 min at room temperature in humid chamber followed by three washings with PBS buffer for 3 min each. Non-specific binding was blocked by incubating sections with ready-to-use power block for 10 min at room temperature in the moist chamber. On one section of each slide, primary polyclonal rabbit anti-rabies antibody of 1:1000 dilution (in PBS) was added, and slide was incubated for 1 h in moist chamber at room temperature, whereas, on the other section of each slide, PBS without primary antibody was added, so as to serve as a negative control. The sections were washed thrice in PBS buffer for 3 min each, and thereafter, incubated with polymer HRP (Super Sensitive label, One Step Polymer-HRPO Reagent) for 30 min at room temperature in the moist chamber, followed by three washing in PBS buffer for 3 min each. The antigen-antibody peroxidase reaction was developed with a freshly prepared 3,3-diaminobenzidine (DAB) solution by mixing two drops of DAB chromogen with 1 ml of DAB buffer supplied by the manufacturer adding 5 ml hydrogen peroxide. Sections were washed in distilled water for 5 min and counterstained with Gill's hematoxylin (Merck, Germany) for 30 s and washed in running tap water for 5 min. Finally, the slides were dehydrated in ascending grades of alcohol, cleared in xylene, mounted in DPX and examined under an advanced microscope (BX 61, Olympus Corporation, USA).

Extraction of viral RNA

Total RNA was extracted from brain tissue using Trizol reagent (Invitrogen, USA) following manufacturer's instructions with minor modifications. Briefly, 0.1 g brain tissue was homogenized with 1 ml Trizol and 200 μl chloroform (Ambion Life Technologies, USA) was added. After centrifugation of the sample at 10,000 rpm for 15 min, the top aqueous layer was recovered, and RNA was precipitated by adding 0.5 ml isopropanol. The sample was spun at 10,000 rpm for 10 min, the liquid removed and the pellet washed with 1 ml of 75% ethanol. The dried RNA pellet was dissolved in 50 μl sterile RNase free water. RNA concentration was measured using Nano Drop Spectrophotometer (Nano Drop Technologies, CA) in ng/μl. The quality of RNA was checked as a ratio of OD 260/280 and stored at −80°C. RNA was converted into cDNA using High-Capacity cDNA Reverse Transcription Kit with RNAse inhibitor (Applied Biosystems, USA).

RNA Amplification

Amplification of 2 µl of reverse-transcribed cDNA template was performed in a final volume of 25 µl; 12.5 µl ×2 PCR mix (GoTaq Green Master Mix, Promega), 1.0 µl of each forward and reverse primer (JW12 and JW6) with 10 pmol concentration, and nuclease free water was added to make final volume of 25 µl. The amplification was performed in a thermal cycler with cycling conditions of initial denaturation at 94°C for 3 min; 35 cycles denaturation at 94°C for 30 seconds; annealing at 56°C for 45 s and elongation at 72°C for 20 s. Final elongation was performed at 72°C for 3 min. For HnRT-PCR, similar quantities of the PCR mixture constituents except 2 µl of the primary PCR product as template and JW12 as forward and JW10 as reverse primer were used (Table-1). Thermocyclic conditions were kept same as that of primary PCR. PCR amplified products were visualized in 1% agarose gel electrophoresis after ethidium bromide staining of 586 bp amplicons.

RIDA kit

A commercial RIDA kit was used the following the manufacturer's direction (Bionote, Korea). Briefly, a swab supplied with the kit was dipped into 10% homogenate of brain samples. The content of swab was shifted to an enclosed proprietary buffer of RIDA kit. A 100 µl aliquot of the sample was transferred to the sample well. The appearance of two lines, 5 min after addition of the brain samples, was considered positive result whereas the formation of one line was considered as a negative result [13].

Calculation of sensitivity, specificity, and accuracy

Sensitivity was calculated as [TP/(TP+FN)] × 100. Specificity was calculated as [TN/(TN+FP)] × 100. Accuracy was calculated as [TP+TN/(TP+FP+FN+TN)] × 100 wherein TP was true-positives; FN was false-negatives; TN was true negatives and FP was false positives as determined by the reference assay, i.e., FAT.

Results

Out of 11 cattle brain samples screened by FAT, only six cows (54.54%) (07RL14, 15RL14, 19RL14, 21RL14, 42RL14 and 02RL15) were confirmed to be rabid (or TP). Same six samples were detected as positive by IHC as well as by HnRT-PCR. However, RIDA could detect rabies only in five samples. Further, the

intensity of the test lines, in positive samples, also varied in different field samples. The sensitivity of detection of rabies by IHC, HnRT-PCR, and RIDA was 100%, 100% and 85.71% respectively (Table-2). Specificity of detection of rabies by IHC, HnRT-PCR, and RIDA was 100% in all the tests. The accuracy of detection of rabies by IHC and HnRT-PCR was 100% and by RIDA, was 91.66% (Tables-3-5).

As such, sensitivity for detection of rabies from brain tissue by RIDA was comparatively lower (85.7%) as compared to IHC as well as HnRT-PCR (100%). Likewise, accuracy for detection of rabies by RIDA was also lesser (91.6%) as compared to IHC and HnRT-PCR (100%), whereas specificity of RIDA (100%) was comparable to IHC and HnRT-PCR (100%) (Table-6).

Discussion

FAT

Direct FAT is gold-standard for rabies diagnosis as recommended by the World Health Organization and Office International des Epizootics [14]. Bright apple-green, round to oval intracellular fluorescent bodies were observed in all the positive brain samples as observed earlier [15].

Histopathology

Neuronal necrosis, Negri bodies (Figure-1), satellitosis, gliosis, neuronophagia, congestion, hemorrhage, and perivascular cuffing observed in brain samples was in accordance with the findings of Singh [16] and Sumedha [17].

IHC

IHC in formalin fixed paraffin embedded tissue sections has been reported to be a sensitive

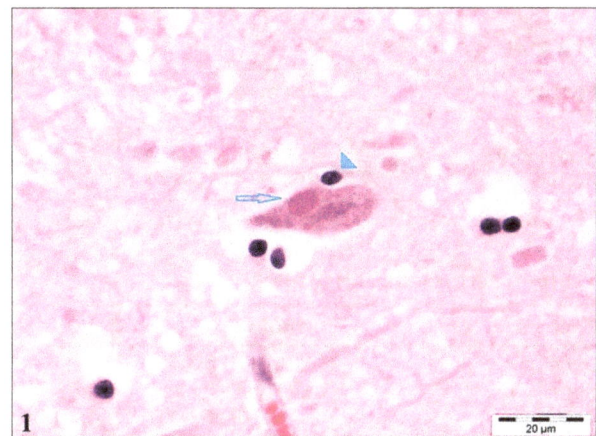

Figure-1: Section of the hippocampus of rabid cattle showing sharply Negri body and neuronophagia (×100).

Table-1: Primers used for HnRT-PCR to target N gene.

Primer	Nucleotide sequences (5'-3')	Nucleotide position	Sense	Size of amplicon (bp)
JW 12	5'ATGTAACACCCCTACAATG3'	55-73	+	586
JW 6	5'CAATTGGCACACATTTTGTGT3'	660-641	−	
JW 10	5'GTCATCAGAGTATGGTGTTC3'	636-617	−	

HnRT-PCR=Hemi-nested reverse transcriptase polymerase chain reaction technique for detection of rabies antigen [18] and has been found to be of immense value for retrospective studies [19,20]. With IHC viral antigens were observed as fine granules in the cytoplasm of the neurons (Figure-2), which were not clearly visible with H and E staining.

HnRT-PCR

In the present study, 100% agreement was observed between FAT and HnRT-PCR targeting N gene of virus (Figure-3). HnRT-PCR using a primer set that amplified the N gene of RABV was able to detect the isolates from six cows confirmed to be rabid by FAT. These isolates were detected only after both primary as well as secondary PCRs were accomplished in the assay of HnRT-PCR as reported earlier [21,22].

RIDA

The present study evaluated the efficacy of RIDA for diagnosis of rabies for use in field condition. RIDA detected rabies (Figure-4) in cattle brain samples with a sensitivity of 85.71%. The result obtained in the present study is comparable to earlier usage of RIDA kit on European mammals wherein the sensitivity of 88% reported [23]. Nevertheless, higher sensitivity of 91%

was also reported, in another study, wherein, 54 brain samples were tested [24]. Despite a comparatively low sensitivity and accuracy of RIDA, it is still of use

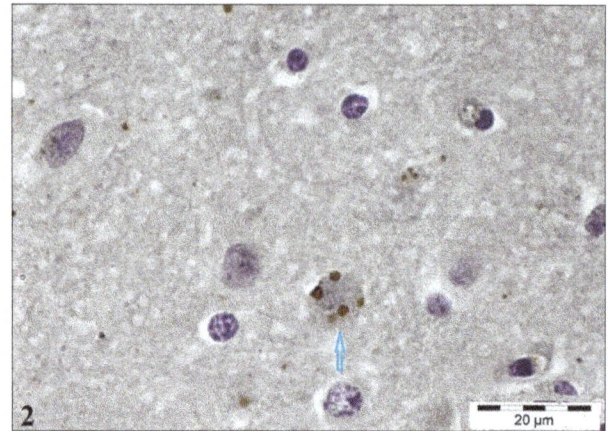

Figure-2: Section of the cerebellum of rabid cattle showing brown colored Negri bodies in the purkinje cells (×100).

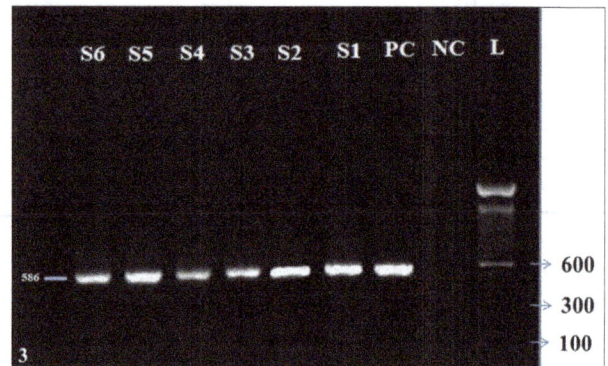

Figure-3: Agarose gel (1%) stained with ethidium bromide. Lane L is the 100 bp ladder, NC is the negative control, PC is a positive control, S1-S6 are the samples that are positive for fluorescent antibody technique.

Table-2: Test results of IHC, HnRT-PCR and RIDA in comparison with FAT.

FAT	IHC		HnRT-PCR		RIDA		Total
	P	N	P	N	P	N	
P	06	00	06	00	05	01	06 [TP]
N	00	05	00	05	00	05	05 [TN]
Total	06	05	06	05	05	06	11

IHC=Immunohistochemistry, HnRT-PCR=Heminested polymerase chain reaction, RIDA=Rapid immunodiagnostic assay, FAT=Fluorescent antibody test, P=Positive, N=Negative, TP=True positive, TN=True negative

Table-3: Test results of RIDA.

Factors	Formula	Calculation	Result (%)
Sensitivity	TP/(TP+FN)]×100	5/5+1=5/6	85.71
Specificity	[TN/(TN+FP)]×100	5/5+0=5/5	100
Accuracy	TP+TN/(TP+FP+FN+TN)]×100	6+5/6+0+1+5	91.66

TP=True positive, TN=True negative, FP=False positive, FN=False negative, RIDA=Rapid immunodiagnostic assay

Table-4: Test results of HnRT-PCR.

Factors	Formula	Calculation	Result (%)
Sensitivity	TP/(TP+FN)]×100	6/6+0=6/6	100
Specificity	[TN/(TN+FP)]×100	5/5+0=5/5	100
Accuracy	TP+TN/(TP+FP+FN+TN)]×100	6+5/6+0+0+5=11/11	100

TP=True positive, TN=True negative, FP=False positive, FN=False negative, HnRT-PCR=Heminested polymerase chain reaction

Table-5: Test results of IHC.

Factors	Formula	Calculation	Result (%)
Sensitivity	TP/(TP+FN)]×100	6/6+0=6/6	100
Specificity	[TN/(TN+FP)]×100	5/5+0=5/5	100
Accuracy	TP+TN/(TP+FP+FN+TN)]×100	6+5/6+0+0+5=11/11	100

TP=True positive, TN=True negative, FP=False positive, FN=False negative, IHC=Immunohistochemistry

Table-6: Comparison of sensitivity, specificity and accuracy of three diagnostic techniques.

Factors	IHC (%)	HnRT-PCR (%)	RIDA (%)
Sensitivity	100.00	100.00	85.71
Specificity	100.00	100.00	100.00
Accuracy	100.00	100.00	91.66

IHC=Immunohistochemistry, HnRT-PCR=Heminested polymerase chain reaction, RIDA=Rapid immunodiagnostic assay

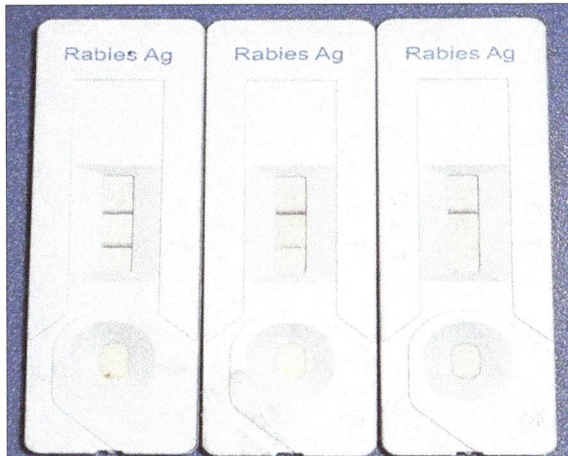

Figure-4: Rapid immunodiagnostic assay A and B are positive and C is negative.

to screen a large number of field samples promptly. It is, however, recommended that any negative result with RIDA should be ruled out by confirmation with a suitable alternative diagnostic approach.

Conclusion

It is possible to use RIDA for prompt diagnosis of rabies in the field conditions. However, the samples found negative by RIDA need to be investigated further by immunofluorescent/molecular approach for authentication/confirmation of the diagnosis of rabies.

Authors' Contributions

CKS designed the experiment, organized sample collection. The experiment was performed by AA under the supervision of CKS. AA collected samples and performed the diagnostic techniques. Both authors read and approved the final manuscript.

Acknowledgments

The authors are thankful to the Director of Research, Guru Angad Dev Veterinary and Animal Sciences University, Ludhiana for providing the necessary facilities and fund for this study.

Competing Interests

The authors declare that they have no competing interests.

References

1. Lembo, T., Niezgoda, M., Velasco-Villa, A., Cleaveland, S., Ernest, E. and Rupprecht, C.E. (2006) Evaluation of a direct, rapid immunohistochemical test for rabies diagnosis. *Emerg. Infect. Dis.,* 12: 310-313.

2. Sharma, P., Singh, C.K., Sood, N.K., Sandhu, B.S., Gupta, K. and Brar, A.P.S. (2014) Diagnosis of rabies from brain: Comparison of histochemical and histopathological approaches. *Indian J. Vet. Pathol.,* 38(4): 269-272.

3. Wahan, S., Sandhu, B.S., Singh, C.K., Gupta, K., Sood, N.K. and Kaw, A. (2012) Comparison of clinico-pathological, immunohistochemical and immunofluorescent techniques for diagnosis of rabies in animals. *Indian J. Anim. Sci.,* 82(1), 3-8..

4. Sandhu, B.S., Sood, N.K., Awahan, S., Singh, C.K. and Gupta, K. (2011) Immunohistochemistry, histopathology, quantitative morphometry of Negri bodies in the brain of rabid animals. *Indian J. Vet. Pathol.,* 35(2): 117-122.

5. David, D., Yakobson, B., Rotenberg, D., Dveres, N., Davidson, I. and Stram, Y. (2002) Rabies virus detection by RT-PCR in decomposed naturally infected brains. *Vet Microbiol.,* 87: 111-118.

6. Yang, J., Hooper, D.C., Wunner, W.H., Koprowski, H. and Dietzschold, B.F. (1998) The specificity of rabies virus RNA encapsidation by nucleoprotein. *Virology,* 242: 107-117.

7. Pranoti, S., Singh, C.K. and Deepti, N. (2015) Comparison of immunochromatographic diagnostic test with heminested reverse transcriptase polymerase chain reaction for detection of rabies virus from brain samples of various species. *Vet. World,* 8(2): 135-138.

8. WHO. (1992) Expert Committee on Rabies. 8th Report. WHO Technical Report Series, No. 824. World Health Organization, Geneva. p7, 8.

9. Meslin, F.X., Kaplan, M.M. and Koprowski, H. (1996) Laboratory Diagnosis of Rabies. WHO, Geneva. p88-95.

10. Luna, L.G. (1968) Manual of Histological Staining Methods of the Armed Forces Institute of Pathology. 3rd ed. The Blakiston Division, McGraw-Hill Book Co., New York.

11. Pranoti, S., Singh, C.K., Sood, N.K., Gupta, K., Sandhu, B.S. and Brar, A.P.S. (2015) Immunohistochemical detection of rabies in dogs from skin. *Indian J. Canine Pract.,* 7(1): 37-40.

12. Pedroso, P.M.O., Pescador, C.A., Bandarra, P.M., Raymundo, D.L., Borba, M.R., Wouters, F., Bezerra-Junior, P.S. and Driemeier, D. (2008) Standardization of immunohistochemistry technique for detection of rabies virus in formalin-fixed and paraffin-embedded tissue samples from central nervous system of cattle. *Pesqui. Vet. Bras.* 28(12): 627.

13. Dong, K.Y., Eun, K.S., Yoon, I.O., Kyung, W.L., Chung, S.L., Seo, Y.K., Jeong, A.L. and Jae, Y.S. (2012) Comparison of four diagnostic methods for detecting rabies viruses circulating in Korea. *J. Vet. Sci.,* 13(1): 43-48.

14. Dean, D.J., Abelseth, M.K. and Atanasiu, P. (1996) The fluorescent antibody test. In: Meslin, F.X., Kaplan, M.M. and Koprowski, H., editors. Laboratory Techniques in Rabies. 4th ed. WHO, Geneva. p88-95.

15. Ehizibolo, D.O., Nwosuh, C., Ehizibolo, E.E. and Kia, G.S.N. (2009) Comparison of the fluorescent antibody test and direct microscopic examination for rabies diagnosis at the National Veterinary Research Institute, Vom, Nigeria. *Afr. J. Biomed. Res.,* 12: 1.

16. Singh, H. (1999) Experimental rabies in buffalo calves with street rabies virus. M.V.Sc. Thesis, Punjab Agricultural University, Ludhiana, India.

17. Sumedha, A. (2010) Anti-mortem and post-mortem detection of rabies virus antigen in natural cases of rabies in animals - An immunopathological study. M.V.Sc. Thesis. Guru Angad Dev Veterinary and Animal Sciences University, Ludhiana, India.

18. Last, R.D., Jardine, J.E., Smit, M.M.E. and Van Der Lugt, J.J. (1994) Application of immunoperoxidase techniques to formalin-fixed brain tissue for the diagnosis of rabies in southern Africa. *J. Vet. Res.,* 61(2): 183-187.

19. Gunawardena, G.S.P. and Blakemore, W.F. (2007) Proceedings of the Peradeniya University Research Sessions, Sri Lanka. Vol. 12. No. 1.p168.

20. Rissi, D.R., Fighera, R.A., Irigoyen, L.F., Kommers, G.D. and Claudio, S.L.B. (2008) Occurrence of rabies in sheep in Rio Grande do Sul, Brazil. *Pesqui. Vet. Bras.,* 28(10): 495.

21. Soares, R.M., Bernardi, F., Sakamoto, S.M., Heinemann, M.B., Cortez, A., Alves, L.M., Meyer, A.D., Ito, F.H. and Richtzenhain, L.J. (2002) A heminested polymerase chain reaction for the detection of Brazilian rabies isolates from vampire bats and herbivores. *Mem. Inst. Oswaldo Cruz,* 97: 109-111.

22. Orłowska, A., Smreczak, M., Trębas, P. and Żmudziński, J.F. (2008) Comparison of real-time PCR and heminested RT-PCR methods in the detection of rabies virus infection in bats and terrestrial animals. *Bull. Vet. Inst. Pulawy,* 52: 313-318.

23. Servat, A., Picard-Meyer, E., Robardet, E., Muzniece, Z., Must, K. and Cliquet, F. (2012) Evaluation of a rapid immunochromatographic diagnostic test for the detection of rabies from brain material of European mammals. *Biologicals,* 40(1): 61-66.

24. Kang, B., Oh, J., Lee, C., Park, B.K., Park, Y., Hong, K., Lee, K., Cho, B. and Song, D. (2007) Evaluation of a rapid immunodiagnostic test kit for rabies virus. *J. Virol. Methods,* 145(1): 30-36.

23

Assessment of motion and kinematic characteristics of frozen-thawed Sirohi goat semen using computer-assisted semen analysis

Mukul Anand and Sarvajeet Yadav

Department of Veterinary Physiology, College of Veterinary Sciences and Animal Husbandry, Uttar Pradesh Pandit Deen Dayal Upadhayaya Pashu Chikitsa Vigyan Vishwavidyalaya Evam Go Anusandhan Sansthan, Mathura - 281 001, Uttar Pradesh, India.
Corresponding author: Mukul Anand, e-mail: drmukulanandvet@gmail.com,
SY: yadavsarvajeet24@gmail.com

Abstract

Aim: The aim was to determine the motion and kinematics characteristic of frozen-thawed spermatozoa in Sirohi goat using computer-assisted semen analysis.

Materials and Methods: A study was carried out in Sirohi buck. Semen collection was made biweekly from each buck with the help of artificial vagina. A total of 12 ejaculates were collected from two bucks (six ejaculates from each buck). Freshly collected semen was pooled and later evaluated. The pooled semen sample was extended with standard glycerolated egg yolk tris extender and later subjected to a process of cryopreservation. The motion and kinematic characteristics of spermatozoa were studied during freez-thawing process.

Results: Significantly ($p < 0.01$) higher value of live percent, hypo-osmotic swelling test, and acrosomal integrity were recorded in neat semen followed by diluted and frozen thaw semen. The proportion of spermatozoa showing slow progression were the highest in the neat and diluted semen followed by rapid and non-progressively motile, while a reverse pattern was observed in the frozen thaw semen where the proportion of non-progressively motile spermatozoa were significantly ($p < 0.01$) higher followed by slow and rapid progression.

Conclusion: This study showed that the best results for motion, vitality, plasma membrane integrity, and acrosome status were obtained in the neat semen followed by diluted and frozen thaw semen. Further, the process of cryopreservation results in a shift of motility from slow to non-progressive in the post-thaw semen with a significant decrease in the path velocities when compared to neat and diluted semen. Hence, it can be concluded that freezing-thawing process reduces the motility and kinematic characters spermatozoa and may be an important factor affecting the fertilizing ability of spermatozoa resulting in poor conception rate after insemination in goats.

Keywords: computer-assisted semen analysis, cryopreservation, motility, semen, Sirohi goat.

Introduction

Goat has been an integral part of animal husbandry system in India. Due to its peculiar feeding habits and low input cost, the majority of goats are kept and reared by small, marginal and landless farmers in country [1]. But with the increase in population and decrease in the pasture land, goat husbandry practice is gaining importance as an alternate food source in our country. There has been a tremendous increase in number of commercial goats farms in recent years [2]. However, due to indiscriminate breeding and unawareness among the animal owners, the productive and reproductive efficiency of goats lags behind and need improvement. Establishment of true line breeds with high proliferacy and fast growth are major challenges

to be addressed. Selective breeding of goats can be alternate for genetic upgradation. Artificial insemination (AI) through the use of cryopreserved semen is an important tool for successful implementation of breeding program to establish pure line breed of goat [3]. The success of AI largely depends on quality of cryopreserved semen that in turns determines the conception rate [4]. Hence, quality assurance through regular monitoring of semen quality has becomes an important component of freez-thawing protocol. Different parameters have been establish for assessment of semen quality, *viz.*, percent live, hypo-osmotic swelling test (HOST), acrosomal integrity, motility, etc. that defines the quality of semen.

Motility is a phenomenon responsible for transport of spermatozoa from site of deposition to site of fertilization. This process peculiar to spermatozoa depends on the physiological and morphological status of a sperm cell and is highly sensitive to stressor encountered during the process of cryopreservation. Earlier the motility was evaluated through visual observation, i.e., mass motility and progressive motility that lack precision. Further, motility characteristic is considered as the parameter of choice to determine the degree of sperm damage inflicted by the cryo-preservation in goats due to the wide range of results found for sperm motility [5].

Hence, taking into account the importance of motility and motion characters exhibited by sperms in determining the fertility, computer-assisted semen analysis (CASA) techniques is now being used to study motion and path velocities of spermatozoa. CASA provides an objective and reproducible data on a number of sperm motion parameters and enhance the value of motility assessment to fertility prognosis resulting in high correlations among several CASA motility parameters [6,7]. Since the identification of ejaculates as suitable, or not suitable is based on fresh and post-thaw semen quality [8], the study was conducted to evaluate the motility and kinematic parameters in the neat, diluted and frozen thaw semen of Sirohi buck.

Materials and Methods

Ethical approval

No ethical approval was necessary to pursue this research work.

Animal and sampling

The study was conducted on 2 Sirohi bucks aged between 3 and 4 years, weighing between 30 and 40 kg, reared in experimental goat shed of Department of Physiology, Pt. Deen Dayal Upadhaya Pashuchikitisha Vigyan Vishwa Vidyalay Evam Go Anusandhan Sansthan (DUVASU), Mathura. The work related to semen analysis was performed in the Department of Veterinary Physiology (Hi-Tech Lab), College of Veterinary Science and Animal Husbandry, DUVASU, Mathura, Uttar Pradesh Semen collection was made biweekly from each buck with the help of artificial vagina. A total of 12 ejaculates were collected from two bucks (six ejaculates from each buck). Freshly collected semen was evaluated and pooled. The pooled semen (spermatozoa with seminal plasma) was extended with standard glycerolated egg yolk tris extender (3% egg yolk and 6% glycerol) and later subjected to process of cryopreservation. Sperm attributes *viz.,* percent live sperms [9], HOST [10] and sperms with intact acrosome [11] were evaluates manually using standard protocol while sperm kinematics were evaluated using the CASA system during the free-thawing process. To assess post-thaw sperm parameters, straws were removed from liquid nitrogen storage container with the help of forceps and dipped in water maintained at 37°C for 30 s in thawing unit (IMV, France). Later straws were withdrawn and wiped with tissue paper to make it moisture free. Sperm motion parameters and sperm kinematics were evaluated using CASA on a plate warmed to 37°C, negative phase contrast and ×10 objective. Settings of the CASA system (Biovis CASA 2000, Version 4.6, India) designed using algorithm based on size, shape, detection of sperm

head and classes for motile, immotile, rapid, slow and non-progressive were as follow: Frames/s - 60, number of frames acquired - 61, max velocity (for tracking): V (um/s) - 150 motility min, curvilinear velocity (VCL): V (um/s) - >25 motility min, average path velocity: V (um/s) - >10 motility min, straight-line velocity: V(um/s) - >1 min, track length (% of frames) - 51, aspect - 0-99,999, area - 2-20, axis (major) - 4-20, axis (minor) - 2-10, compactness - 0-50, perimeter ratio - 0-99,999, minimum cell size on major axis - 20, minimum cell size on min axis - 10 magnification - ×10 phase, calibration × (pixels/unit) - 1.905 μ, Y (pixels/unit) - 1.905 μ, size of image - 1280 × 960 pixels. Semen was diluted and adjusted to a concentration of about 50×10^6 spermatozoa per ml for computer aided motility analysis. A 4 μl of diluted semen sample was loaded in metallic sperm counting chamber and a range of 3-6 fields were acquired for motility analysis.

Statistical analysis

Statistical analyses were performed using Statistical Package for Social Science (SPSS® Version 20.0 for Windows®, SPSS Inc., Chicago, USA). The means were compared using Analysis of Variance, Duncan's multiple range test and presented as mean ± standard error (SE).

Results and Discussion

The effects of freeze-thawing process on live percent, HOST and percent sperms with intact acrosome has been shown in Figure-1. The observed mean (±SE) values different seminal attributes were well within the normal range at all the three steps evaluated during the experiment. A significant difference (p<0.01) was observed in all the three steps studied during the freez-thawing process with highest values observed in the neat followed by dilution and post-thaw semen. Significantly (p<0.01) lower value recorded for diluted semen compared to the neat may be the result of lethal interaction between the seminal plasma and egg yolk in semen extender [12] supplemented with osmotic disturbance. Buck seminal

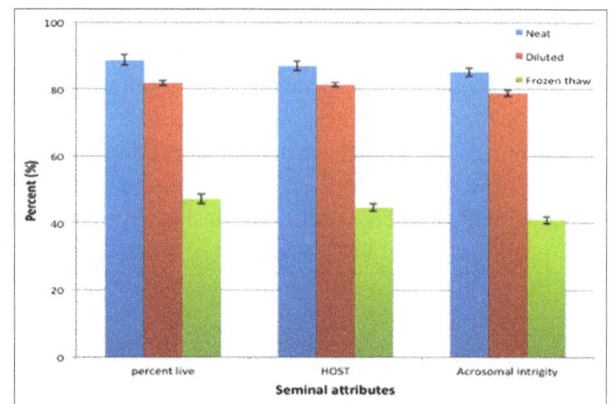

Figure-1: Different seminal attributes in Sirohi goat subjected to freezing-thawing process. Significance level (p<0.01).

plasma contains an enzyme secreted by the bulbo-urethral glands, which in the presence of egg yolk, by hydrolysis, leads to the formation of lysophosphatidylcholines – which are toxic to sperm [12,13]. Exposure of sperm to extracellular solute concentration leads to transport of water and solutes, including ions into or out of the cell, that affects the sperm osmotic tolerance limits above and below affecting motility and viability of spermatozoa [14]. Significantly (p<0.01) lower values recorded in the frozen thaw semen compared to neat and diluted semen may be the result of cryogenic stress incurred by spermatozoa during freezing-thawing process. During the process of semen cryopreservation spermatozoa are subjected cooling, freezing-thawing, and the addition of cryoprotectants. Spermatozoa subjected to cryopreservation are very sensitive to a rapid reduction in temperature from room temperature to 5°C [15] this produces cold shock, freezing-induced dehydration of the cells causes a more severe phase transition to a highly ordered gel phase resulting in a loss of selective permeability and integrity of the plasma membrane [16] leading to loss of motility and diminished metabolism.

Different motility patterns exhibited by spermatozoa during the freez-thawing process have been presented in Table-1. Significantly (p<0.01) higher number of motile spermatozoa was observed in the neat semen followed by diluted and frozen thaw semen. The proportion of spermatozoa showing slow progression were significantly (p<0.01) higher in the neat and diluted semen followed by rapid and non-progressive, while a reverse pattern was observed in the frozen thaw semen where the proportion of spermatozoa with non-progressive motility were significantly (p<0.01) higher followed by slow and rapid progression. The difference in the motility pattern exhibited by the spermatozoa may be the result of semen dilution resulting in hypertonic stress during the addition of cryoprotective agents [17], effect of egg yolk [18], disturbed plasma membrane integrity and mitochondrial activity that influenced the sperm morphology and physiology after dilution. Further, freezing-thawing result in overproduction of reactive oxygen species (ROS) [19]. ROS affects the membrane structure, leads to a change in permeability and probably influence integrity of cellular organelles (e.g. mitochondria, endoplasmic reticulum, etc.),

impairs cellular structure and destroys membranes by interacting with biomolecules that affects the viability and motility of spermatozoa and can also induce oxidative stress [20].

The different path velocities and kinematic characters exhibited by spermatozoa at different time interval have been presented in Table-2. Non-significantly higher values were recorded for all the path velocities except for VCL which was significantly (p<0.01) higher in the neat semen as compared to diluted semen. This difference in the velocity patterns of spermatozoa may be the result of reduced tolerance to hypotonic stress, a decreased intracellular pH and increased intracellular potassium affecting mitochondrial function and cell physiology [21]. Significantly (p<0.01) lower values of different path velocities were observed in post-thaw semen when compared to the neat and diluted semen. The results recorded during the study are comparable with those observed by Amidi et al., [22] and Bezerra et al., [23] in cryopreserved goat semen. The spermatozoa during the process of freez-thawing undergo stress. This leads to production of ROS, movement of proteins and cholesterol leading to change in membrane permeability accompanied by osmotic stress and ice crystal formation. The formation of intracellular ice crystals and ROS production result in the concentration of solutes remaining in the unfrozen fraction increases, thereby both depressing the freezing point and increasing the osmotic pressure altering sperm function [24,25]. Induction of premature acrosomal reaction, altered mitochondrial function and failure of chromatin decondensation, during the process of cryopreservation which influences the motility, viability and fertility of the sperm cells [26].

Conclusion

From the findings of the present study, it can be concluded process of cryopreservation results in shift of motility pattern of spermatozoa from slow progression to non-progression in the post-thaw semen with a significant (p<0.01) decrease in the path velocities when compared to neat and diluted semen. Further, the freezing-thawing process that reduces the motility and kinematic characters spermatozoa may be an important factor influencing the fertilizing ability of spermatozoa resulting in poor conception rate after insemination in goats.

Authors' Contributions

SV and MA designed and conducted the study. MA drafted and revised the manuscript. Both authors read and approved the final manuscript.

Acknowledgments

The authors are thankful to Vice Chancellor, DUVASU and Dean, College of Veterinary Sciences and Animal Husbandry for providing funds and facilities to pursue this research work.

Table-1: Motility pattern exhibited by spermatozoa during freezing-thawing process.

Parameter (%)	Neat semen	Diluted semen (tris-glycerol)	Frozen thaw semen
Motility	83.80[c]±0.949	79.15[b]±0.625	41.70[a]±0.819
Rapid	16.87[b]±0.970	13.40[b]±1.434	1.10[a]±0.331
Slow	57.00[b]±0.544	56.10[b]±0.821	12.12[a]±1.205
Non-progressive	9.92[b]±0.975	9.70[b]±0.481	28.42[a]±1.647

Means with different superscript letters (a, b, c) differ significantly (p<0.01) within a row

Table-2: Different path velocities exhibited by spermatozoa during freeing-thawing process.

Parameter	Units	Neat semen	Diluted semen (tris-glycerol)	Frozen thaw semen
VCL	µm/s	102.00[a]±1.08	96.75[b]±1.10	63.75[c]±0.47
VAP	µm/s	42.25[b]±0.478	41.00[b]±0.707	30.35[a]±0.478
VSL	µm/s	35.75[b]±0.629	34.50[b]±0.645	18.50[a]±0.288
LIN	%	34.95[b]±0.184	35.72[b]±0.221	29.60[a]±0.470
STR	%	83.37[b]±0.449	83.07[b]±0.469	61.62[a]±1.291
WOB	%	41.62[a]±0.209	42.60[a]±0.168	47.65[b]±0.518
BCF	hz	19.00[b]±0.108	18.25[b]±0.366	12.65[a]±0.087
ALH	µm	5.15[b]±0.028	5.07[b]±0.062	3.57[a]±0.047
DNC	µm²/sec	422.00[b]±8.348	393.00[b]±5.922	173.77[a]±0.667

Means with different superscript letters (a, b, c) differ significantly (p<0.01) within a row. VLC=Curvilinear velocity, VAP=Average path velocity, VSL=Straight line velocity, LIN=Linearity, STR=Straightness, WOB=Wobble, BCF=Beat cross frequency, ALH=Amplitude-lateral head displacement, DNC=Dance

Competing Interests

The authors declare that they have no competing interests.

References

1. Jayashree, R., Jayashankar, M.R., Nagaraja, C.S., Satyanarayana, K. and Isloor, S. (2014) Goat rearing practices in southern Karnataka. *Int. J. Sci. Environ. Technol.,* 3(4): 1328-1335.
2. Kumar, S. (2007) Commercial goat farming in India: An emerging agri-business opportunity. *Agric. Econ. Res. Rev.,* 20: 503-520.
3. Nimbkar, C. and van Arendonk, J. (2010) Recent Trends in Global Organization of Animal Breeding "Paper for the International Technical Expert Workshop" Exploring the Need for Specific Measures for Access and Benefit Sharing of Animals Genetic Resource for Food and Agriculture. Wageningen, Netherlands, Dec. 8-10.
4. Mittal, P.K., Anand, M., Madan, A.K., Yadav, S. and Kumar, J. (2014) Antioxidative capacity of vitamin E, vitamin C and their combination in cryopreserved Bhadawari bull semen. *Vet. World,* 7(12): 1127-1131.
5. Kathiravan, P., Kalatharan, J., Karthikeya, G., Rengarajan, K. and Kadirvel, G. (2011) Objective sperm motion analysis to assess dairy bull fertility using computer aided system – A review. *Reprod. Domest. Anim.,* 46: 165-172.
6. Mortimer, S.T. (2000) CASA-practical aspects. *J. Androl.,* 21: 515-524.
7. Foote, R.H. (2003) Fertility estimation: A review of past experience and future prospects. *Anim. Reprod. Sci.,* 75: 119-139.
8. Dorado, J., Munoz-Serrano, A. and Hidalgo, M. (2010) The effect of cryopreservation on goat semen characteristics related to sperm freezability. *Anim. Reprod. Sci.,* 121: 115-123.
9. Hancock, J.L. (1952) The morphology of bull spermatozoa. *J. Exp. Biol.,* 29: 445-453.
10. Jeyendran, R.S., Vander-Ven, H.H., Perez-Pelaez, M., Crabo, B.G. and Zanevld, L.J.D. (1984) Development of an assay to assess the functional integrity of the human sperm membrane and its relationship to other semen characters. *J. Repord. Fertil.,* 70: 219-228.
11. Watson, P.F. (1975) Use of giemsa stain to detect changes in acrosomes of frozen ram spermatozoa. *Vet. Res.,* 97: 12-15.
12. Leboeuf, B., Restall, B. and Salomon, S. (2000) Production and storage of goat semen for artificial insemination. *Anim. Reprod. Sci.,* 62: 113-141.
13. Roy, A. (1957) Egg yolk-coagulation enzyme in the semen and Cowper's gland of the goat. *Nature,* 179: 318-319.
14. Gilmore, J.A., Du, J., Tao, J., Peter, A.T. and Critser, J.K.

(1996) Osmotic properties of boar spermatozoa and their relevance to cryopreservation. *J. Reprod. Fertil.,* 107: 87-95.
15. Rodenas, C., Parrilla, I., Roca, J., Martinez, E.A. and Lucas, X. (2014) Effects of rapid cooling prior to freezing on the quality of canine cryopreserved spermatozoa. *J. Reprod. Dev.,* 60(5): 355-361.
16. Oldenhof, H., Friedel, K., Akhoondi, M., Gojowsky, M., Wolkers, W.F. and Sieme, H. (2012) Membrane phase behavior during cooling of stallion sperm and its correlation with freezability. *Mol. Membr. Biol.,* 29(4): 95-106.
17. Mazur, P. (2010) A biologist's view of the relevance of thermodynamics and physical chemistry to cryobiology. *Cryobiology,* 60: 4-10.
18. Qureshi, M.S., Khan, D., Mushtaq, A. and Afridi, S.S. (2013) Effect of extenders, postdilution intervals, and seasons on semen quality in dairy goats. *Turk. J. Vet. Anim. Sci.,* 37: 147-152.
19. Agarwal, A., Saleh, R.A. and Bedaiwy, M.A. (2003) Role of reactive oxygen species in the patho-physiology of human reproduction. *Fertil. Steril.,* 79: 829-843.
20. Zhu, H., Luo, H.L., Meng, H. and Zhang, G.J. (2009) Effect of vitamin E supplementation on development of reproductive organs in Boer goat. *Anim. Reprod. Sci.,* 113: 93-101.
21. Blassea, A.K., Oldenhofb, H., Ekhlasi-Hundriesera, M., Wolkersc, W.F., Siemeb, H. and Bollweina, H. (2012) Osmotic tolerance and intracellular ion concentrations of bovine sperm are affected by cryopreservation. *Theriogenology,* 78: 1312-1320.
22. Amidi, F., Farshad, A. and Khor, A.K. (2010) Effects of cholesterol-loaded cyclodextrin during freezing step of cryopreservation with TCGY extender containing bovine serum albumin on quality of goat spermatozoa. *Cryobiology,* 61: 94-99.
23. Bezerra, F.S.B., Castelo, T.S., Alves, H.M., Oliveira, I.R.S., Lima, G.L., Gislayne, C.X., Peixoto, G.C.X., Bezerra, A.C.S. and Silva, A.R. (2011) Objective assessment of the cryoprotective effects of dimethylformamide for freezing goat semen. *Cryobiology,* 63: 263-266.
24. Alvarez, J.G. (2012) Male Infertility: Loss of Intracellular Antioxidative Enzymes Activity during Sperm Cryopreservation: Effect of Sperm Function after Thawing. Springer, New York. p237-244.
25. Munoz, O.V., Briand, L.A., Bancharif, D., Anton, M., Deserches, S., Shmitt, E., Thorin, C. and Tainturier, D. (2010) Effect of low density, spermatozoon concentration and glycerol on functional and motility parameter of Bull spermatozoa during storage at 4°C. *Asian J. Androl.,* 13(2): 281-286.
26. Wongtawan, T., Saravia, F., Wallgren, M., Caballero, A. and Rodriguez-Martinez, H. (2006) Fertility after deep intra-uterine artificial insemination of concentrated low-volume boar semen doses. *Theriogenology,* 65: 773-787.

24

Conjugation of ampicillin and enrofloxacin residues with bovine serum albumin and raising of polyclonal antibodies against them

B. Sampath Kumar, Vasili Ashok, P. Kalyani and G. Remya Nair

Department of Veterinary Biochemistry, College of Veterinary Science, Sri Venkateswara Veterinary University, Korutla, Karimnagar, Telangana, Andhra Pradesh, India.
Corresponding author: B. Sampath Kumar, e-mail: samkum85@gmail.com,
VA: vasiliashok@gmail.com, PK: parvathalakalyani@gmail.com, GRN: remyagnair10@gmail.com

Abstract

Aim: The aim of this study is to test the potency of bovine serum albumin (BSA) conjugated ampicillin (AMP) and enrofloxacin (ENR) antigens in eliciting an immune response in rats using indirect competitive enzyme-linked immunosorbent assay (icELISA).

Materials and Methods: AMP and ENR antibiotics were conjugated with BSA by carbodiimide reaction using 1-ethyl-3-(3-dimethylaminopropyl) carbodiimide (EDC) as a cross-linker. The successful conjugation was confirmed by sodium dodecyl sulfate polyacrylamide gel electrophoresis. Sprague-Dawley rats were immunized with the conjugates and blood samples were collected serially at 15 days time interval after first immunization plus first booster, second booster, third booster, and the fourth sampling was done 1½ month after the third booster. The antibody titres in the antisera of each antibiotic in all the four immunization cycles (ICs) were determined by an icELISA at various serum dilutions ranging from 1/100 to 1/6400.

Results: Analysis of antibiotic-BSA conjugates by sodium dodecyl sulfate polyacrylamide gel electrophoresis and coomassie blue staining revealed high molecular weight bands of 85 kDa and 74 kDa for AMP-BSA and ENR-BSA respectively when compared to 68 kDa band of BSA. Both the antibiotic conjugates elicited a good immune response in rats but comparatively the response was more with AMP-BSA conjugate than ENR-BSA conjugate. Maximum optical density 450 value of 2.577 was recorded for AMP-BSA antisera, and 1.723 was recorded for ENR-BSA antisera at 1/100th antiserum dilution in third IC.

Conclusion: AMP and ENR antibiotics proved to be good immunogens when conjugated to BSA by carbodiimide reaction with EDC as crosslinker. The polyclonal antibodies produced can be employed for detecting AMP and ENR residues in milk and urine samples.

Keywords: 1-ethyl-3-(3-dimethylaminopropyl) carbodiimide, antibodies against antibiotics, conjugation, indirect competitive enzyme linked immunosorbent assay.

Introduction

Antibiotics are being used extensively in the treatment of sick animals. They are also being used as growth promoters and prophylactic agents in lactating animals which is responsible for the presence of their residues in the milk [1]. Beta-lactam antibiotics like penicillin are the most frequently used, the residues of which can produce detrimental effects such as allergic reactions in humans who are sensitive to beta-lactams [2]. It may also lead to the development of antibiotic-resistant strains of bacteria [3]. Antibiotics when used inappropriately and irrationally it provides favorable conditions for the development of a resistant group of microbes that can spread very easily [4]. Enrofloxacin (ENR) is widely used in the treatment of infectious diseases because of its broad spectrum activity, and this may result in persistence of ENR residues in animal body which in turn might lead to the development of drug-resistant bacterial strains or allergies in the animal [5]. Dinki and Balcha [6] reported antibiotic residues in 28 samples with 23.3% detection rate in cattle milk samples collected from six different milk collection centres in Guwahati city in India. Gentamycin and streptomycin residues were estimated to be 90 µg/L and 80 µg/L respectively by Zeina *et al.* [7]. in cattle milk in Lebanon which were below the maximum residue limit of 200 µg/L set by FAO/WHO. A study conducted in Nepal by Dhakal *et al.* [8] revealed that mastitis pathogens have developed resistance to ampicillin (AMP) and penicillin. Gentamycin and streptomycin are found to be developing resistance. All these results emphasize the need to have strict control measures on the use of antibiotics in veterinary practice both as therapeutic as well as prophylactic agents and also the need to have rapid and sensitive screening methods to detect antibiotic residues in milk.

Antibiotics are small molecules with molecular weights of <1 kDa (haptens) and to elicit an immune response, they have to be conjugated with carrier molecules such as bovine serum albumin (BSA) [9].

Antibodies are utilized for analysis, purification, and enrichment, and to mediate or modulate physiological responses. The ability of antibodies to bind an antigen with a high degree of affinity and specificity has led to their ubiquitous use in a variety of scientific and medical disciplines. Their use in diagnostic assays and as therapeutics has had a profound impact on the improvement of health and welfare in both humans and animals [10].

This study was undertaken with the objective of producing polyclonal antibodies (pAbs) against AMP and ENR antibiotics by conjugating them with BSA and detection of these pAbs by a sensitive indirect competitive enzyme linked immunosorbent assay (icELISA) in antibiotic specific antisera.

Materials and Methods

Ethical approval

The experimental protocol was approved by the Institutional Animal Ethics Committee under order No. 8/i/10.

Animals

The rats (Sprague-Dawley) for the experiment were procured from the National Institute of Nutrition, Hyderabad (No. DBT/LAISC 2455). The Sprague-Dawley rats aged 7-8 weeks were kept under well lighted experimental house and maintained on standard rat feed with *ad libitum* water. A total three groups with three rats in each were maintained, two test groups (for AMP and ENR) and one control group.

Conjugation of AMP and ENR with BSA

AMP was conjugated with BSA as per the method described by Samsonova *et al.* [11] with slight modifications whereas ENR was conjugated by the method described by Sui *et al.* [12]. For conjugation 2.5 ml of AMP (100 mg/ml) and 20 mg of BSA were taken in a clean beaker and 2.5 ml of ENR (100 mg/ml) and 20 mg of BSA were taken in another clean beaker. 580 mg of 1-ethyl-3-(3-dimethylaminopropyl) carbodiimide (EDC) was dissolved in 2 ml of distilled water and was added drop-wise to each of the above mixtures separately, accompanied by continuous stirring on a magnetic stirrer. The pH of the solutions was adjusted to 5.0-6.0 by adding 0.1 N HCl.

The above reaction mixtures of AMP-EDC-BSA and ENR-EDC-BSA were incubated at room temperature (RT) in separate beakers with continuous stirring for 2 h. After the reaction time of 2 h, uncoupled antibiotic and EDC were removed by dialysis. Dialysis membrane having the cut-off molecular weight of 12-14 kDa was procured from Hi-Media (Cat.No.DM003). Dialysis was performed according to the method described by Bollag *et al.* [13]. The samples were dialyzed against phosphate buffer saline (PBS) (pH – 7.4) with four changes, each for 8 h. The conjugated samples were analyzed by sodium dodecyl sulfate polyacrylamide gel electrophoresis (SDS-PAGE) to confirm successful conjugation [14]. SDS-PAGE was performed according to the method described by Christoph [14]. The images of the stained gels were taken in the gel documentation system (G-box-Syngene).

Immunogen preparation

For primary immunization, AMP and ENR immunogens were prepared by adding 40 µl of each of the two conjugates separately to 460 µl PBS and 500 µl of complete Freund's adjuvant. AMP and ENR booster immunogens were prepared by adding 40 µl of the conjugate to 460 µl of PBS buffer and 500 µl of incomplete Freund's adjuvant as described by Dykman *et al.* [15].

The immunogen was mixed thoroughly, and 300 µl was injected to each rat (test group) subcutaneously at two different sites (150 µl at each site) according to the immunization schedule as described by Dykman *et al.* [15].

Collection of blood from rats

The blood was collected by orbital sinus venipuncture method described by Oruganti and Gaidhani [16]. A total of four blood collections were made in each group at different time intervals according to the schedule given in Table-1.

Estimation of total protein, albumin, and A/G ratio

The serum samples of rats from test and control groups collected after second booster (third immunization cycle [IC]) were analyzed for total protein, albumin and A/G ratio by using ensure biotech total protein and albumin teaching kit.

Preparation of ELISA antigens (casein-antibiotic conjugates)

0.83 µmol of casein was dissolved in 2 ml of distilled water in the presence of small amount of sodium-bi-carbonate to maintain alkaline condition. 83 µmol of antibiotic and 83 µmol of EDC were added to the above protein solution. The reaction mixture was stirred on a magnetic stirrer continuously for 2 h at RT. The pH of the solution was adjusted to 5.0.

Table-1: Immunization schedule.

Immunization schedule	Procedure
Day 0	1st immunization antigen+CFA
Day 15	1st boost antigen+ICFA
Day 30	1st test bleed
Day 37	2nd boost antigen+ICFA
Day 52	2nd test bleed
Day 59	3rd boost antigen+ICFA
Day 74	3rd test bleed
Day 104	4th test bleed

CFA=Complete Freund's adjuvant, ICFA=Incomplete Freund's adjuvant

Reaction mixtures of both the antibiotics were then incubated overnight at 4°C. Conjugates were dialyzed against distilled water as per the method given by Samsonova et al. [11].

Standardization of icELISA

The serum samples collected after the second booster (third IC) were used for the standardization. Checkerboard titration was performed using different dilutions of antigens against different serum dilutions of test groups and negative control at constant secondary antibody-horseradish peroxidase (HRP) conjugate dilution of 1/10,000 (manufacturer's instruction). Serial antigen dilutions (from 2×10^6 ng/ml to 2 ng/ml) were taken from rows B to H in 96 well polystyrene plates and serial primary antibody dilutions (from 1/50 to 1/1600) were taken from columns 1 to 6 for test group samples and columns 7 to 12 for control group samples. The dilution of antigen which showed, maximum absorbance reading and started to maintain almost a stationary phase was taken as the optimum according to the procedure described by Fan et al. [17].

Indirect ELISA

96 well flat bottom polystyrene ELISA plates (Nunc, Denmark) were coated with 250 µl of antigen (antibiotic-casein conjugate) in 0.01 M carbonate buffer (pH - 9.6). The plates were incubated overnight at 4°C. The wells were washed 3 times with 250 µl/well of PBS that contained 0.05% tween 20 (PBST). The free (unbound) sites were blocked with 250 µl/well of blocking buffer containing 2% casein. The plates were incubated at 37°C for 1 h. The wells were washed 3 times with PBS, 250 µl/well. 100 µl of antiserum samples with two-fold dilutions from 1/100 to 1/6400 in PBST were added to each well and the plate was incubated for 1 h at 37°C. The wells were washed 3 times with PBST (250 µl/well per wash cycle). 100 µl of a conjugate of secondary antibodies with HRP in PBST was added to each well and the plate was incubated for 1 h at 37°C. The wells were washed 3 times with PBST (250 µl/well per wash cycle). 100 µl of the substrate (3, 3', 5, 5' tetramethylbenzidine) in PBST (1 in 20 dilution) was added to each well. The reaction was stopped after 10-15 min by adding 50 µl/well of 4M H_2SO_4 as the method described by Samsonova et al. [11]. Optical density (OD) was measured by using ELISA microtitre plate reader at 450 nm (Biotech instrument-µquant).

Testing the antiserum samples for antibody titres

The antibody titres in the serum samples collected from immunized rats were tested by icELISA standardized as described above. The optimum antigen concentrations and primary antibody dilutions obtained for all the four antibiotics by the above-described method were used for the test. The antisera of all the three animals in each group collected during all the three ICs and 4th sampling were tested at various serum dilutions ranging from 1/100 to 1/1600. Each

sample was tested in duplicate including the control serum samples. In the reagent blank, PBST was added instead of antiserum. In the negative control wells, serum samples of control group rats were added. The mean OD_{450} of various serum dilutions at each IC for each group of rats were used to plot a graph with absorbance on Y-axis and serum dilutions on X-axis.

Construction of PNT baseline

The mean and the standard deviation (SD) values of the control group at each dilution ranging from 1/100 to 1/6400 were calculated for each of the two different antigen coated plates used in this study. Three units of SD was added to the corresponding mean absorbance value and a graph was plotted with values of mean plus 3 times SD (M + 3SD) on Y-axis and serum dilutions on X-axis. This was considered as positive, negative threshold (PNT) baseline [18]. Separate PNT baselines were constructed for each test group.

Prediction of antibody titres

The positive antibody titres were determined based on the cut-off value obtained from PNT baseline constructed. The highest OD_{450} value of the PNT baseline rounded off to the nearest single digit decimal was taken as cut-off value. The OD_{450} value over and above the cut-off value was considered positive antibody titer [18].

Results and Discussion

Determination of successful conjugation

Analysis of antibiotic conjugates by SDS-PAGE and coomassie blue staining revealed higher molecular weights of antibiotic-BSA conjugates when compared to normal BSA (Figure-1). Before conjugation with antibiotic, the molecular weight of BSA was 68 KDa. After conjugation, the molecular weights of conjugates were 85 kDa, 74 kDa for AMP-BSA and ENR-BSA, respectively. These results clearly indicate the successful conjugation of antibiotics with BSA and

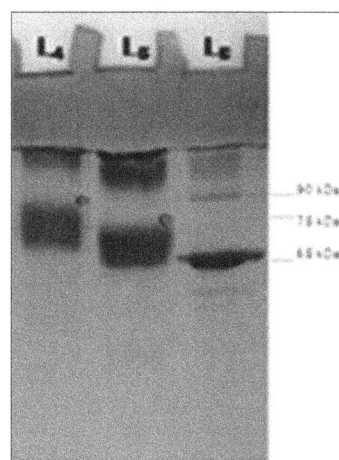

Figure-1: Coomassie blue stained sodium dodecyl sulfate polyacrylamide gel electrophoresis gel of antibiotic conjugates: L_4: Ampillicin conjugate, L_5: Enrofloxacin conjugate, L_6: Bovine serum albumin (*) conjugates.

are similar to those obtained by Jiang *et al.* [19] who analyzed sarafloxacin-BSA conjugate by SDS-PAGE and observed an increase in the molecular weight of the conjugate when compared to the carrier protein BSA.

Estimation of total protein, albumin and A/G ratio

The mean values of total protein, albumin, globulin, and A/G ratio of serum samples collected during third IC. The mean total protein concentration was 12 ± 1.15 g/dL and 24 ± 1.73 g/dL for AMP and ENR antisera, respectively and in the control group, it was 6.66 ± 0.01 g/dL. The mean albumin concentration was 3.36 ± 0.173 g/dL, 3.21 ± 0.003 g/dL for AMP and ENR antisera are respectively compared to 3.36 ± 0.173 g/dL in the control group. The mean globulin concentration was 8.64 ± 0.10 g/dL and 20.79 ± 0.08 g/dL for AMP and ENR antisera, respectively, whereas it was 3.30 ± 0.04 g/dL in the control group. The mean A/G ratio was 0.38 ± 0.008 and 0.15 ± 0.017 for AMP and ENR antisera, respectively. The mean A/G ratio in the control group serum was 1.02 ± 0.012. Increased globulin concentration and decreased A/G ratio indicates the presence of antibodies in the antisera.

Standardization of antigen concentration and antiserum dilution for indirect ELISA

The checker board titration results are presented in Table-2 for AMP-casein conjugate and in Table-3

for ENR-casein conjugate. In all the titrations, the OD_{450} values of the test wells increased suddenly from the coated antigen concentration of 2 to 20 ng/ml and continued to maintain a steady phase at higher concentrations. So, 20 ng/ml was chosen as optimum antigen concentration. The absorbance values of the negative control wells dropped suddenly from serum dilution of 1/50 to 1/100 and continued to maintain similar range at higher dilutions and at all antigen concentrations. The test wells continued to maintain higher absorbance values at corresponding dilutions. Hence, 1/100 was chosen as optimum serum dilution. The highest M + 3SD values obtained for negative sera were 0.213 (Table-4) and 0.209 (Table-5) for AMP-casein and ENR-casein coated plates, respectively. Hence, the cut-off value was selected as 0.3 for antibiotics.

Detection of antibody titres in the AMP antisera

The mean of the corrected OD values of the three animals in AMP test group and M + 3SD of the three animals in each control group at various serum dilutions and various ICs are depicted in Table-4. The highest M + 3SD value was 0.213. The cut-off value was selected as 0.3 (nearest single digit decimal above 0.213). The mean OD_{450} values of the serum samples from immunized rats were above the cut-off value up to serum dilution of 1/3200 in all the three ICs and

Table-2: Checker board titration to standardize optimum casein-AMP conjugate and antiserum dilution.

Concentration of antigen (ng/ml)	Well	Test serum sample						Negative control					
		Dilutions of antisera						Dilutions of antisera					
		1/50	1/100	1/200	1/400	1/800	1/1600	1/50	1/100	1/200	1/400	1/800	1/1600
		1	2	3	4	5	6	7	8	9	10	11	12
Blank	A	0.148	0.159	0.078	0.190	0.111	0.178	0.091	0.163	0.143	0.155	0.140	0.147
2×10^6	B	2.983	2.545	2.068	1.976	1.587	1.057	0.624	0.192	0.187	0.189	0.195	0.116
2×10^5	C	2.745	2.451	1.987	1.852	1.456	0.958	0.525	0.112	0.185	0.165	0.159	0.112
2×10^4	D	2.415	2.316	1.886	1.689	1.321	0.845	0.656	0.184	0.158	0.195	0.188	0.159
2×10^3	E	2.221	2.215	1.769	1.521	1.205	0.833	0.587	0.156	0.165	0.189	0.125	0.141
200	F	2.115	2.110	1.645	1.361	1.124	0.782	0.495	0.121	0.198	0.156	0.151	0.128
20	G	2.021	1.994	1.607	1.246	0.972	0.759	0.458	0.184	0.185	0.136	0.102	0.196
2	H	1.498	1.331	1.026	0.752	0.578	0.396	0.321	0.146	0.175	0.117	0.085	0.129

AMP=Ampicillin

Table-3: Checker board titration to standardize optimum casein-ENR conjugate and antiserum dilution.

Concentration of antigen (ng/ml)	Well	Test serum sample						Negative control					
		Dilutions of antisera						Dilutions of antisera					
		1/50	1/100	1/200	1/400	1/800	1/1600	1/50	1/100	1/200	1/400	1/800	1/1600
		1	2	3	4	5	6	7	8	9	10	11	12
Blank	A	0.109	0.103	0.100	0.088	0.125	0.109	0.134	0.126	0.154	0.163	0.128	0.133
2×10^6	B	2.598	2.326	2.159	1.998	1.652	1.450	0.556	0.116	0.185	0.156	0.149	0.112
2×10^5	C	2.441	2.236	2.079	1.789	1.536	1.241	0.531	0.121	0.186	0.152	0.145	0.198
2×10^4	D	2.326	2.187	1.969	1.656	1.324	1.105	0.401	0.178	0.156	0.123	0.189	0.119
2×10^3	E	2.158	2.056	1.851	1.523	1.121	0.959	0.459	0.189	0.187	0.125	0.197	0.157
200	F	2.103	1.925	1.754	1.386	0.956	0.843	0.358	0.142	0.195	0.178	0.185	0.139
20	G	2.044	1.889	1.595	1.027	0.819	0.775	0.338	0.196	0.183	0.138	0.118	0.141
2	H	1.156	0.721	0.521	0.495	0.352	0.229	0.352	0.185	0.189	0.119	0.158	0.176

ENR=Enrofloxacin

Table-4: Mean OD_{450} values of indirect ELISA of AMP antisera.

ICs	Serum dilutions						
	1/100	1/200	1/400	1/800	1/1600	1/3200	1/6400
1st IC	1.499	1.156	0.840	**0.668**	0.458	0.323	0.281
2nd IC	1.781	1.607	1.429	1.225	**0.924**	0.568	0.436
3rd IC	2.577	2.195	1.841	1.619	1.453	1.417	**1.184**
4th collection	1.944	1.601	1.267	**0.932**	0.756	0.642	0.558
Negative control (M+3SD)	0.213	0.199	0.157	0.12	0.107	0.105	0.107

Bold numbers indicate 50% titres. IC=Immunization cycle, OD=Optical density, ELISA=Enzyme linked immunosorbent assay, AMP=Ampicillin

Table-5: Mean OD_{450} values of indirect ELISA of ENR antisera.

IC	Serum dilutions						
	1/100	1/200	1/400	1/800	1/1600	1/3200	1/6400
1st IC	1.018	0.735	**0.447**	0.297	0.148	0.099	0.065
2nd IC	1.252	1.046	0.759	**0.628**	0.445	0.302	0.272
3rd IC	1.723	1.476	1.241	1.091	0.94	**0.893**	0.755
4th Sampling	1.04	0.783	**0.565**	0.461	0.399	0.275	0.191
Negative control (M+3SD)	0.209	0.216	0.158	0.16	0.115	0.105	0.099

Bold numbers indicate 50% titres. IC=Immunization cycle, OD=Optical density, ELISA=Enzyme linked immunosorbent assay, ENR=Enrofloxacin, SD=Standard deviation

fourth collection which indicated positive antibody titers (Figure-2). The values of 50% antibody titres increased from the antiserum dilution of 1/800 in first IC to 1/6400 in third IC as depicted in Table-4. The AMP antisera gave positive antibody titers up to a dilution of 1/3200 in first IC and 1/6400 in second and third ICs and fourth sampling. Maximum OD_{450} value of 2.577 was obtained at 1/100 antiserum dilution in third IC which clearly indicated that the immune response was the highest in third IC. The immune response significantly increased from first IC to third IC at 1/100 antiserum dilution and decreased in fourth collection (Figure-3). Anti-AMP antibodies were successfully produced by Strasser et al. [20] in rabbits which were confirmed by double antibody solid phase ELISA. The maximum antibody titer of 1:550,000 was obtained after third booster injection (fourth IC) at working antiserum dilution of 1:1000 which is much higher than 1/6400 in this study. The difference could be attributed to species variations in the ability to produce antibodies. Competitive ELISA used by McConnell et al. [21] for AMP antisera yielded positive antibody titers indicating clearly that AMP-carrier protein conjugate was immunopotent and capable of eliciting specific immune response.

Detection of antibody titres in the ENR antisera

The results of corrected mean OD_{450} values of the test group (three animals) and M + 3SD values of the control group (three animals) at various serum dilutions and various ICs are depicted in Table-5. The highest M + 3SD value was 0.209. The cut-off value was selected as 0.3 (nearest single digit decimal above 0.209). The mean OD_{450} values of the ENR antisera were above the cut-off value up to a dilution of 1/400 in first IC and up to dilution of 1/1600 in second and third and ICs and fourtth collection which indicated

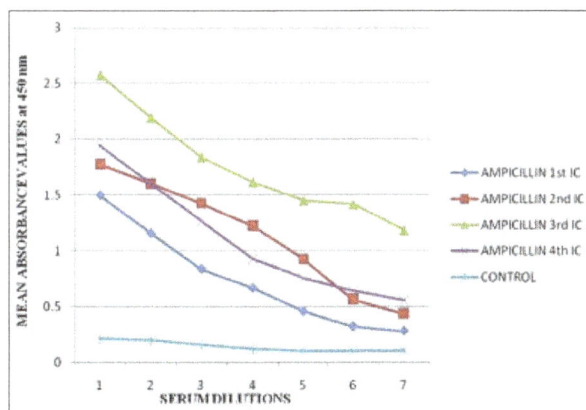

Figure-2: Calibration curve for indirect enzyme linked immunosorbent assay of bovine serum albumin-ampicillin antisera at various immunization cycles (1, 2, 3, 4, 5, 6, 7 represents serum dilutions of 1/100, 1/200, 1/400, 4/800, 1/1600, 1/3200, and 1/6400 respectively).

positive antibody titres (Figure-4). The immune response significantly increased from first IC to third IC at 1/100 antiserum dilution and decreased in fourth sampling (Figure-5). The values of 50% antibody titres increased from the antiserum dilution of 1/400 in first IC to 1/3200 in third IC as depicted in Table-5. The ENR antisera gave positive antibody titres up to a dilution of 1/400 in first IC, 1/3200 in second IC, 1/6400 in third IC and 1/1600 in fourth sampling. Maximum OD_{450} value of 1.723 was obtained at 1/100 antiserum dilution in third IC which clearly indicated that the immune response was the highest in third IC. Liu et al. [22] used ELISA and competitive inhibition ELISA to determine antibody titers in ENR antisera and obtained antibody titre as high as 1:250,000 for three analogs of ENR belonging to fluoroquinolone family.

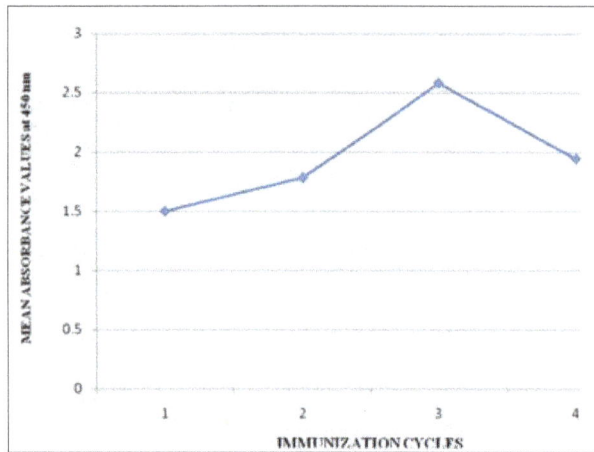

Figure-3: Calibration curve for indirect enzyme linked immunosorbent assay of bovine serum albumin-ampicillin antisera at 1/100th serum dilution of various immunization cycles (ICs) (1, 2, 3, 4 represents serum dilutions of 1st, 2nd, 3rd, 4th ICs respectively at 1/100th serum dilation).

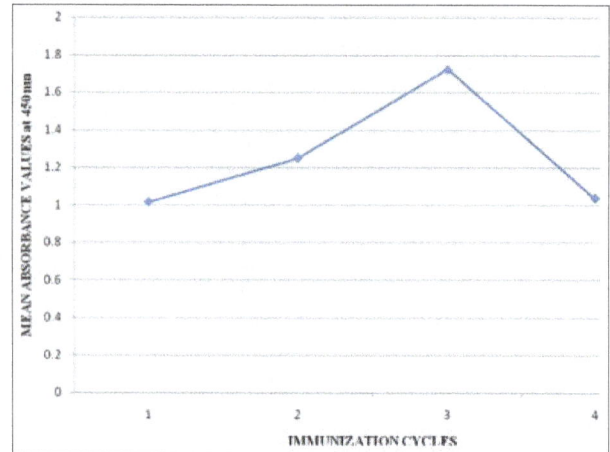

Figure-5: Calibration curve for indirect enzyme linked immunosorbent assay of bovine serum albumin-enrofloxacin antisera at 1/100th serum dilution of various immunization cycles (IC) (1, 2, 3, 4 represents serum dilutions of 1st, 2nd, 3rd, 4th ICs respectively at 1/100th serum dilation).

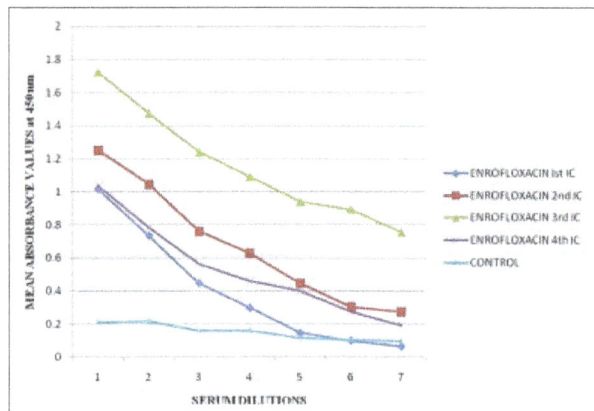

Figure-4: Calibration curve for indirect enzyme linked immunosorbent assay of bovine serum albumin-enrofloxacin antisera at various immunization cycles (1, 2, 3, 4, 5, 6, 7 represents serum dilutions of 1/100, 1/200, 1/400, 4/800, 1/1600, 1/3200, and 1/6400 respectively).

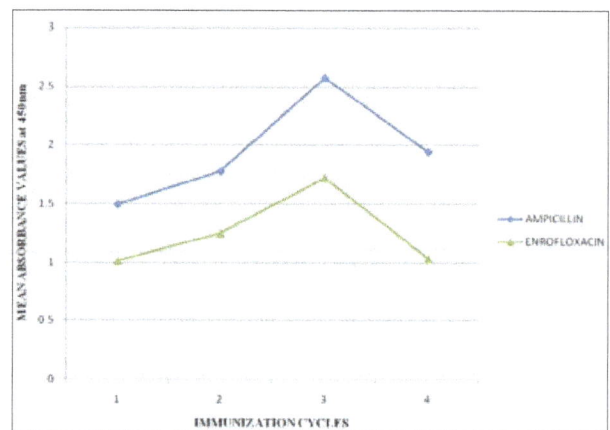

Figure-6: Comparative calibration curves for indirect enzyme linked immunosorbent assay of bovine serum albumin-antibiotic antisera at 1/100th serum dilution of various immunization cycles (ICs) (1, 2, 3, 4 represents serum dilutions of 1st, 2nd, 3rd, 4th ICs respectively at 1/100th serum dilation).

Comparative immunogenic potency of AMP-BSA and ENR-BSA antisera

Highest immune response was seen in AMP antiserum followed by ENR evidenced by OD_{450} values of 2.577, 1.723 for AMP and ENR antisera respectively at 1/100 serum dilution in third IC (Figure-6).

Raised antibodies to detect the AMP and ENR in milk samples

To use produces antibodies for the detection of antibiotics in milk samples, we need large quantities of antibodies for which the work has to be scaled up and large number of animals have to be maintained to obtain sufficient antiserum for harvesting antibodies. This is the first part of work done to test the efficacy of BSA conjugates of AMP and ENR in eliciting immune response in rats. The second part of work is to scale up the process and use the antibodies in developing quantitative assay or lateral flow through assay to detect antibiotic residues in milk samples.

Novelty and contribution to the animal health

This work mostly concerned with the public health importance. Antibiotics residues in milk higher than maximum residue levels are of great concern to dairy farmers, milk processors, regulatory agencies, and consumers due to their possible adverse effects on people allergic to antibiotics, potential buildup of antibiotic-resistant organisms in humans [23]. The novelty of this work lies in using BSA as a suitable conjugating agent with EDC as coupler for AMP and ENR which are otherwise haptens and hence incapable of eliciting immune response.

Conclusion

In this study, the antibiotics (AMP and ENR) were successfully conjugated with carrier protein BSA by carbodiimide reaction using EDC as a cross linker. These conjugated antibiotics were capable of producing pAbs which was confirmed by indirect ELISA.

Authors' Contributions

BSK and PK collected the blood samples from rats for the study. BSK carried out the current investigation under the guidance of VA. BSK drafted and revised the manuscript under the guidance of PK. GRN helped in carry out the ELISA part of work. All the authors have read and approved the manuscript.

Acknowledgments

The authors gratefully acknowledge Sri Venkateswara Veterinary University, Tirupati for providing facilities and funds to do research work as part of the M.V.Sc. thesis work.

Competing Interests

The authors declare that they have no competing interests.

References

1. Singh, S., Shukla, S., Tandia, N., Kumar, N. and Paliwal, R. (2014) Antibiotic residues: A global challenge. *Pharm. Sci. Monitor*, 5(3): 184-197.

2. Fitzgerald, S.P., Loan, N., Connell, R.M., Benchi, E.KH. and Kane, N. (2007) stable competitive Enzyme-Linked immunosorbent assay kit for rapid measurement of 11 active beta-lactams in milk, tissue, urine and serum. *J.AOAC. Int.*, 90 (1):334-342.

3. Kebede, G., Zenebe, T., Disassa, H. and Tolosa, T. (2014) Review on detection of antimicrobial residues in raw bulk milk in dairy farms. *AJBAS.*, 6(4): 87-97.

4. Padol, A.R., Malapure, C.D., Domple, V.D. and Kamdi, B.P. (2015) Occurance, public health implications and detection of antibacterial drug residues in cow milk. *Environ. We Int. J. Sci. Tech.*, 10: 7-28.

5. Yan, H., Wang, H., Qin, X., Liu, B. and Du, J. (2011) Ultra sound-assisted dispersive liquid-liquid micro extraction for determination of fluroquinolones in pharmaceutical waste water. *J. Pharm. Biomed. Anal.*, 54(1): 53-57.

6. Dinki, N. and Balcha, E. (2013) Detection of antibiotic residues and determination of microbial quality of raw milk from milk collection centres. *Adv. Anim. Vet. Sci.*, 1(3): 80-83.

7. Zeina, K., Pamela, A.K. and Fawwak, S. (2013) Quantification of antibiotic residues and determination of antimicrobial resistance profiles of microorganisms isolated from bovine milk in Lebanon. *Food Nutr. Sci.*, 4: 1-9.

8. Dhakal, I.P., Dhakal, P., Koshihara, T. and Nagahata, H. (2007) Epidemiological and bacteriological survey of buffalo mastitis in Nepal. *J. Vet. Med. Sci.*, 69(12): 1241-1245.

9. Suzanne, N.S. and Lioyd, E.M. (2003) In: Food Analysis. Kluwer Academic/Plenum Publishers, New York. p35-49.

10. Lipman, N.S., Jackson, L.R., Trudel, L.J. and Weis-Garcia, F. (2005) Monoclonal versus polyclonal antibodies: Distinguishing characteristics, applications, and information resources. *ILAR J.*, 46(3): 258-268.

11. Samsonova, Z.V., Shchelokova, O.S., Ivanova, N.L., Rubtsova, M.Y. and Egorov, A.M. (2005) Enzyme-linked immunosorbent assay of ampicillin in milk. *J. Appl. Biochem. Microbiol.*, 41: 589-595.

12. Sui, J., Hong, L., Limin, C. and Zhenxing, L. (2009) Dot-immunogold filtration assay for rapid screening of three fluroquinolones. *J. Food Agric. Immunol.*, 20: 125-137.

13. Bollag, D., Micheal, D.R. and Stuart, J.E. (1996) In: Protein Methods. 2nd ed. Ch. 3, 4, 5. Wiley-Liss Publication, USA. p68, 86, 91, 103, 108.

14. Christoph, K. (2002) Posttranslational modifications of proteins: tools for proteomics. In: methods in molecular biologypp.

15. Dykman, L.A., Sumaroka, M.V., Staroverou, S.A., Zaltseva, I.S. and Bogatyrev, V.A. (2004) Immunogenic properties of colloidal gold. *Biol. Bull.*, 31: 75-79.

16. Oruganti, M. and Gaidhani, S. (2011) Routine bleeding techniques in laboratory rodents. *IJPSR.*, 2(3): 516-524.

17. Fan, G.Y., Yang, R.S., Jiang, J.Q., Chang, X.Y., Chen, J.J., Qi, Y.H., Wu, S.X. and Yang, X.F. (2012) Development of a class-specific polyclonal antibody based indirect competitive ELISA for detecting fluoroquinolone residues in milk. *J. Zhejiang Univ. Sci. B.* 13(7): 545-554.

18. Ramadass, P., Parthiban, M., Thiagarajan, V., Chandrasekar, M., Vidhya, M. and Raj, G.D. (2008) Development of single serum dilution ELISA for detection of infectious bursal disease virus antibodies. *J. Vet. Arch.*, 78: 23-30.

19. Jiang, J., Zhang, H. and Wang, Z. (2011) Development of an immunoassay for determination of fluroquinolones pollutant in environmental water sample. International conference on nanotechnology and biosensors. *IPCBEE.*, 2: 1-4.

20. Strasser, A., Usleber, E., Schneider, E., Dietrich, R., Burk, C. and Martlbauer, E. (2003) Improved enzyme immune assay for group-specific determination of penicillins in milk. *J. Food Agric. Immunol.*, 15: 135-143.

21. McConnell, R.I., Elouard, B., Stephen, P.F. and John, V.L. (2003) Method and kit for detecting, or determining the quantity of beta-lactam penicillins. United States Patent, Patent No. US 6960653 B2.

22. Liu, C., Hong, L., Limin, C. and Jie, J. (2005) Anti-ENR antibody production by using ENR-screened HSA as an immunogen. *J. Ocean U China*, 4(3): 262-266.

23. Tiwari, R., Chakraborty, S., Dharma, K., Rajagunalan, S. and Singh, S.V. (2013) Antibiotic resistance - An emerging health problem: Causes, worries, challenges and solutions − A review. *Int. J. Curr. Res.*, 5(7): 1880-1892.

25

Prevalence, type, and prognosis of ocular lesions in shelter and owned-client dogs naturally infected by *Leishmania infantum*

Simona Di Pietro[1], Valentina Rita Francesca Bosco[2], Chiara Crinò[1], Francesco Francaviglia[3] and Elisabetta Giudice[4]

1. Department of Veterinary Science, University of Messina, Polo Universitario Annunziata, 98168 Messina, Italy; 2. DVM, Veterinary Medical Centre S. Chiara, Viale Vittorio Veneto, 96014 Floridia (SR), Italy; 3. DVM, Local Public Health Unit (ASP) of Palermo, Via G. Cusmano 24, 90141, Palermo, Italy; 4. Department of Chemical, Biological, Pharmaceutical and Environmental Sciences, University of Messina, Viale F. Stagno d'Alcontres 31, 98168 Messina, Italy.
Corresponding author: Simona Di Pietro, e-mail: dipietros@unime.it,
VRFB: valentina1022000@hotmail.com, CC: chiaracrino@gmail.com, FF: vetcanile@asppalermo.org,
EG: egiudice@unime.it

Abstract

Aim: The point prevalence of ocular lesions due to leishmaniasis was evaluated in 127 dogs living in a municipal shelter placed in a highly endemic area (Sicily, Italy). Moreover, the period prevalence, the type, and prognosis of lesions due to leishmaniasis were evaluated in 132 dogs with ocular pathologies referred to a Veterinary Teaching Hospital (VTH) in the same endemic area over a 3-year period.

Materials and Methods: All the dogs were submitted to ophthalmological examination. The diagnosis of leishmaniasis was made by cytological, serological (immune-fluorescent antibody test), and molecular (quantitative polymerase chain reaction) tests.

Results: The point prevalence of ocular lesions in 45 shelter dogs with leishmaniasis was 71.11% (45/127 dogs). The most frequent ocular lesion was blepharitis (50%) while anterior uveitis was observed in only 9.37% of cases. The period prevalence of ocular lesions due to leishmaniasis in the VTH group was 36.36% (48/132 dogs). In both groups, most of the lesions were bilateral and involved the anterior segment. Anterior uveitis was the most frequent ophthalmic finding in client-owned dogs (37.50%), but it occurred in only 9.37% of the shelter dogs. Keratouveitis often occurred during or after antiprotozoal treatment (14.58%; 7/48). In this study, the healing of eye injury following systemic antiprotozoal treatment was recorded in about half of cases (48%; 12/25 dogs), in which follow-up was possible. In more than 1/3 of cases (36%; 9/25), there was an improvement, but it was necessary to associate a long-term topical treatment; most of them, as well as those who had not responded to systemic therapy (16%; 4/25), had anterior uveitis or keratoconjunctivitis sicca.

Conclusions: Ocular manifestations involve up to 2/3 of animals affected by canine leishmaniasis and lesions account for over 1/3 of ophthalmic pathologies observed at a referral clinic in an endemic area. The occurrence of anterior uveitis is more frequent in client-owned dogs than in shelter dogs. The onset of keratouveitis during or after antiprotozoal treatment could be attributed to the treatment or to a recurrence of the systemic form. The post-treatment uveal immune reaction, already observed in humans, could explain the difference in the frequency of keratouveitis between client-owned and shelter dogs, which have never been treated.

Keywords: dog, follow-up, leishmaniasis, ocular lesions, post-treatment uveitis.

Introduction

Many endo- or ecto-parasites may affect animals and their adverse effects on health, production, and welfare have been repeatedly documented [1,2]. Furthermore, many parasitic diseases are zoonoses and thus a severe public health concern [3,4].

Canine leishmaniasis is a chronic and severe systemic disease caused by the protozoan parasite *Leishmania infantum*. It is endemic in the Mediterranean area, and the infection vectors are sand flies (*Phlebotomus* spp.).

Clinical signs associated with leishmaniasis are highly variable as the consequence of numerous different pathogenic mechanisms and different immune responses of individual hosts [5]. Ocular signs occur in 16-80% of affected dogs [5-7]. Blepharitis, keratoconjunctivitis, and anterior uveitis were described as the most frequent signs [6]. Adnexal lesions such as periocular alopecia, eyelid nodule, and keratoconjunctivitis sicca (KCS) are also common. Previous clinical studies have reported the occurrence of KCS in dogs with leishmaniasis varying from 2.8% to 26.43% [6-8]. Other reported ocular manifestations include cyclitis, chorioretinitis, retinal detachment, cataract, glaucoma, and orbital cellulitis [5].

In literature, there is a considerable variability in the prevalence of eye lesions observed during canine leishmaniasis, likely due to differences in the canine population and the clinical approach (generic or specialist) evaluated. Although studies conducted on both shelter and client-owned dogs are numerous, there is a lack of knowledge in the comparison between these types of population.

The aim of this study was to evaluate the point prevalence of ocular lesions in shelter dogs and the period prevalence, type, and prognosis of ocular lesions associated to leishmaniasis in dogs referred to a specialty clinic both from the same endemic area.

Materials and Methods

Ethical approval

All treatments, housing, and animal care reported in this study were reviewed and approved in accordance with the standards recommended by the Guide for the Care and Use of the Laboratory Animals and the EU Directive 2010/63/EU for animal experiments. The pet owners consented to have their animals involved in this study.

Canine population

A total of 259 dogs, of various breeds, sex, and age (Table-1), were enrolled in the study: 127 dogs living in a municipal shelter in Palermo (Northern Sicily, Italy) and visited in September 2007; 132 dogs referred to the ophthalmology unit of the Veterinary Teaching Hospital (VTH) of the Department of Veterinary Sciences of the University of Messina (Northern Sicily) over a 3-year period (2004-2007). All animals were submitted to general physical examination and ophthalmological assessment.

Canine samples

Popliteal lymph node aspirates were obtained from each dog using a thin biopsy needle. A thin smear was performed immediately after collection. When occurred, smears were performed on nodular and/or ulcerative lesions. Smears were stained with May-Grünwald Giemsa and examined under an optical microscope to determine whether amastigote forms of *L. infantum* were present. Each smear was examined for 10 min (100 microscopic fields) under a 100× oil immersion objective lens.

On each dog, peripheral blood was obtained from the jugular vein and equally distributed into tubes with and without ethylenediaminetetraacetic acid, for biomolecular testing (quantitative polymerase chain reaction [qPCR]) and serologic (immune-fluorescent antibody test [IFAT]), respectively. For the former tests, samples were also collected from left popliteal lymph node and conjunctival swabs (exfoliative epithelial cells collected using sterile cotton swabs rubbed robustly back and forth once in the lower conjunctival sac).

All serological and molecular tests were performed at the Italian National Reference Centre for Leishmaniasis (CReNaL) of the Istituto Zooprofilattico Sperimentale della Sicilia, Palermo, Italy.

The IPT1 ZMON1 *L. infantum* promastigotes were used as antigen for IFAT assay and to construct the standard curve for qPCR. The IPT1, taken from the collection of CReNaL, were grown in Tobie agar medium Evans modified [9,10].

In the IFAT assay, the antigen was fixed on multispot microscope slides (Bio-Merieux, Marcy L'Etoile, France) in acetone bath. The dog sera were serially diluted (1:40-1:5120) in pH 7.2 phosphate-buffered saline (PBS) and added to the antigen-coated wells. The slides were incubated for 30 min at 37°C. Positive and negative controls were included in each series of analyzed samples. Fluorescent staining was performed using an anti-dog immunoglobulin G labeled with fluorescein isothiocyanate (Sigma-Aldrich, Saint Louis, MO, USA) diluted 1:200 in PBS. The slides were examined using a fluorescence microscope (Leica DM 4000B, Heerbrugg, Switzerland). The IFAT results were regarded as positive when dilutions of the sera gave an evident yellowish-green fluorescent signal on microscopic observation while non-reactive samples showed no color. The cutoff value was established at a serum dilution of 1:40. The positive control consisted in a known title serum of a dog with positive cultural isolation. The negative control consisted in serum from a dog which was negative to cultural test.

In tissue samples, the DNA was extracted using EZNA. Tissue DNA Kit (Omega Biotech VWR) according to the manufacturer's instructions. The PCR test was targeted on a 123 bp fragment inner the constant region in the minicircle kinetoplast DNA (NCBI accession number AF291093) and was carried out as previously described [11]. The primers and probe were chosen with the assistance of Primer Express Software (Applied Biosystems). The primer sequences were: QLK2-U 5'-GGCGTTCTGCGAAAACCG-3'; QLK2-D 5'-AAAATGGCATTTTCGGGCC-3'; while the associated probe was: 5'-TGGGTGCAGAAATCCCGTTCA-3' 5'FAM and 3' BHQ labeled. Each amplification was performed in duplicate. The thermal cycling conditions comprised an initial incubation for 2' at 50°C for uracil-N-glycosylase activity. This step was followed by a 10' denaturation at 95°C and 45 cycles at 95°C for 15" and 60°C for 1' each. The quantity of DNA in the samples examined was detected by comparison with a standard curve. The DNA concentration was estimated by spectrophotometric determination of A260 and A280 and by gel electrophoresis. On the basis of the linearity in the fluorescent signal through the serial standard DNA dilutions, PCR test and dedicated software (SDS Applied Biosystems) permitted detection of parasitic charge lower than 1 cell/mL of the tissue matrices. Two replicates of six different concentrations of *L. infantum* DNA were tested in the same run. In this

Table-1: Signalment of canine population.

Group	Dogs	Sex		Age (years)		
		Male	Female	<1	1-4	>4
Shelter group	127	53	74	25	42	60
VTH group	132	86	46	12	28	92
Total	259	139	12	37	70	152

VTH=Veterinary teaching hospital

way, we performed intra- and inter-assay comparison of the obtained signal for each DNA concentration.

Results

Shelter group

Out of the 127 examined dogs, 45 (35.43%) were affected by leishmaniasis. The diagnosis was made on the basis of the positivity of serology (IFAT, ≥1:640), microscopy and at least lymph node qPCR. 32 of these animals (point prevalence: 71.11%) showed ocular and periocular lesions referable to the disease. Ocular lesions were bilateral in 27 dogs (84.37%), 20 of which had more than one ocular sign. In all animals and eyes (100%), the lesions involved the anterior segment and in one dog the lesion involved the anterior segment in one eye and both segments in the other eye. The type and frequency of ocular lesions in 32 shelter dogs with leishmaniasis (59 affected eyes) are reported in Table-2 and Figure-1. The most frequent ocular lesion was blepharitis (16/32, 50%); anterior uveitis was observed in only 3 dogs (9.37%).

VTH group

Out of the 132 dogs with ocular pathologies referred to the ophthalmology unit of the VTH, 58 (43.94%) were affected by leishmaniasis, resulting positive to the diagnostic tests. 48 of these animals showed ocular and periocular lesions referable to the disease (period prevalence: 36.36%). Ocular lesions were bilateral in 42 cases (87.50%); 28 dogs (58.33%) had more than one ocular sign. The ocular lesions involved the anterior segment in 46 dogs (95.83%) and the posterior segment in 8 dogs (16.67%). In 4 dogs (8.33%), the lesions involved both segments. The distribution of the ocular lesions in 48 referred dogs with leishmaniasis (90 eyes) is reported in Table-2 and Figure-1. The most common lesions were anterior uveitis which occurred in 18 dogs (37.50%).

In 41 dogs (85.42%), the ocular lesions were recorded when leishmaniasis was diagnosed, whereas

in the other 7 dogs (14.58%) the lesions (keratouveitis) occurred during or after the specific treatment; in 1 case, uveitis developed on the 15th day of therapy; in 6 cases, the lesions appeared several weeks after the beginning of a previous cycle of antimonial therapy (mean 132.5±31.2 days; median: 129 days; range: 90-179 days).

Follow-up study

About 25 cases of the VTH group were evaluated to ascertain response and prognosis of ocular lesions to antiprotozoal therapy, with N-methylglucamine antimoniate (100 mg/kg daily for 60 days, subcutaneously), combined with allopurinol (10 mg/kg twice daily for 6-12 months orally). The mean follow-up was 8.7 months (range: From 2 months to 2 years).

In 12 dogs (48%), a complete resolution of ocular lesions was obtained after antiprotozoal therapy alone (mean: 14.5±10.4 days; median: 12.5 days; range: 5-45 days). The lesions were as follows: Nodular blepharitis (n=2 cases), keratoconjunctivitis (n=2), keratitis (n=2), and keratouveitis (n=6). In 9

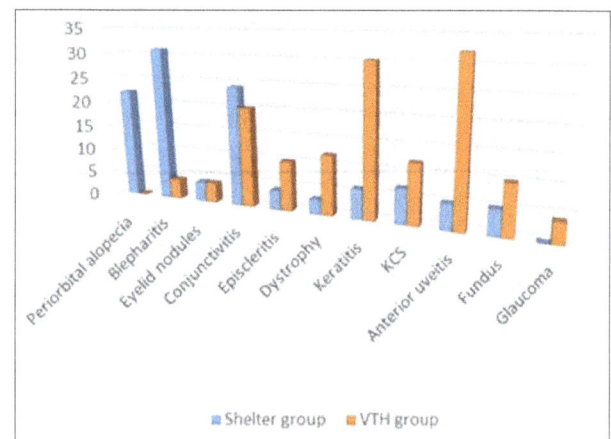

Figure-1: Type and frequency of ocular lesions in 80 leishmaniotic dogs (shelter group and Veterinary Teaching Hospital group).

Table-2: Type and frequency of ocular lesions in 48 client-owned dogs (VTH group) and in 32 shelter dogs (shelter group) with leishmaniasis.

Ocular lesion	VTH group		Shelter group	
	Dogs (%)	Eyes (%)	Dogs (%)	Eyes (%)
Periorbital alopecia	0	0	11 (34.37)	22 (37.29)
Blepharitis	2 (4.17)	4 (4.44)	16 (50.00)	31 (52.54)
Eyelid nodules	4 (8.33)	4 (4.44)	3 (9.37)	4 (6.78)
Conjunctivitis	10 (20.83)	20 (22.22)	12 (37.50)	24 (40.68)
Episcleritis	6 (12.50)	10 (11.11)	2 (6.25)	4 (6.78)
Dystrophy	6 (12.50)	12 (13.33)	2 (6.25)	3 (5.08)
Keratitis	16 (33.33)	30 (33.33)	4 (12.50)	6 (10.17)
KCS	6 (12.50)	12 (13.33)	4 (12.50)	7 (11.86)
Anterior uveitis	18 (37.50)	32 (35.55)	3 (9.37)	5 (8.47)
Fundus	6 (12.50)	10 (11.11)	3 (9.37)	5 (8.47)
Glaucoma	2 (4.17)	4 (4.44)	-	-
Anterior district	46 (95.83)	84 (93.33)	32 (100)	59 (100)
Posterior district	8 (16.67)	14 (15.55)	3 (9.37)	5 (8.47)
Sub total	48 (100)	90 (93.75)	32 (100)	59 (92.19)
No lesion	-	6 (6.25)	-	5 (7.81)
Total	48 (100)	96 (100)	32 (100)	64 (100)

VTH=Veterinary teaching hospital, KCS=Keratoconjunctivitis sicca

dogs (36%), the antiprotozoal treatment determined an improvement of ocular lesions, while healing was achieved only after a long topical therapy (14-56 days) with non-steroidal or steroidal anti-inflammatory, cyclosporine, artificial tears, midriatic/cycloplegics, and/or antiglaucoma medications, whether or not associated with systemic anti-inflammatories. The lesions were: KCS (n=3), keratouveitis (n=2), anterior uveitis (n=3), and post-uveitic glaucoma (n=1). In the other 4 dogs (16%), the combined treatment did not lead to healing but produced only a slight improvement. All the dogs had serious and inveterate lesions: Blepharoconjunctivitis associated to keratouveitis (n=1), glaucoma (n=1), and KCS (n=2) (Table-3).

Discussion

The present research was carried out in two different areas of Sicily (Southern Italy) with a similar high-endemicity for leishmaniasis [12].

During canine leishmaniasis, ocular manifestations involved up to 2/3 of the affected animals (shelter group), and the lesions due to leishmaniasis are more than 1/3 of the ophthalmic pathologies observed in a referral clinic in an endemic area.

Anterior uveitis was the most frequent ophthalmic finding in client-owned dogs (37.50%), but it occurred in only 9.37% of the shelter dogs. As the operators and research methodology as well as the geographical area of study were the same, the only variable that may explain the different percentages of occurrence is the type of sample, client-owned dogs being well cared for while shelter dogs are almost never treated.

The occurrence of anterior uveitis in seven animals (28%) during or after the antiprotozoal treatment could be attributed to the treatment itself or to a recurrence of the systemic form. The nodular form of uveitis, which often develops after initiation of antiprotozoal therapy, may have an allergic basis resulting from the death of the organism in tissues [6], similarly to what is observed for post-kala-azar anterior uveitis in humans [13].

The post-treatment uveal immune reaction may explain the difference in the frequency of uveitis between client-owned dogs and shelter dogs.

Periocular lesions, such as blepharitis and periocular alopecia, are more frequent in shelter dogs (50% and 34.37%, respectively) than in VTH group (33.33% and 0%, respectively). Eyelid lesions are also often considered as dermatological signs (periocular dermatitis), and they are not referred to an ophthalmologist.

Granulomatous nodular lesions were recorded in both VTH and shelter groups. In two client-owned dogs, this kind of lesion was found in lateral corneal limbus (Figure-2) and also described in previous papers [6] and similar to granulomatous episcleritis observed in Collies and other breeds [14]. Nodular lesions in cornea, conjunctiva, and eyelids were also found in five client-owned dogs and three shelter dogs (Figure-3). The microscopic examination of granulomas always showed the parasite (Figure-4). This suggests that cytology is useful in these lesions but also that inflammation of the conjunctiva and cornea could be directly related to the protozoan rather than to an altered immune response due to infection [6]. The granulomas on the eyelid margin could also be a reaction at the vector biting site, as hypothesized by other researchers [6,11].

In this study, the healing of eye injury following systemic antiprotozoal treatment was recorded in about

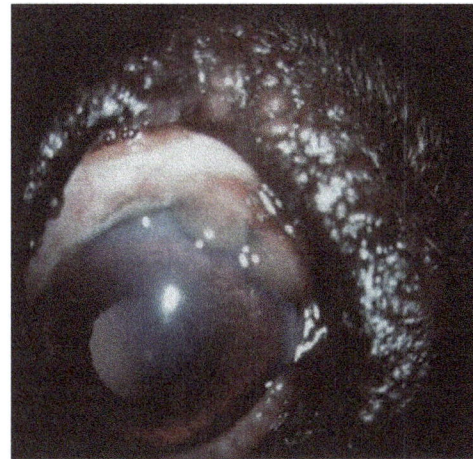

Figure-2: Granulomatous lesions at lateral corneal limbus due to *Leishmania* spp.

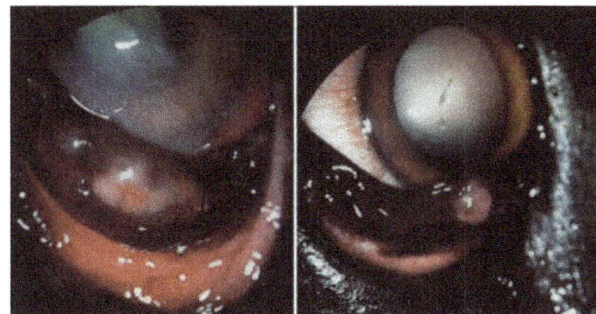

Figure-3: Nodular lesions on cornea, conjunctiva, and eyelids due to *Leishmania* spp.

Table-3: Response of ocular lesions to antiprotozoal treatment alone or combined with ocular therapy and healing times of in 25 leishmaniotic dogs referred to a Veterinary Teaching Hospital.

Response to treatment	Antiprotozoal therapy		Follow-up (days)			Total N (%)
	Alone (%)	Plus ocular therapy (%)	Mean	Median	Range	
Complete healing	12 (48)		14.5±10.4	12.5	5-45	21 (84)
		9 (36)	31.1±14.5	28.0	14-56	
No healing		4 (16)	403.7±219	365	180-705	4 (16)
Total	12 (48)	13 (52)				25 (100)

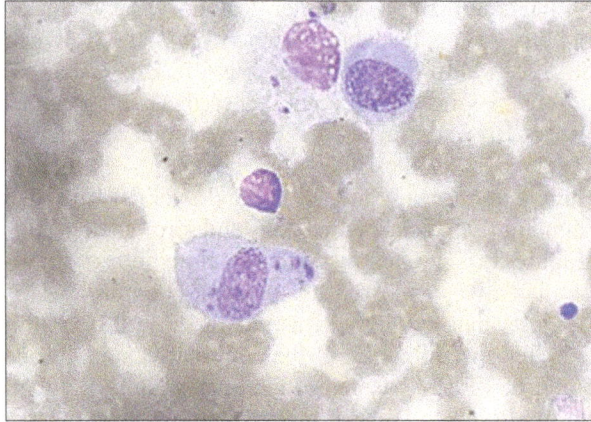

Figure-4: Microscopic examination of an ocular nodule that showed the presence of amastigote parasites.

half the cases (48%), in which follow-up was possible. In over 1/3 of cases (36%), there was an improvement, but it was necessary to associate a long-term (months) topical treatment; most of them, as well as those which had not responded to combined therapy (16%), had anterior uveitis or KCS. These findings agree with previous observations [6,15], in which a favorable prognosis for the lesions of the adnexa and for most inflammatory intraocular lesions was envisaged, except for anterior uveitis which is often refractory to antiprotozoal therapy and much more difficult to treat.

Conclusion

Many aspects of leishmaniasis have not yet been clarified, and ocular involvement can direct toward a diagnosis of the disease, especially when it is the only clinical sign or in the case of the specific granulomatous lesions. Special attention should also be paid to uveal lesions that may be particularly severe and difficult to treat and whose appearance may be linked to causal therapy.

Given the complexity of ocular lesions and their varied response to therapy, we need an earlier and accurate diagnosis, obtained by appropriate means, the use of which may require the expertise of a specialist.

Authors' Contributions

SDP, VRFB, and EG designed the study. The experiment was done by SDP, VRFB, CC, FF, and EG, whereas laboratory work was done by EG and VRFB. All the authors participated in data analysis, draft, and revision of the manuscript. All authors read and approved the final manuscript.

Acknowledgments

The authors acknowledge the Italian National Reference Centre for Leishmaniasis (CReNaL), Istituto Zooprofilattico Sperimentale Della Sicilia (Italy), for providing necessary laboratory facilities to carry out the research work. Particularly, we thank the chief of CReNaL, Dr. Fabrizio Vitale, for his technical and scientific assistance. In addition, we are grateful to Ms. Caroline Keir for assistance with language and for her careful review of the manuscript. This research received no specific grant from any funding.

Competing Interests

The authors declare that they have no competing interests.

References

1.   Pugliese, A., Di Pietro, S. and Giudice, E. (2006) Clinical and diagnostic patterns of leishmaniasis in the dog. *Vet. Res. Commun.*, 30 Suppl 1: 39-43.

2.   Giudice, E., Domina, F., Britti, D., Di Pietro, S. and Pugliese, A. (2003) Clinical findings associated with *Borrelia burgdorferi* infection in the dog. *Vet. Res. Commun.*, 27 Suppl 1: 767-770.

3.   Giudice, E., Di Pietro, S., Alaimo, A., Blanda, V., Lelli, R., Francaviglia, F., Caracappa, S. and Torina, A. (2014) Molecular survey of *Rickettsia felis* in fleas from cats and dogs in Sicily (Southern Italy). *PLoS One*, 9(9): e106820.

4.   Giudice, E., Di Pietro, S., Gaglio, G., Di Giacomo, L., Bazzano, M. and Mazzullo, G. (2013) Adult of *Dirofilaria repens* in a dog with recurrent multiple subcutaneous nodular lesions. *Parasitol. Res.*, 113(2): 711-716.

5.   Peña, M.T., Naranjo, C., Klauss, G., Fondevila, D., Leiva, M., Roura, X., Davidson, M.G. and Dubielzig, R.R. (2008) Histopathological features of ocular leishmaniasis in the dog. *J. Comp. Pathol.*, 138: 32-39.

6.   Peña, M.T., Roura, X. and Davidson, M.G. (2000) Ocular and periocular manifestations of leishmaniasis in dogs: 105 cases (1993-1998), *Vet. Ophthalmol*, 3: 35-41.

7.   Naranjo, C., Fondevila, D., Altet, L., Francino, O., Rios, J., Roura, X. and Peña, T. (2012) Evaluation of the presence of *Leishmania spp.* by real-time PCR in the lacrimal glands of dogs with leishmaniasis. *Vet. J.*, 193, 168-173.

8.   Ciaramella, P., Oliva, G., De Luna, R., Ambrosio, R., Cortese, L., Persechino, A., Gradoni, L. and Scalone, A. (1997) A retrospective clinical study of canine leishmaniasis in 150 dogs naturally infected by *Leishmania infantum*. *Vet. Rec.*, 141: 539-543.

9.   Titus, R.G., Marchand, M., Boon, T. and Louis, J.A. (1985) A limiting dilution assay for quantifying *Leishmania* major in tissues of infected mice. *Parasite Immunol.*, 7: 545-555.

10. Tobie, E.J., Von Brand, T. and Mehelman, B. (1950) Cultural and physiological observations on *Trypanosoma rhodiense* and *Trypanosoma gambiense*. *J. Parasitol.*, 36: 48-54.

11. Manna, L., Reale, S., Vitale, F., Picillo, E., Pavone, L.M. and Gravino, A.E. (2008) Realtime PCR assay in *Leishmania*-infected dogs treated with meglumine antimoniate and allopurinol. *Vet. J.*, 177: 279-282.

12. Lombardo, G., Pennisi, M.G., Lupo, T., Chicharro, C. and Solano-Gallego, L. (2014) Papular dermatitis due to *Leishmania infantum* infection in seventeen dogs: Diagnostic features, extent of the infection and treatment outcome. *Parasit. Vectors*, 7: 120.

13. el Hassan, A.M., Khalil, E.A., el Sheikh, E.A., Zijlstra, E.E., Osman, A. and Ibrahim, M.E. (1998) Post kala-azar ocular leishmaniasis. *Trans. R. Soc. Trop. Med. Hyg.*, 92: 177-179.

14. Esson, D.W. (2015) Clinical Atlas of Canine and Feline Ophthalmic Disease. 1st ed. John Wiley & Sons Ed., Wiley Blackwell, Ames, IA. p122-4.

15. Roze, M. (2004) Ocular manifestations of canine leishmaniasis. Diagnosis and treatment. In: Proceedings from the 27th World Small Animal Veterinary Association (WSAVA) World Congress, 2002 October 3-6, Granada, Spain. Available from: http://www.vin.com/proceedings/Proceedings.plx-?CID=WSAVA 2002. Accessed on 19-04-2004.

26

Estimates of genetic parameters for fat yield in Murrah buffaloes

Manoj Kumar[1], Vikas Vohra[2], Poonam Ratwan[1], Jamuna Valsalan[1], C. S. Patil[3] and A. K. Chakravarty[1]

1. Division of Dairy Cattle Breeding, ICAR-National Dairy Research Institute, Karnal - 132 001, Haryana, India;
2. Department of Animal Genetic Resources, ICAR-National Bureau of Animal Genetic Resources, Karnal - 132 001, Haryana, India; 3. Department of Animal Genetics and Breeding, Lala Lajpat Rai University of Veterinary & Animal Sciences, Hisar, Haryana, India.
Corresponding author: Vikas Vohra, e-mail: vohravikas@gmail.com,
MK: drmanojneemwal@gmail.com, PR: punam.ratwan@gmail.com, JV: jamunavalsalan@gmail.com,
CSP: dr.cspatil03@gmail.com, AKC: ak_chakravarty@yahoo.co.in

Abstract

Aim: The present study was performed to investigate the effect of genetic and non-genetic factors affecting milk fat yield and to estimate genetic parameters of monthly test day fat yields (MTDFY) and lactation 305-day fat yield (L305FY) in Murrah buffaloes.

Materials and Methods: The data on total of 10381 MTDFY records comprising the first four lactations of 470 Murrah buffaloes calved from 1993 to 2014 were assessed. These buffaloes were sired by 75 bulls maintained in an organized farm at ICAR-National Dairy Research Institute, Karnal. Least squares maximum likelihood program was used to estimate genetic and non-genetic parameters. Heritability estimates were obtained using paternal half-sib correlation method. Genetic and phenotypic correlations among MTDFY, and 305-day fat yield were calculated from the analysis of variance and covariance matrix among sire groups.

Results: The overall least squares mean of L305FY was found to be 175.74±4.12 kg. The least squares mean of overall MTDFY ranged from 3.33±0.14 kg (TD-11) to 7.06±0.17 kg (TD-3). The h^2 estimate of L305FY was found to be 0.33±0.16 in this study. The estimates of phenotypic and genetic correlations between 305-day fat yield and different MTDFY ranged from 0.32 to 0.48 and 0.51 to 0.99, respectively.

Conclusions: In this study, all the genetic and non-genetic factors except age at the first calving group, significantly affected the traits under study. The estimates of phenotypic and genetic correlations of MTDFY with 305-day fat yield was generally higher in the MTDFY-5 of lactation suggesting that this TD yields could be used as the selection criteria for early evaluation and selection of Murrah buffaloes.

Keywords: genetic factors, Murrah buffalo, non-genetic factors, test-day fat yields.

Introduction

India has about 51 million milch buffaloes [1] contributing about 51% [2] of the total milk produced in the country. Compared with cow's milk, buffalo's milk has a higher percentage of fat percentage. The reported values of fat percentage for buffalo's milk varies from 6.87% to 8.59% [3,4]. In spite of its higher fat percentage, milk cholesterol content is lower in buffalo's milk compared to cow's milk, which is 275 mg versus 330 mg as reported by Zicarelli [5]. Milk fat plays a significant role in the nutritive value and physical properties of milk and milk products. Besides serving as a rich source of energy, fat contains significant amounts of essential fatty acids-linolenic and arachidonic acid. The most distinctive role which milk fat plays in dairy products concerns flavor.

Nowadays, milk pricing system is also based on the percentage of fat in milk, therefore, higher milk fat yield fetches better economic returns. Murrah is the most important buffalo breed with superior genetic potential for milk fat yield production.

To find out an alternative to daily milk yield recording, which is a costly and time-consuming proposition under field conditions, some studies have been made in the past in buffaloes on test day (TD) milk yields [6,7]. Various advantages of using TD milk yield records are individual test date effects, and the number of records per animal as well as the interval between records can be accounted for better adjustment of non-genetic factors influencing the milk yield leading to more accurate genetic evaluation. Today, in many countries across the continents, multi trait evaluations are employed in genetic evaluations. TD milk fat yield records can be used in combination for more accurate genetic evaluation. Although TD fat yield records offer greater advantage compared to 305-day fat yield in selection schemes, information on estimation of genetic parameters based on TD records particularly, monthly records are limited.

The present investigation was undertaken with the objective to study the influence of various non-genetic and genetic factors on monthly TD and lactation 305-day fat yields (L305FY) and to estimate the genetic parameters for milk fat yield, which could be used for selecting Murrah buffaloes for higher fat yield.

Materials and Methods

Ethical approval

The experiment was conducted following the code of ethics for animal experimentation with approval from the Institute's Animal Ethics Committee.

Data

A total of 10381 monthly TD fat yield (MTDFY) records comprised first four lactations of 470 Murrah buffaloes calved during 1993-2014 at the ICAR-National Dairy Research Institute, Karnal were collected from the history-cum-pedigree sheets and monthly record of milk yield and fat percentage register. The traits considered for analysis were MTDFY and L305FY. Culling in the middle of lactation, abortion, stillbirth, or any other pathological causes affecting the lactation yield were considered as abnormalities and thus, such records were not taken for the study. Records of buffaloes with <500 kg of milk production and covered <100 days of lactation, were not considered, a set practice at our herd, as usually such animals had shown good average daily milk yield. To ensure the normal distribution, the outliers ($\mu \pm 3$ standard deviation) were removed, and data set was standardized. The data were analyzed to study the effect of non-genetic factors (parity, season, period and age at first calving [AFC] groups) on 11 MTDFY records (from 6th, 36th, 66th, and 300th day of lactation) and L305FY records. The data were classified into different seasons, periods and AFC groups. Each year was classified into four seasons on the basis of rainfall, temperature and humidity over the years-winter (December-March), summer (April-June), rainy (July-August), and autumn (September-November). The data spread over 22 years were classified into 10 periods. The data were classified into 9 AFC sub-groups using Sturges' formula [8]. Fat percentage was determined by Lacto Star apparatus (German equipment produced by Funke-Gerber). For calibration of Lacto Star apparatus, fat percentage of milk was tested by Gerber method [9].

Statistical methods

The least squares maximum likelihood program of Harvey [10] was used to estimate and study the effect of genetic and non-genetic factors on MTDFY and L305FY records of Murrah buffaloes:

$$Y_{ijklmn} = \mu + PA_i + S_j + P_k + A_l + B_m + e_{ijklmn}$$

Where, Y_{ijklmn} = Observation on the nth individual in ith parity, jth season, kth period, lth AFC group and sired by mth bull, μ = Overall population mean, PA_i = Effect of ith parity (1-4), S_j = Effect of jth season (1-4) four seasons: Winter (December to March), summer (April to June), rainy (July to August), autumn

(September to November) were considered for analysis, P_k = Fixed effect of kth period of study (1-10) a period in a block of 2 years was considered, A_l = Fixed effect of lth AFC group, B_m = Random effect of mth bull (sire), e_{ijklmn} = Random error, NID (0, σ^2_e).

Estimation of heritability

Paternal half-sib correlation method given by Becker, 1975 [11] was used to estimate the heritability of different characters and their genetic correlations. A total of 75 bulls having three or more number of progeny were included for the estimation of heritability. The data were adjusted for those non-genetic factors showing significant effects and further used for estimation of heritability. The standard error of heritability was estimated as per Swiger et al. [12].

Genetic and phenotypic correlations

The genetic and phenotypic correlations among MTDFY and 305-days fat yield were calculated from the analysis of variance and covariance among sire groups as given by Becker [11] and shown in below.

$$r_{g(XY)} = Cov\ S_{xy}/\sqrt{\sigma^2_{s(x)} \cdot \sigma^2_{s(y)}}$$

Results and Discussion

The least squares mean along with their standard errors for MTDFY and L305FY are shown in Table-1. The highest MTDFY was observed in MTDFY-3 (7.06 kg), and the lowest was observed in MTDFY-11 (3.33 kg). In general, MTDFY increased until MTDFY-3 and thereafter a gradual decline was noticed until the end of lactation. The overall mean of average 305-day fat yield was 175.74±4.12 kg. Ibrahim et al. [13] and Tonhati et al. [14] reported overall mean of 305-day fat yield as 147.67 kg and 90.1 kg in Egyptian buffaloes and Murrah buffaloes herd in Sao population, respectively, which was comparatively lower than Murrah breed in this study.

Effect of non-genetic factors

Parity

The effect of parity was highly significant (p<0.01) up to MTDFY-6 and L305FY; non-significant

Table-1: Least squares means of L305FY and different MTDFY (in kg).

Trait	N	Mean±SE	CV (%)
MTDFY1	1049	6.81±0.184	39.44
MTDFY2	1049	7.05±0.18	33.41
MTDFY3	1049	7.06±0.17	31.72
MTDFY4	1049	6.55±0.14	31.34
MTDFY5	1048	6.11±0.13	33.12
MTDFY6	1028	5.56±0.16	34.33
MTDFY7	1002	5.15±0.17	36.80
MTDFY8	949	4.56±016	38.42
MTDFY9	869	4.73±0.13	42.76
MTDFY10	722	3.74±0.15	44.01
MTDFY11	567	3.33±0.14	48.09
L305FY	1049	175.74±4.12	26.55

N=Number of observation, L305FY=Lactation 305-fat yield, MTDFY=Monthly test day fat yields, SE=Standard error, CV=Coefficient of variation in percentage

Table-2: Mixed model ANOVA showing mean sum of squares for factors affecting MTDFY and L305FY.

Traits	Sire	Parity	Season	Period	AFC group	Error
d. f.	74	3	3	9	8	951
MTDFY1	7.38*	154.86**	22.90**	11.56*	7.67NS	5.37
MTDFY2	6.88**	85.91**	30.84**	10.91*	9.97*	4.625
MTDFY3	6.19**	70.12**	40.11**	8.05*	11.69**	4.03
MTDFY4	4.80NS	35.96**	2.78NS	6.18NS	7.16NS	3.86
MTDFY5	4.51NS	28.21**	3.54NS	8.90*	9.19*	3.66
MTDFY6	5.91**	23.46**	6.47NS	6.85NS	7.99*	3.93
MTDFY7	6.46**	9.97NS	9.48NS	9.11*	4.47NS	4.36
MTDFY8	5.83*	3.60NS	15.24*	7.97NS	4.51NS	4.35
MTDFY9	4.93NS	7.99NS	19.435**	10.58*	4.87NS	4.66
MTDFY10	5.40NS	3.06NS	22.53**	11.75**	3.06NS	4.58
MTDFY11	4.67NS	2.98NS	21.20**	11.68**	2.55NS	3.89
L305FY	3521.85**	44925.29**	16778.69**	11805.05**	1353.61NS	2301.15

*$p \leq 0.05$, **$p \leq 0.01$. NS=Non-significant, L305FY=Lactation 305-fat yield, MTDFY=Monthly test day fat yields, AFC=Age at first calving

effect of parity was observed in rest TD (Table-2). Singh et al. [15] observed the non-significant effect of parity on fat percentage in Murrah buffaloes. Similar results were shown by Shah and Schermerhorn [16] in Nilli-Ravi buffaloes.

Season

The effect of season of calving was highly significant ($p<0.01$) up to MTDFY-3 then MTDFY-9 to MTDFY-11 and L305FY; significant ($p<0.05$) for MTDFY-8. Non-significant effect of season of calving was observed MTDFY-4 to MTDFY-7 (Table-2). Ibrahim et al. [13] and Mourad et al. [17] reported significant effect of season of calving on lactation fat yield in Egyptian buffaloes. Khan et al. [18] also reported a significant effect of season of calving on fat yield in Nilli Ravi buffaloes. In Murrah buffaloes, Hatwar [19] found significant effect of season of calving on fat yield and fat percentages.

Period

Highly significant effect ($p<0.01$) of the period of calving was observed for L305FY and MTDFY-10 and MTDFY-11; significant ($p<0.05$) for MTDFY-1, MTDFY-2, MTDFY-3, MTDFY-5, MTDFY-7, and MTDFY-9. Non-significant effect of period of calving was observed MTDFY-4, MTDFY-6, and TDFY-8 (Table-2). Ibrahim et al. [13] and Mourad et al. [17] observed significant effect of period of calving on lactation fat yield in Egyptian buffaloes. Khan et al. [18] also found a significant effect of period of calving of fat yield in Nili Ravi buffaloes.

AFC groups

The effect of AFC groups on MTDFY is presented in Table-2. A significant effect ($p<0.01$) of the AFC was observed on MTDFY-3; significant ($p<0.05$) for MTDFY-2, MTDFY-5, MTDFY-6 and rest TD have non-significant effect of AFC groups. Non-significant effect of AFC groups was also observed on L305FY. Shah and Schermerhorn [16] reported non-significant effect of AFC on fat percentage in Nilli-Ravi buffaloes.

Table-3: Heritability estimates along with their standard error for L305FY and different MTDFY.

Trait	N	h²±SE	Trait	N	h²±SE
MTDFY1	1049	0.28±0.16	MTDFY7	1002	0.29±0.16
MTDFY2	1049	0.37±0.17	MTDFY8	949	0.06±0.14
MTDFY3	1049	0.43±0.18	MTDFY9	869	0.22±0.12
MTDFY4	1049	0.30±0.17	MTDFY10	722	0.18±0.15
MTDFY5	1048	0.41±0.18	MTDFY11	567	0.13±0.15
MTDFY6	1028	0.40±0.18	L305FY	1049	0.33±0.16

N=Number of observation, L305FY=Lactation 305-fat yield, MTDFY=Monthly test day fat yields, SE=Standard error

Genetic and phenotypic parameters

Heritability

The heritability of the MTDFY is shown in Table-3. The h² estimate of MTDFY was the lowest (0.06) for MTDFY-8 and the highest (0.43) for MTDFY-3 and L305FY heritability was 0.33. Madad et al. [20] observed that heritability estimates ranged from 0.03 to 0.24 for TD fat percentages in Iranian buffaloes. Ibrahim et al. [13] reported heritability of lactation fat yield in Egyptian buffaloes as 0.19. Aspilcueta-Borquis et al. [21] found heritability estimate as 0.23 for L305FY in buffaloes. In Murrah buffaloes, Tonhati et al. [14] observed heritability estimate of lactation fat yield as 0.21.

Genetic and phenotypic correlations

The estimates of genetic and phenotypic correlations among 305-day fat yield and MTDFY are shown in Table-4. The estimates of genetic and phenotypic correlations between 305-day fat yield and MTDFY ranged from 0.51 to 0.99 and 0.32 to 0.48, respectively. Estimate of genotypic and phenotypic correlation between traits was similar to Sahoo et al., 2014 [22]. MTDFY-5 had the highest genetic (0.99) and phenotypic (0.48) correlation with L305FY. Records up to five months can provide the similar results to lactation fat yield with almost 99% accuracy. Therefore, instead of 11 months with L305FY analysis can be made based on MTDFY-5.

Table-4: Genetic and phenotypic correlations among L305FY and different MTDFY.

Trait 1	Trait 2	Genetic correlations	Phenotypic correlations
L305FY	MTDFY1	0.87±0.28	0.32
	MTDFY2	0.63±0.26	0.39
	MTDFY3	0.92±0.20	0.42
	MTDFY4	0.90±0.30	0.45
	MTDFY5	0.99±0.30	0.48
	MTDFY6	0.99±0.18	0.46
	MTDFY7	0.99±0.19	0.47
	MTDFY8	0.88±0.24	0.46
	MTDFY9	0.99±0.19	0.46
	MTDFY10	0.51±0.41	0.45
	MTDFY11	0.73±0.36	0.43

L305FY=Lactation 305-fat yield, MTDFY=Monthly test day fat yields

Conclusions

In this study, all the genetic and non-genetic factors except AFC group significantly affected the considered traits. The h^2 estimate of lactation milk fat yield was around 0.33 and it ranged from 0.06 (MTDFY-8) to 0.43 (MTDFY-3). The estimates of phenotypic and genetic correlations of monthly TD yields with 305-day fat yield were generally higher in MTDFY-5 of lactation suggesting that this 5th TD fat yields could be used as the selection criteria for early evaluation and selection of Murrah buffaloes.

Authors' Contributions

Research work was done by MK. The experiment was designed and supervised by VV. PR, JV and CSP assisted MK in data recording, literature collection and data analysis, respectively. AKC provided valuable suggestion regarding design of experiment and data analysis. VV and MK compiled the results as well as the manuscript. All authors read and approved the final manuscript.

Acknowledgments

The authors are thankful to the Director cum Vice Chancellor NDRI & Director, NBAGR, Karnal (Haryana) for providing the necessary facilities and ICAR for providing financial support. Thanks to In-charge LRC, and In-charge computer center, NDRI for their help.

Competing Interests

The authors declare that they have no competing interests.

References

1. 19th Livestock Census. (2012) Available from: http://www.dahd.nic.in/dahd/writeread data/livestock.pdf. Accessed on 05-11-2014.
2. BAHS. (2013) Basic Animal Husbandry Statistics. Department of Animal Husbandry, Dairying and Fisheries. Ministry of Agriculture, Government of India.
3. Rosati, A. and Van Vleck, L.D. (2002) Estimation of genetic parameters for milk, fat, protein and mozzarella cheese production for the Italian river buffalo *Bubalus bubalis* population. *Livest. Prod. Sci.,* 74: 185-190.
4. Tonhati, H., Vasconcellors, F.B. and Albuquerque, L.G. (2000) Genetic aspects of productive and reproductive traits in a Murrah buffaloes herd in Sao population. *J. Anim. Breed Genet.,* 117: 331-336.
5. Zicarelli, L. (2004) Buffalo milk: Its properties, dairy yield and mozzarella production. *Vet. Res. Common.,* 1(28): 127-135.
6. Chakraborty, D., Dhaka, S.S., Pander, B.L., Yadav, A.S., Singh, S. and Malik, P.K. (2010) Prediction of lactation milk yield from test day records in Murrah buffaloes. *Indian J. Anim. Sci.,* 80(3): 244-245.
7. Singh, S. and Tailor, S.P. (2013) Prediction of 305 days first lactation milk yield from fortnightly test day and part yields. *Indian. J. Anim. Sci.,* 83(2): 166-169.
8. Sturges, H.A. (1926) The choice of a class interval. *J. Am. Stat. Assoc.,* 21(153): 65-66.
9. Indian Standard, IS: 1224 (Part I). (1977) Determination of Fat by Gerber Method. Part I. Milk (First Revision). Indian Standard Institution, Manak Bhavan, New Delhi.
10. Harvey, W.R. (1990) User's Guide for LSMLMW, Mixed Model Least-Squares and Maximum Likelihood Computer Programme. Ohio State University, Columbus, Mimeo.
11. Becker, W.A. (1975) Manual of Quantitative Genetics. 3rd ed. Washington State University, Washington, USA.
12. Swiger, L.A., Harvey, W.R., Everson, D.O. and Gregory, K.E. (1964) The variance of interclass correlation involving group with one observation. *Biometrics,* 20: 818-826.
13. Ibrahim, M.A., Khattab, A.S., Habaeib, S.E., Awad, S. and Tızser, J. (2012) Genetic parameters for buffalo milk yield and milk quality traits using animal model. *AWETH,* 8(2): 175-182.
14. Tonhati, H., Ceron, M.F., Oliveira, J.A.M. and El Faro, L. (2008) Test-day milk yield as a selection criterion for dairy buffaloes (*Bubalus bubalis Artiodactyla, Bovidae*). *Genet. Mol. Biol.,* 31: 674-679.
15. Singh, A., Basu, S.B. and Bathia, K.L. (1979) Milk fat and SNF percentages of Murrah buffaloes. *Indian J. Anim. Sci.,* 32: 446-449.
16. Shah, S.K. and Schermerhorn, E.C. (1983) Factors affecting milk fat percent of Nili-Ravi buffaloes in Pakistan. *J. Dairy Sci.,* 66: 573-577.
17. Mourad, A.K., Mohamed, M.M. and Khattab, A.S. (1991) Genetic parameters for milk production traits in a closed herd of Egyptian buffaloes. *Egypt. J. Anim. Prod.,* 28: 11-20.
18. Khan, M.S., Hassan, F.U., Saif-ur-Rehman, M., Hyder, A.U. and Bajwa, I.R. (2007) Genetic control of milk yield from lactations of different duration in Nili-Ravi buffaloes. *Arch. Tierz. Dummerstorf.,* 50(3): 227-239.
19. Hatwar, R.K. (1986) M.Sc. Thesis, NDRI, Kurukshetra University, Kamal, India.
20. Madad, M., Hossein-Zadeh, N.G., Shadparvar, A.A. and Kianzad, D. (2013) Random regression models to estimate genetic parameters for test-day milk yield and composition in Iranian buffaloes. *Arch. Tierz. Dummerstorf.,* 56(27): 276-284.
21. Aspilcueta-Borquis, R.R., Araujo Neto, F.R., Baldi, F., Bignardi, A.B., Albuquerque, L.G. and Tonhati, H. (2010) Genetic parameters for buffalo milk yield and milk quality traits using Bayesian. *J. Dairy Sci.,* 93: 2195-2201.
22. Sahoo, S.K., Singh, A., Gupta, A.K., Chakravarty, A.K., Singh, M. and Ambhore, G.S. (2014) Estimates of genetic parameters of weekly test day milk yields and first lactation 305 day milk yield in Murrah buffaloes. *Vet. World,* 7(12): 1094-1098.

27

Optimization of dry period in Karan Fries cow

K. Puhle Japheth[1], R. K. Mehla[1], Mahendra Singh[2], A. K. Gupta[3], Ramendra Das[3], Pranay Bharti[1] and T. Chandrasekar[1]

1. Division of Livestock Production Management, ICAR-National Dairy Research Institute, Karnal - 132 001, Haryana, India; 2. Division of Dairy Cattle Physiology, ICAR-National Dairy Research Institute, Karnal - 132 001, Haryana, India; 3. Division of Dairy Cattle Breeding, ICAR-National Dairy Research Institute, Karnal - 132 001, Haryana, India.
Corresponding author: K. Puhle Japheth, e-mail: puhleveto7@gmail.com,
RKM: mehla1954@gmail.com, MS: chhokar.ms@gmail.com, AKG: guptaak2009@gmail.com,
RD: ramenvets@gmail.com, PB: dr12pranay@gmail.com, TC: chandrulpm1986@gmail.com

Abstract

Aim: The objective of this study was to optimize dry period (DP) length that can maximize the production across adjacent lactations and overall lifetime yield.

Materials and Methods: Performance records with respect to DP spread over a period of 15-year in Karan Fries (KF) cattle maintained at Livestock Research Centre (National Dairy Research Institute), were collected for the study. Data of 681 KF cows were analyzed by least square technique to examine the effect of non-genetic factors on DP. Season of calving was classified into four seasons: Winter season (December-March), summer season (April-June), rainy season (July-September), and autumn season (October-November); period of calving into five periods: 1998-2000 (1-period), 2001-2003 (II-period), 2004-2006 (III-period), 2007-2009 (IV-period), and 2010-2012 (V-period), and parity into six parities, i.e., 1st, 2nd, 3rd, 4th, 5th, and >6th parities to see the effect of non-genetic factors on DP.

Results: Period of calving, season of calving, and parity did not affect the DP significantly ($p < 0.05$). The overall least square mean of DP was 67.93±2.12 days. For the optimization of DP with regard to milk productivity, analysis was carried out by class interval method. DP was classified into eight classes (<22, 23-45, 46-67, 68-89, 90-111, 112-133, 134-155, and >156 days), and optimum level was obtained at 46-67 days (3rd class) with the following respective milk yield (MY) of 305 daily MY (4016.44±43.68 kg), total MY (4704.21±61.51 kg), MY per day of lactation length (13.03±0.13 kg), and MY per day of calving interval (11.68±0.41 kg).

Conclusion: From the study, it was concluded that this optimal DP length (46-67 days) is suitable for maximizing the production. Hence, one should aim to dry off pregnant cows to achieve a DP of appropriate length to enhance productivity in the next lactation, as very short and very long DP reduces the economic profitability in dairy animals.

Keywords: dry period, economic trait, Karan Fries cow, non-genetic factors, optimization.

Introduction

The economic survey 2011 analyzed the dairy situation in India, considering that the requirement of milk in 2021-2022 is expected to be 180 million tons as against the current level of milk production of 127.3 million tons [1]. Dairy managers aim to dry off pregnant cows to achieve a dry period (DP) of appropriate length to maximize productivity in the next lactation [2]. A DP of 60 days is considered as ideal [3]. DP <30 days (in US Holstein cow) are detrimental to lifetime yield and should be avoided [4]. The fetus completes almost two-thirds of its growth during the last 2 months of gestation. This fetal growth takes priority over the cow's own needs for body tissue maintenance. The rumen papilla and microflora must adapt to the change from an energy dense lactating ration to one that meets basic maintenance requirements, and then prepare again during the transition period to adjust back to the lactating ration.

So, this is a period of anatomical and physiological challenging time for the cow and her udder [5]. It is a time of nutritional, metabolic, and mammary change that will profoundly impact health and productivity in the next lactation. Another principle factor for causing the variation in milk yield (MY) and calving interval (CI) is DP thus, influencing the efficiency of MY in dairy cow. A reasonable length of DP is necessary because this period provides time to regain the energy lost during the previous lactation and to regenerate the secretory cells of animal for next lactation. Despite many remarkable performances, there is a wide range of variability in the range of DP of Karan Fries (KF) cattle that hampered the productive as well as reproductive performance of the cows.

Therefore, the study was conducted with the objective to find out the optimum level of DP in a narrower range which would be considered as optimum so as to improve milk production not only in the particular lactation but also in the overall performance of the animal by enhancing genetic gain.

Materials and Methods

Ethical approval

The present study was carried out after getting approval by the Research Committee and Institutional Animal Ethic Committee of National Dairy Research Institute.

Experimental site

The study was conducted at the National Dairy Research Institute (NDRI), Karnal, India. The farm is located at an altitude of 245 m above the sea level, in the Indo-Gangetic alluvial plains at 29° 42'N and latitude 72° 54' E longitude. The climate of this region is subtropical in nature with temperature ranging between 2°C in winter and 45°C in summer. The area receives an annual rainfall of 760-960 mm mostly during July and August with relative humidity ranging from 41% to 85%. Thus, it is obvious the cattle maintained at NDRI farm were exposed to extreme climate conditions due wide range of meteorological variation.

Housing management

The KF cattle in the farm were kept under loose housing system. The open paddocks are brick on edge flooring system with large space available to provide adequate exercises. The pregnant cows were transferred to the maternal pen 2 weeks before the actual date of calving. Pregnant cows were provided single pen with ample space 12 m² × 12 m² for covered and opened area (Bureau of Indian Standards standard), proper ventilation, and drainage system. During summer season, cows were provided with provision of fan and water sprinklers to mitigate heat stress.

Feeding and other management

The nutritional requirement of KF cattle was met through both roughages and concentrate. The farm practices *ad libitum* feeding thrice a day (i.e. morning, afternoon, and evening) with good quality green fodder throughout the year such as berseem, lucern, cowpea, maize, jowar, bajra, and wheat. Silage and hay were also used during the lean season. Concentrate was provided to the cows as per their milk production at the time of milking (i.e. morning, afternoon, and evening). The cows accessed to *ad libitum* fresh drinking water day and night.

Both hand milking and machine milking were practice in the farm. Milking is done thrice a day, i.e. early morning, afternoon, and evening. The average MY in a lactation and MY per day were 4677.84±50.35 kg and 12.93±0.99 kg, respectively [6]. All the sanitary care and measure were taken before, during, and after milking. All types of veterinary aids, prophylactic, and sanitary measures were taken care.

Collection of data

The data of production traits of 681 KF cow were collected and utilized for the study from the period of 1998 to 2012 (15 years). The record of cows with abnormal calvings such as premature calving, abortion, and shorter lactation length (LL) was omitted in the study. The lactation records of 250 days and above were considered as normal and included in the study to see the effects of season of calving, period of calving, and parity on the DP. The data were classified and coded according to different seasons: Winter season (December-March), summer season (April-June), rainy season (July-September), and autumn season (October-November). For period of calving, it was classified into five periods: 1998-2000 (I-period), 2001-2003 (II-period), 2004-2006 (III-period), 2007-2009 (IV-period), and 2010-2012 (V-period). Finally for parities, the data are classified into six classes: 1st, 2nd, 3rd, 4th, 5th, and >6th (parities six and above were combined due to lesser animal number of observation) to observe the effect of non-genetic factors on DP.

Statistical analysis

The data were subjected to least-squares technique [7] to see the effects of season of calving, period of calving, and parity on DP. Duncan's multiple range test was used to test the significance of differences between treatments' means. The least squares analysis model is given as:

$$Y_{ijkl} = \mu + S_i + P_j + A_k + e_{ijkl}$$

Where,

Y_{ijkl}=Dependent trait (DP) of Ith cow born in i^{th} season, j^{th} period, and k^{th} parity,

μ=Overall mean,

S_i=Effect of ith season of calving (i=1-4),

P_j=Effect of jth period of calving (j=1-5),

A_k=Effect of kth parity (k=1-6),

e_{ijkl}=Random error, NID with zero and constant variance $(0, \sigma_e^2)$.

Optimization of DP

For optimization of DP with regard to milk productivity, the various DP lengths were classified into eight (1-8) classes (Table-1). Class interval for DP was calculated with the help of Sturges formula.

$$C = R/1 + 3.322 \log 10N$$

Where,

C=Width of class/class interval,

N=Number of observations,

R=Range (maximum-minimum),

1+3.322 log10N=Number of classes.

The average MYof different classes of the DP was studied using least squares analysis. The model used is given below:

$$Y_{ij} = \mu + C_i + e_{ij}$$

Where,

Y_{ij}= j^{th} observation of ith class of DP,

C_i= Effect of ith class of DP,

I = 1, 2., 8 class of DP,

e_{ij}= Random error, assumed to be normally and independently distributed with mean zero and constant variance, i.e. NID (0, σe2).

Results

Effect of non-genetic factors on DP

In the study, the overall least squares means of DP was 67.93±2.12 days (Table-2). It was observed that season of calving, period of calving, and parity had no statistically significant effect on the DP. The longest DP was observed in those cows which calved during autumn season (70.03±2.67 days), whereas, the shortest DP was observed in rainy season (66.42±2.38 days). For the period of calving, the longest DP was observed in the III-period (71.32±2.11 days), whereas shortest average mean of DP was observed in I-period (62.46±2.96 days). In case of parity, there is no much variation in the average mean DP length across the different lactations.

Optimization of DP

DP was divided into eight different classes by the use class interval method (Table-1a and b). The last two classes (i.e., 8th and 9th class) had been combined due to lesser numbers of animal observations. The average means of 305 days or less MY (305 daily MY [DMY]), total MY (TMY), MY per day of LL (MY/LL), and MY per day of CI (MY/CI) for each class of DP were estimated and presented (Table-1a and b).

DP and 305 days or less MY and TMY

The estimated averages of 305 days or less MY and TMY for each class of DP were presented (Table-1a). The maximum 305 DMY (4171.07±209.16 kg) and TMY (5268.21±294.53 kg) were observed in the 7th class (134-155 days). More than majority of the number of animal observations (60.94%) was observed in 3rd class (46-67 days), while minimum numbers of animal observations are falls in

1st and 8th class, respectively with the same number of animal observations (2.86%) each. There is no significant effect of DP on 305 days or less MY and TMY.

DP and MY/LL

The average MY/LL for each class of DP was estimated and presented (Table-1b). The animal group in the 3rd class (46-67 days) showed the highest MY/LL (13.03±0.13 kg), whereas those animals in the 8th class (134-155 days) revealed the least MY/LL (10.83±0.63 kg). Maximum number of animal observation (60.94%) was observed in 3rd class (46-67 days), whereas minimum number of animal observation (2.86%) was found in 1st and 8th class, respectively (<22 and >156 days).

DP and MY/CI

The averages of MY/CI for each class of DP were estimated and presented (Table-1b). The maximum MY/CI (11.72±1.11 kg) was observed in 2nd class (23-45 days), whereas minimum MY/CI (8.99±1.86 kg) was found in 6th class (112-133 days). The majority number of animal observations (60.94%) was in 3rd class group (46-67 days), whereas the minimum number of animals (2.86%) observation was fall in 1st class and 8th class group (<22 and >156 days). There was a significant effect of DP on MY/LL and MY/CI.

Discussion

From the study, the overall least squares means of DP was 67.93±2.12 days (Table-2), which was in agreement with Singh and Tomar [8], Singh [9], who also reported similar observation in KF cattle. Higher average DP was also reported by Nayak and

Table-1a: Average 305 DMY and TMY (kg) for different classes of DP in KF cow.

Class of DP (days)	Number of observation	Percentage of animals	Cumulative (%)	Average 305 DMY (kg)	Average TMY (kg)
<22	28	2.86	2.86	4037.0±201.55	4705.34±283.82
23-45	84	8.58	11.44	4050.25±116.36	4686.48±163.86
46-67	596	60.94	72.38	4016.44±43.68	4704.21±61.51
68-89	114	11.65	84.03	3879.8±99.89	4497.0±140.66
90-111	72	7.36	91.39	3833.98±125.69	4391.97±176.99
112-133	30	3.06	94.45	3939.77±194.72	4788.77±274.19
134-155	26	2.65	97.10	4171.07±209.16	5268.21±294.53
>156	28	2.86	100	3489.79±201.55	4319.0±283.82

DP=Dry period, KF=Karan Fries, TMY=Total milk yield, DMY=Daily milk yield

Table-1b: Average MY/LL and MY/CI (kg) for different classes of DP in KF cow.

Class of DP (in days)	Number of observation	Percentage of animals	Cumulative (%)	MY/LL (kg)*	MY/CI (kg)*
<22	28	2.86	2.86	11.79±0.63^{abc}	12.93±1.93^{b}
23-45	84	8.58	11.44	12.98±0.36^{bc}	11.72±1.11^{ab}
46-67	596	60.94	72.38	13.03±0.13^{c}	11.68±0.41^{b}
68-89	114	11.65	84.03	12.12±0.31^{ab}	10.02±0.95^{ab}
90-111	72	7.36	91.39	11.86±0.39^{a}	9.30±1.20^{ab}
112-133	30	3.06	94.45	11.82±0.61^{abc}	8.99±1.86^{ab}
134-155	26	2.65	97.10	12.23±0.65^{abc}	9.09±2.00^{ab}
>156	28	2.86	100	10.83±0.63^{a}	7.45±1.93^{a}

*Significant at 5% level (p<0.05) and the values with different superscripts within a column differ significantly. DP=Dry period, KF=Karan Fries, MY/LL=Milk yield per day of lactation length, MY/CI=Milk yield per day of calving interval

Table-2: Least square means±SE value and effects of non-genetic factors on DP in KF cow.

Parameters	Number of observation	Average means of dry period (days)
Overall means	965	67.93±2.12
Season of calving		
Winter season	356	67.46±1.99
Summer season	250	67.80±2.18
Rainy season	205	66.42±2.38
Autumn season	154	70.03±2.67
Period of calving		
I-period	136	62.46±2.96
II-period	207	68.03±2.38
III-period	240	71.32±2.11
IV-period	272	67.63±2.11
V-period	110	70.20±3.08
Parity		
1st lactation	405	65.31±1.61
2nd lactation	247	69.93±1.97
3rd lactation	147	65.74±2.55
4th lactation	83	69.11±3.40
5th lactation	46	69.10±4.58
6th and above lactation	37	68.37±5.07

SE=Standard error, DP=Dry period, KF=Karan Fries

Raheja [10], Singh *et al.* [11] in various HF cross with Zebu cows. It was observed that season of calving, period of calving, and parity had no significant effect on the DP. Similar results are also reported by Singh and Tomar [8], Singh [9] in HF crossbred. However, significant effects of the period of calving are reported by Thalkari *et al.* [12] and Javed *et al.* [13] in HF crossbred and indigenous cows. Furthermore, researchers such as Javed *et al.* [13,14] reported a significant effect of season of calving on DP in HF crossed with indigenous cows. The non-significant effect of parity on DP was reported by Rehman *et al.* [15] in indigenous cattle and Gatchearle *et al.* [16] in HF crossed with Deoni cattle. On the other hand, significant effects of parity on DP are reported in Friesian crossbred [17].

The rate of change of milk production in relations to change in length of DP shows that there was increase in milk production with increase in DP length till 3rd class and then shows a slight decrease in the subsequent classes. Season of calving and lactation number did not influence on 305 DMY, TMY, MY/LL, and MY/CI as reported by Nehra and Divya *et al.* [18,19] while there was report of the significant effect of period of calving on 305 DMY in KF cattle [20]. However, various important factors (i.e., calving year, calving season, age groups, and parity) affect not only TMY but also the rate of milk production throughout the length of lactation [21]. The average mean of DP length for different parities was almost more or less the same.

Conclusion

From the study, it was concluded that the production performance was better in the animal group which falls under the 3rd class (46-67 days) with more than majority numbers of animal observations (60.94%).

As in economical point of view, too short DP are not favorable, as it does not give proper rest to regain cows body condition for next lactation. However, very lengthy DP is also not profitable as it shortens the LL. Since DP is a crucial stage in the lactation cycle of a dairy cow, therefore, one should aim to dry off pregnant cows to achieve a DP of appropriate length to maximize productivity in the next lactation.

Authors' Contributions

KPJ, RKM, MS, and AKG designed the work. KPJ and RKM conducted the research work. Data analysis and manuscript were written by KPJ with the help of RD, PB, and TC under the guidance of RKM, MS, and AKG. All the authors have read and approved the final manuscript.

Acknowledgment

The authors are highly thankful to the Director of NDRI, Karnal, for providing the necessary facilities. Furthermore, sincere thanks and gratitude are given to Dr. U. S. Narwaria, Shri. Gian Singh, Dr. Ulfina Galmessa and Livestock Record Unit, for their help and support during the research work.

Competing of Interests

The authors declare that they have no competing interests.

References

1. MOA, (Ministry of Agriculture). (2012) The Economic Survey of the Dairy Situation in India. Government of India, Statistical Report.

2. Enevoldesn, C. and Sorensen, J.T. (1991) The effect of dry period length on milk production in the next lactation. *J. Dairy Sci.*, 74: 1277-1283.

3. Dingwell, R.T., Kelton, D.F., Leslie, K.E. and Edge, V.L. (2001) Deciding to dry-off: Does level of production matter? National Mastitis Council Annual Meeting Proceedings. p69-79.

4. Kuhn, M.T., Hutchison, J.L. and Norman, H.D. (2006) Dry period length to maximize production across adjacent lactations and lifetime production. *J. Dairy Sci.*, 89: 1713-1722.

5. Oetzel, G.R. (1998) Nutritional management of dry dairy cows. The compendium on continuing education for practicing veterinarians. *Vet. Learn. Syst.*, 20(3): 391-396.

6. Japheth, K.P., Mehla, R.K., Imtiwati. and Bhat, S.A. (2015) Effect of non-genetic factors on various economic traits in Karan Fries crossbred cattle. *Indian J. Dairy Sci.*, 68(2): 163-169.

7. Harvey, W.R. (1975) Least Squares Analysis of Data with Unequal Subclass Numbers. ARS, USDA, Washington, DC. p2-28.

8. Singh, R. and Tomar, S.S. (1990) Inheritance of first lactation production traits and their inter-relationship in crossbred cattle. *Indian J. Dairy Sci.*, 43(2): 147-151.

9. Singh, M.K. (1995) Factors Affecting Trends in Performance Karan Swiss and Karan Fries cattle. Ph.D. Thesis. National Dairy Research Institute, Karnal, India.

10. Nayak, S.K. and Raheja, K.L. (1996) Performance of half-bred and three breed crosses of Hariana with exotic dairy breeds. *Indian J. Anim. Sci.*, 66(2): 154-158.

11. Singh, A., Gandhi, R.S., Chakarvarty, A.K., Sharma, R.C. and Gurnani, M. (2001) Effect of postpartum breeding interval on milk production and reproduction traits in Karan Fries cattle. *Indian J. Anim. Res.*, 35(2): 83-87.

12. Thalkari, B.T., Biradar, U.S. and Rotte, S.G. (1995) Performance of Holstein Friesian-Deoni and Jersey – Deoni halfbred cattle. *Indian J. Dairy Sci.*, 48(4): 309-310.

13. Javed, K., Mohiuddin, G. and Abdullah, M. (2000) Environmental factors affecting various productive traits in Sahiwal cattle. *Pak. Vet. J.,* 20(4): 187-192.

14. Jadhav, K.L., Tripathi, V.N. and Kale, M.M. (1991) Performance of crossbred cows for production and reproduction traits in different production level groups. *Indian J. Dairy Sci.,* 45(11): 620-622.

15. Rehman, S.U., Amad, M. and Shafiq, M. (2008) Comparative performance of Sahiwal cows at the livestock experiment station Bahadurnagar, Okara vs Patadar's herd. *Pak. Vet. J.,* 26: 179-183.

16. Gatchearle, P.L., Mitkari, K.R., Mule, R.S., Baswade, S.V. and Bhadekar, S.V. (2010) Effects of season of calving and parity on dry period and inter-calving period in inter- se progeny of HF X Deoni. *Vet. World,* 3(2): 85-87.

17. Ogundipe, R.I., Adeoye, A.A. and Muritala, I. (2011) Effect of genetic and non-genetic factors on the diary production traits of Friesian, Wadara and their crossbreds. *Adv. Agric. Biotechnol.,* 1: 43-48.

18. Nehra, M. (2011) Genetic Analysis of Performance Trends in Karan Fries Cattle. M.V.Sc. Thesis. National Dairy Research Institute, Karnal, India.

19. Divya, P., Singh, A. and Alex, R. (2014) Standardization of voluntary waiting period and evaluation of production and reproduction traits in Karan Fries cows. *Haryana Vet.,* 53(2): 113-116.

20. Kokate, L.S. (2009) Genetic Evaluation of Karan Fries Sires Based on Test Day Milk Yield Records. M.V.Sc., Thesis. National Dairy Research Institute, Karnal, India.

21. Dongre, V.B., Gandhi R.S., Singh, A. and Gupta, A. (2011) A brief review on lactation curve models for predicting milk yield and different factors affecting lactation curve in dairy cattle. *Int. J. Agric.,* 1(1): 6-15.

28

Ultrastructural study on the granulocytes of Uttara fowl (*Gallus domesticus*)

Khan Idrees Mohd, Meena Mrigesh, Balwinder Singh and Ishwar Singh

Department of Veterinary Anatomy, College of Veterinary & Animal Sciences, G.B. Pant University of Agriculture and Technology, Pantnagar, Uttarakhand, India.
Corresponding author: Meena Mrigesh, e-mail: meenamrigesh@gmail.com,
KIM: idrees413@gmail.com, BS: dhot_balwinder@yahoo.co.in, IS: singh_iswar@yahoo.co.in

Abstract

Aim: The present study was conducted to know the ultrastructural detail of the blood cells of Uttara fowl (native fowl of Uttarakhand).

Materials and Methods: The experiment was conducted on 10 apparently healthy adult birds of either sex reared at the Instructional Poultry Farm, G.B. Pant University of Agriculture and Technology, Pantnagar, Uttarakhand. The blood was collected from wing vein using ethylenediamine tetraacetic acid as anticoagulant. The blood was further processed for scanning and transmission electron microscopic (TEM) studies separately.

Results: Ultrastructurally, the heterophils were irregularly round in shape. The cytoplasm was laden with pleomorphic membrane-bound granules, *viz.*, large elliptical-, medium oval-, large round-, and medium round-shaped granules. The eosinophils under TEM were irregularly circular in outline showing pseudopodia and finger-like cytoplasmic processes. The cytoplasmic granules were pleomorphic with elliptical-, round-, and rod-shaped granules. The basophils were irregularly circular in outline containing small hook-like cytoplasmic processes. The cytoplasm contained electron dense and electron lucent round-shaped granules.

Conclusion: Granulocytes contained pleomorphic cytoplasmic granules. However, the shape and electron density of granules varied among the different granulocytes and helped in the characterization of different granulocytes.

Keywords: blood cells, cytoplasmic granules, ultrastructure, Uttara fowl.

Introduction

India has emerged as the third largest egg producer and fifth largest poultry meat producer in the world. The total chicken population has registered an annual growth of 7.3% in the last decade. Farm chicken grows at 12.4%, whereas Desi chicken showed much lower growth rate of about 2% [1]. Backyard poultry farming has over the years contributed to a great extent to the agrarian economy of India. An important part of the poultry meat and eggs consumed in the country comes from these small-scale producers. Backyard poultry farming offers a great scope and has immense potentials in hills of Uttarakhand. The indigenous hill fowl is the backbone of the backyard poultry farming in hills. The Uttara fowl (local hill fowl) is said to be descended from the Red Jungle fowl. Most of the hill fowls are unique in their adaptation to the agro-climatic conditions of their habitat [2].

The mammalian analog of neutrophil in the bird is called heterophil. These are the first line of defense in the body and play an indispensable role in the immune defense of the avian host. To accomplish this defense, heterophils use sophisticated mechanisms such as phagocytosis, degranulation, and oxidative burst to destroy pathogenic microbes [3]. Their cytoplasmic granules contain several lysosomal and non-lysosomal enzymes including acid phosphatase, arylsulfatase, β-glucuronidase, phosphorylase, neutral and acid α-glucosidases, acid trimetaphosphatase, and lysozyme [4].

Keeping in view, the use of granules in the defense function of the cells, the present study was undertaken to study the general ultrastructural details of the granules present in different granulocytes. Although the reports on granulocyte ultrastructure in other birds such as guinea fowl, ostrich, and painted stork are available. However, the reports on ultrastructural features of granulocyte cells in Uttara fowl are not available. Keeping it in view the above facts, the present study was conducted using scanning electron microscope (SEM) and transmission electron microscope (TEM).

Materials and Methods

Ethical approval

The experimental plan of the study was duly approved by the Animal Ethics Committee G. B. Pant University of Agriculture and Technology (GBPUAT), Pantnagar, Uttarakhand, India.

Resource population

The study was conducted on 10 adults apparently healthy Uttara fowl of either sex reared at instructional poultry farm, College of Veterinary and Animal Sciences, GBPUAT, Pantnagar.

Sample processing

TEM

The blood samples from the bird were collected in 5 ml syringe using ethylenediamine tetraacetic acid (EDTA) as anticoagulant, transferred into siliconized centrifuge tubes and spun at 3000 rpm for 45 min. The plasma was drained off and the buffy coat was fixed for 5 h at 5°C in the standard fixative (5% glutaraldehyde in 0.1 M phosphate buffer, pH 7.4). The fixative was gently removed. Fragile buffy coat disc was carefully removed with the help of a sharp pointed scalpel. After removal, the disc was put in a petridish containing phosphate buffered saline (pH 7.4). The disc was cut into several blocks of about 1-2 mm size. The blocks were washed three times with 0.1 M phosphate buffer (pH 7.4) for 15 min each. The blocks were again fixed at room temperature for 1 h using 1% osmium tetraoxide.

The blocks were dehydrated using graded alcohol. They were then placed into two changes of 100% toluene for 5 min each, before being transferred to a mixture of equal parts of araldite and toluene for overnight at room temperature. Impregnation was carried out in the fresh changes of araldite and continued for 2 days at room temperature. The blocks were finally embedded in another change of fresh araldite and polymerized for 3 days at room temperature.

The thin sections (60-70 nm) were cut on an ultramicrotome and placed on copper grids. The sections were stained in a saturated solution of uranyl acetate in 50% alcohol for 15 min, followed by lead citrate for 15 min and examined under TEM (JEOL JEM-1011) operated at 60-80 KV at TEM laboratory facility at GBPUAT, Pantnagar.

SEM

Samples of venous blood from the birds were collected from the wing vein in 5 ml syringe using EDTA as anticoagulant. Few drops of blood were transferred into siliconized centrifuge tubes, equal amount of 5% glutaraldehyde was added and the blood was fixed for 1 h. The mix was spun at 3000 rpm for 30 min. The plasma was decanted and buffy coat was taken out in another tube. The blood cells were washed three times with 0.1 M phosphate buffer solution (pH 7.4) by centrifuging at 2000 rpm for 2 min. These samples of fixed cells were processed in SEM laboratory facility, GBPUAT, Pantnagar. There the cells were resuspended in distilled water and repeated washings were performed. The film of the blood cells was made on a clean circular glass coverslip. The blood film was coated with gold sputter coating using JFC-1600 Auto Fine Coater and observed under JEOL JSM-6610 LV SEM.

Results

TEM

Heterophils

Ultrastructurally, the heterophils were irregularly round in shape. The nucleus was bilobed or trilobed. The nuclear lobes contained more amount of heterochromatin than euchromatin. The euchromatin occupied a major central portion of the nucleus, whereas heterochromatin was distributed mainly toward periphery in the form of large and small patches (Figure-1). The cytoplasm was laden with membrane-bound cytoplasmic granules showing pleomorphism (Figure-2). The cytoplasmic granules varied greatly in shape, size, and density. The largest granules were electron dense and elliptical in shape, measuring 0.4-1.6 μm in length. The second types of granules were medium electron dense and oval in shape measuring 0.6-0.8 μm in

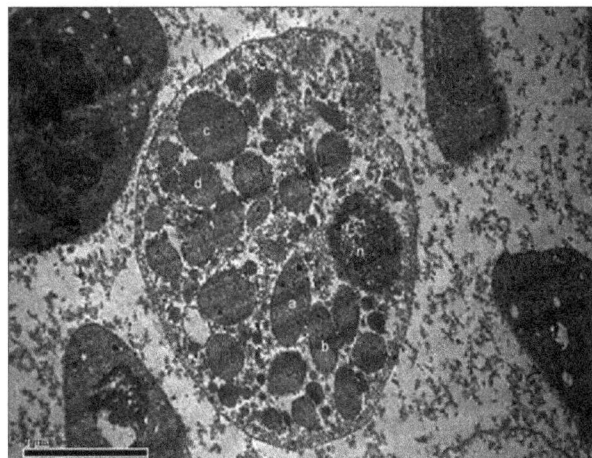

Figure-1: Transmission electron photomicrograph showing heterophil with large electron dense elliptical granule (a), medium electron dense oval granule (b), large electron dense round granule (c), medium electron dense round granule (d) and nucleus (n). Uranyl acetate and lead citrate ×19,900.

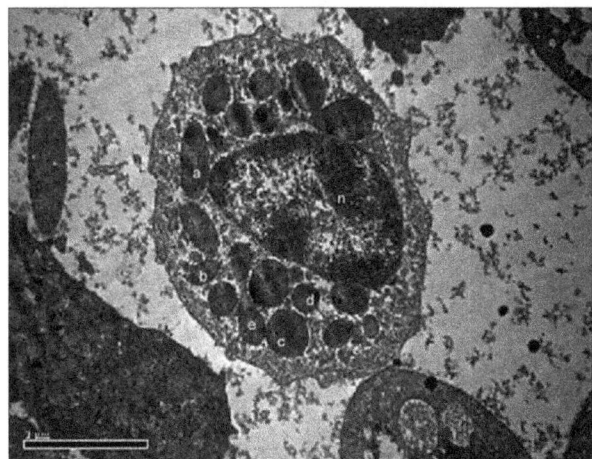

Figure-2: Transmission electron photomicrograph showing heterophil with large electron dense elliptical granule (a), medium electron dense oval granule (b), large electron dense round granule (c), medium electron dense round granule (d), dumbbell-shaped granule (e) and nucleus (n). Uranyl acetate and lead citrate ×19,900.

length. The third types of granules were large electron dense and round in shape. Fourth types of granules were medium electron dense and round in shape. In few heterophils, electron dense dumbbell-shaped granule was also seen and that may be due to fusion of two oval granules. The Golgi apparatus, mitochondria, and endoplasmic reticulum were seen in the cytoplasm. Mitochondria were oval to round in shape. Few vacuoles were observed at periphery which contained phagocytized material inside.

Eosinophils

The eosinophils under TEM were irregularly circular in outline showing pseudopodia and finger-like cytoplasmic processes. The nucleus was usually bilobed (Figure-3). There was a distinct nuclear membrane. The heterochromatin was concentrated toward the periphery in the form of large and small patches. The euchromatin was centralized. The cytoplasmic granules were distributed throughout the cytoplasm and varied greatly in shape and size. The first types of granules were electron dense and elliptical in shape. The second types of granules were large electron dense and round in shape. The third types of granules were medium electron dense and round in shape. The fourth types of granules were small electron dense and round in appearance (Figure-4). In few eosinophils, long rod-shaped electron dense granule was visible.

Basophils

The basophils were irregularly circular in outline containing small hook-like cytoplasmic processes (Figure-5). The majority of basophils contained a single, non-lobulated, eccentrically placed, indented nucleus. The nuclear membrane was distinct. The heterochromatin was distributed toward the periphery as well as in the center in the form of small and large patches. The cytoplasm was laden with cytoplasmic granules showing pleomorphism. Most of the cytoplasmic granules were electron dense and round in shape. Few granules were electron lucent showing a loose honeycomb-like stippling in the interior (Figure-6). The other cell organelles observed in the cytoplasm were mitochondria, Golgi apparatus, vesicles, and smooth as well as rough endoplasmic reticulum. Few small vacuoles were also seen toward the periphery of the cytoplasm. Few loop-like cytoplasmic processes were observed toward the nuclear end of the cell.

SEM

In the present study, four types of leukocytes were observed under SEM. First types of leukocytes were small in size and showed blunt, irregularly round mushroom type outgrowth on their surface. These types of leukocytes also had a varying number of microvilli on their surface (Figure-7). The second types of leukocytes were medium in size having irregularly round mulberry-like surface outgrowths (Figure-8). The third types of leukocytes were large

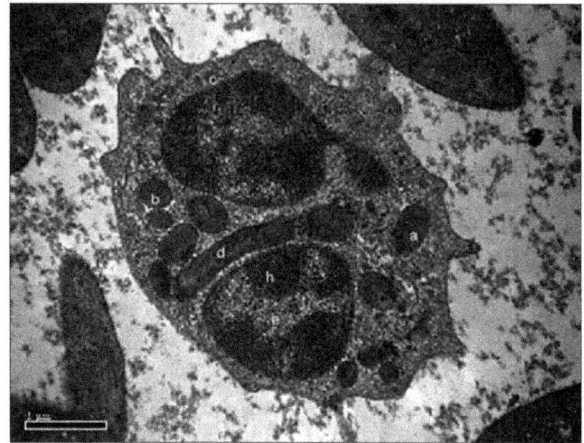

Figure-3: Transmission electron photomicrograph showing eosinophil with large electron dense elliptical granule (a), medium electron dense round granule (b), small electron dense round granule (c), long electron dense rod-shaped granule (d), euchromatin (e) and heterochromatin (h). Uranyl acetate and lead citrate ×26,500.

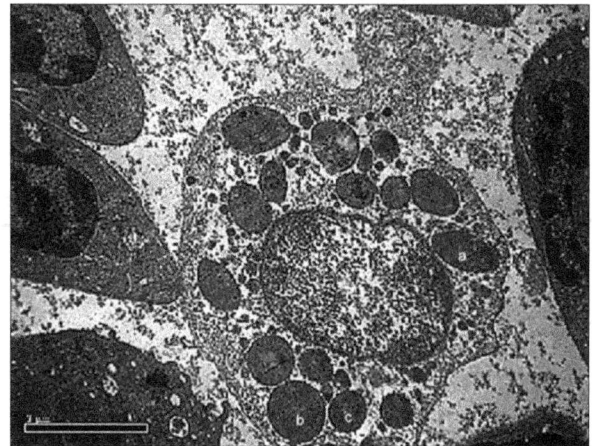

Figure-4: Transmission electron photomicrograph showing eosinophil with large electron dense elliptical granule (a), large electron dense round granule (b), medium electron dense round granule (c), small electron dense round-shaped granule (d) and nucleus (n). Uranyl acetate and lead citrate ×19,900.

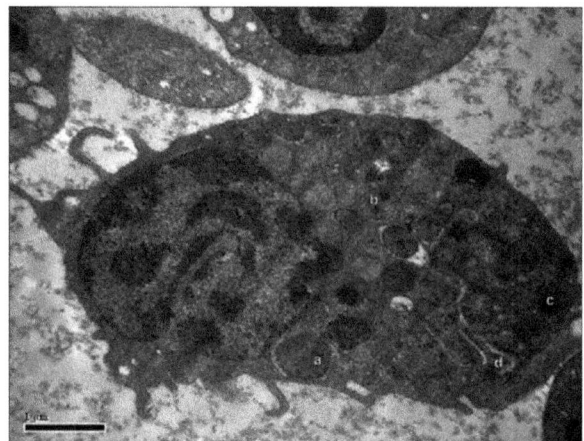

Figure-5: Transmission electron photomicrograph of basophil showing large electron dense round granule (a), round honeycomb-like granule (b), small electron dense round granule (c), and cytoplasmic process (cp). Uranyl acetate and lead citrate ×26,500.

in size and showed cauliflower-like appearance. Their cell surface showed narrow ridge-like profiles

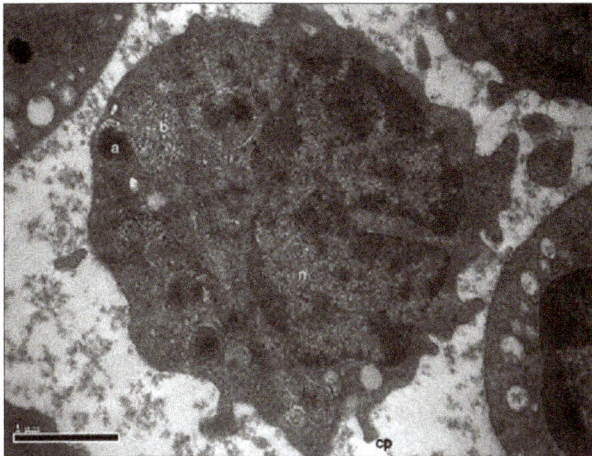

Figure-6: Transmission electron photomicrograph of basophil showing electron-dense round granule (a), electron lucent round honeycomb-like granule (b), cytoplasmic process (cp) and nucleus (n). Uranyl acetate and lead citrate ×33,200.

and small ruffles (Figure-9). The fourth types of leukocytes were also large with more prominent, membrane-like ruffles (Figure-10).

Discussion

The nucleus of the heterophil in the Uttar fowl was multilobulated in appearance. The euchromatin was distributed in the central portion of the nucleus and heterochromatin toward periphery in the form of patches. Heterophils with lobulated nucleus with heterochromatin distributed in the periphery were reported in ostrich [5]. Lobulated nuclei with 2-5 lobes [6] were reported in pig neutrophils in which the heterochromatin occupied a major peripheral portion of the nuclear lobes, whereas the euchromatin was comparatively less and centrally located in the form of patches. The cytoplasmic granules of pleomorphic nature in the Uttara fowl were in collaboration with the findings in painted storks [7] in which numerous membrane-bound pleomorphic granules were seen in the cytoplasm of the heterophil. In place of four types of granules observed in Uttara fowl heterophil,

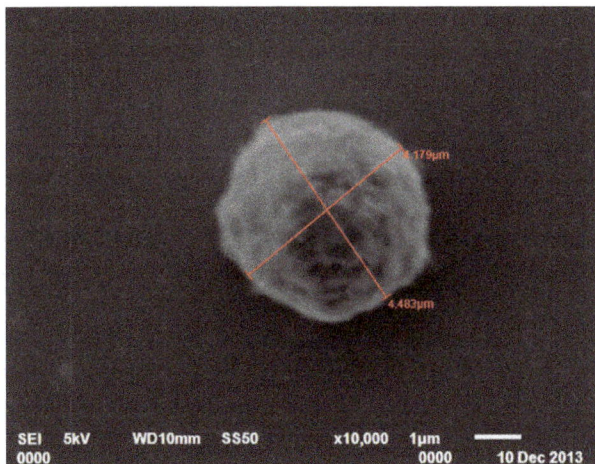

Figure-7: Scanning electron photomicrograph of blood cells showing small leukocyte with mushroom-like appearance ×10,000.

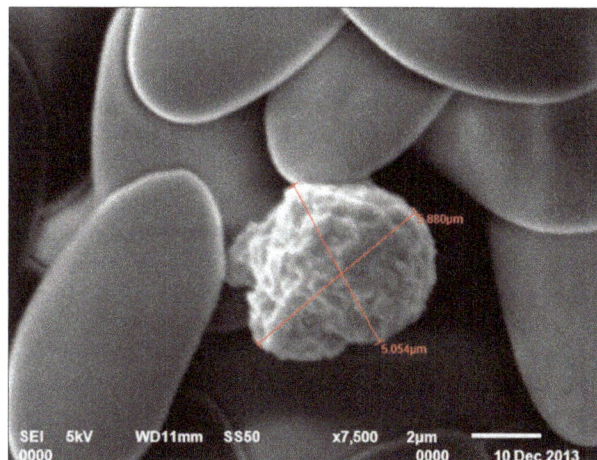

Figure-9: Scanning electron photomicrograph of blood cells showing large leukocyte with cauliflower-like appearance ×7500.

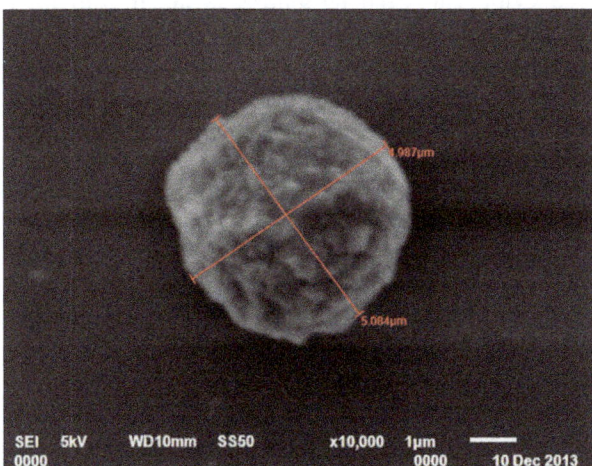

Figure-8: Scanning electron photomicrograph of blood cells showing medium leukocyte with mulberry-like appearance ×10,000.

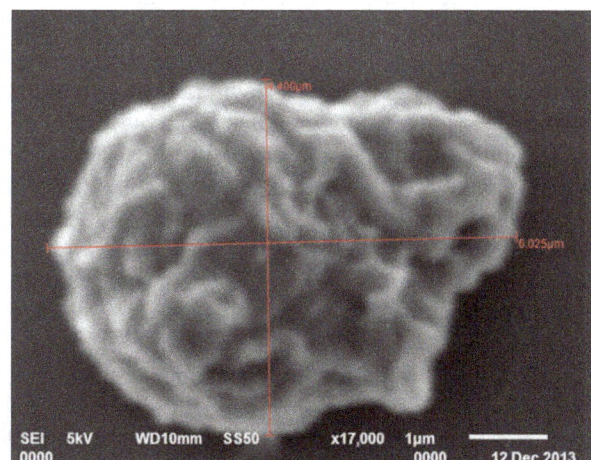

Figure-10: Scanning electron photomicrograph of blood cells showing large leukocyte with membrane-like ruffles ×17,000.

three types of granules were reported in chicken [8], pigeon [9], and aves [10]. There were only two types of granules reported in ostrich heterophil [5]. Type I granules were fusiform with different size and Type II were smaller with varied electron density. Reports also suggested [11] large elliptical-shaped electron dense cytoplasmic granules in Kadaknath fowl. Slightly different findings of granules in avian heterophils were reported [12]. Their primary granules appeared electron-dense fusiform rods (1.5 μm × 0.5 μm), secondary granules (diameter, 0.5 μm) were less dense containing eccentric inclusions, and tertiary granules (0.1 μm) had a dense core that was separated from a membranous envelope of an electron-lucent area. However, the primary granules were almost similar in size to elliptical-shaped granules of the present study. In few heterophils, electron dense dumbbell-shaped granule was also seen, that may be due to fusion of two oval granules. The Golgi apparatus, mitochondria, and endoplasmic reticulum were seen in the cytoplasm. Mitochondria were oval to round in shape. Few vacuoles were observed at periphery which contained phagocytized material inside. However, in Kadaknath fowl [11], vesicles were observed.

The eosinophils contained usually bilobed nucleus with central euchromatin and peripheral heterochromatin arrangement. Similar observations of the bilobed nucleus with similar chromatin pattern [11] were reported in eosinophil of Kadaknath fowl. The eosinophils contained lobed nuclei in painted storks [7]. The eosinophils appeared round to oval shaped with long and narrow cytoplasmic processes in the horse [13]. The cytoplasmic granules were distributed throughout the cytoplasm and were pleomorphic in appearance in the Uttara fowl. These findings were somewhat similar to the findings of duck eosinophil in which round, oval, or elongated granules were observed but the findings were slightly different from goose (oval and round granules), quail (oval and round granules), fantail and homing pigeon (dense large round, less dense round and round granule with empty area within), and turkey (large irregular-shaped granules) eosinophils [14]. The round-shaped eosinophilic granule characteristics were similar as in guinea fowl [15] and in painted storks [7]. Rod-shaped granules along with spherical granules were also observed in birds [10]. The reports suggested that granules in fowl eosinophils were round to oval in shape, but some granules had appearance of vacuoles [16].

The majority of basophils contained a single, non-lobulated, eccentrically placed, indented nucleus. Similarly, the basophils with single non-lobulated nucleus were found in the duck, goose, and turkey [9]. Most of the basophilic cytoplasmic granules of Uttara fowl were electron dense and round in shape. However, few granules were electron lucent showing a loose honeycomb-like stippling in the interior. The basophils contained four types of

double membrane-bound cytoplasmic granules in guinea fowl [15]. Electron dense oval or elongated granules were reported in the Kadaknath fowl [11]. The membrane-bound pleomorphic cytoplasmic granules were reported in painted stork [7] and sheep [17]. In pig basophils, the cytoplasmic granules were comparatively less when compared with neutrophils and eosinophils [6]. The cell organelles observed under TEM in the cytoplasm of basophil in the Uttara fowl were mitochondria, Golgi apparatus, vesicles, and smooth as well as rough endoplasmic reticulum. The cell organelles such as mitochondria, very small empty vesicles, scarce, and poorly developed endoplasmic reticulum were observed in the basophil of domestic fowl [16]. Reports suggest the presence of mitochondria and ribosomes in painted stork [7].

In the present study, four types of leukocytes were observed under SEM. These types of leukocytes had varying number of microvilli on their surface. The leukocytes with microvillus on the surface were also reported [18] in guinea fowl. Four types of leukocytes were also observed in Kadaknath fowl [19] but with different surface morphology as compared to present findings of Uttara fowl. In our findings, cells had different cellular processes such as blunt, irregularly round, mushroom type; mulberry type; cauliflower type, and membrane-ruffled type. However, in Kadaknath fowl, the leukocytes with only coarse wafer-like processes and mushroom-like processes on the surface were observed. In the present study, the leukocytes cannot be conclusively divided into granulocytes and agranulocytes. However in chicken [20], the cells, with ridge-like profiles having membrane ruffles, were considered as polymorphonuclear leukocytes and cells with more prominent membrane ruffles as monocytes.

Conclusions

Ultrastructurally, the heterophils were irregularly round in shape. The nucleus was bilobed or trilobed. The cytoplasm of heterophil was laden with pleomorphic membrane-bound granules. The cytoplasmic granules varied greatly in size and shape, viz., large elliptical-, medium oval-, large round-, and medium round-shaped granules. The eosinophils under TEM were irregularly circular in outline showing pseudopodia and finger-like cytoplasmic processes. The cytoplasmic granules of eosinophils showed pleomorphism with elliptical-, round-, and rod-shaped granules. The basophils were irregularly circular in outline containing small hook-like cytoplasmic processes. The majority of basophils contained a single, non-lobulated, eccentrically placed, indented nucleus. Most of the cytoplasmic granules were electron dense and round in shape. Few granules were electron lucent showing a loose honeycomb-like stippling in the interior. The SEM revealed four different types of leukocytes in the blood.

Authors' Contributions

MKI carried out this study and wrote this manuscript. MM planned, guided, and helped in interpreting and finalizing the results in this research work. BS helped in the processing of samples in this study. IS guided in the interpretation of electron microscopic photomicrographs. All authors have read and approved the final version of the manuscript.

Acknowledgments

The authors are thankful to Indian council of agricultural research, ICAR-PUSA (New Delhi) for providing the necessary financial assistantship. Help extended by the staff of Electron microscopic laboratory, Pantnagar is greatly acknowledged.

Competing Interests

The authors declare that they have no competing interests.

References

1. Planning Commission of India. (2012) Report of the Working Group on Animal Husbandry and Dairying 12th Five Year Plan, (2012-17). Government of India.

2. Kaur, N., Kumar, S., Singh, B., Pandey, A.K. and Somvanshi, S.P. (2010) Morphological characterization of feathered shank local hill fowl of Central Himalayan Region of India. *Indian J. Anim. Sci.*, 80(9): 934-936.

3. Genovese, K.J., He, H., Swaggetry, C.L. and Kogut, M.H. (2013) The avian heterophil. *Dev. Comp. Immunol.*, 41(3): 334-340.

4. Maxwell, M.H. and Robertson, G.W. (1998) The avian heterophil leucocyte: A review. *World's Poult. Sci. J.*, 54(2): 155-178.

5. Bonadiman, S.F., Stratievsky, G.C., Machado, J.A., Albernaz, A.P., Rabelo, G.R. and DaMatta, R.A. (2009) Leukocyte ultrastructure, hematological and serum biochemical profiles of ostriches (*Struthiocamelus*). *Poult. Sci.*, 88(11): 2298-2306.

6. Mehta, S., Singh, I. and Mrigesh, M. (2012) Transmission electron microscopic characterization of granulocytes of pig (*Susscrofa*). *Indian J. Anim. Sci.*, 82: 48.

7. Salakij, C., Salakij, J., Narkkong, N., Pitakkingthong, D. and Poothong, S. (2003) Hematology, morphology, cytochemistry and ultrastructure of blood cells in painted stork (*Mycteria leucocephala*). *Kasetsart J. (Nat. Sci.)*, 37: 506-513.

8. Daimon, T. and Caxton-Martin, A.E. (1977) Electron microscopic and enzyme cytochemical studies on granules of mature chicken granular leukocytes. *J. Anat.*, 123(3): 553-562.

9. Maxwell, M.H. (1973) Comparison of heterophil and basophil ultrastructure in six species of domestic birds. *J. Anat.*, 115(2): 187-202.

10. Dieterein Lievre, F. (1988) Birds. In: Rewley, A.F. and Rat Cliff, N.A., editors. Vertebrate Blood Cells. Cambridge University Press, Cambridge, UK. p257-336.

11. Yadav, G.C. (2011) Light and ultrastructural studies on the blood cells of Kadaknath fowl. M.V.Sc. Thesis, GBPUAT, Pantnagar.

12. Thrall, M.A., Baker, D.C., Campbell, T.W., Fettman, M.J., Lassen, E.D., Rebar, A., Weiser, G. and DeNicola, D. (2004) Hematology of Birds. Veterinary Hematology and Clinical Chemistry. Lippincott Williams and Willkins, A Wolters Kluwer Company, Philadelphia, USA, p529-553.

13. Mehta, S., Guha, K., Dhote, B.S., Shalini, S. and Kumar, C. (2014) Transmission electron microscopic studies on agranulocytes and granulocytes of horse (*Equuscaballus*). *Indian J. Vet. Anat.*, 26(1): 43-46.

14. Maxwell, M.H. and Siller, W.G. (1972) The ultrastructural characteristics of the eosinophil granules in six species of domestic bird. *J. Anat.*, 112(2): 289-303.

15. Gupta, V. and Singh, I. (2008) Transmission electron microscopic studies on the granular leucocytes of guinea fowl (*Numidameleagris*). *Indian J. Anim. Sci.*, 78(11): 1265-1267.

16. Maxwell, M.H. and Trezo, F. (1970) The ultrastructure of white blood cells and thrombocytes of the domestic fowl. *Br. Vet. J.*, 126: 583-592.

17. Kumar, A., Singh, I. and Mrigesh, M. (2012) Ultrastructural studies on the blood cells of sheep. *Vet. Pract.*, 13(2): 209-212.

18. Gupta, V. and Singh, I. (2008) Scanning and transmission electron microscopic studies of the agranulocytes of guinea fowl (*Numidameleagris*). *J. Immunol. Immunopathol.*, 10(2): 107-109.

19. Yadav, G.C., Singh, I. and Mrigesh, M. (2013) Scanning electron microscopic studies on blood cells of Kadaknath fowl. *Indian J. Poult. Sci.*, 48(1): 82-84.

20. Burkhardt, E. (1979) Scanning electron microscopy of peripheral blood leukocyte of the chicken. *J. Cell Tissue Res.*, 204: 147-153.

29

Influence of season and sex on hemato-biochemical traits in adult turkeys under arid tropical environment

Anil Gattani[1], Arti Pathak[2], Ajeet Kumar[1], Vaibhav Mishra[2] and Jitendra Singh Bhatia[2]

1. Department of Veterinary Biochemistry, Bihar Veterinary College, Patna, Bihar, India; 2. Department of Veterinary Physiology & Biochemistry, Apollo College of Veterinary Medicine, Jaipur, Rajasthan, India.
Corresponding author: Anil Gattani, e-mail: gattanianil@gmail.com,
AP: vaibhavmisradr@rediffmail.com, AK: ajeet18@gmail.com, VM: vaibhavmisradr@rediffmail.com,
JSB: bhatiajs05@rediffmail.com

Abstract

Aim: The objective of this study was to evaluate the effect of season and sex on hemato-biochemical parameters of turkey (*Meleagris gallopavo*) in the arid tropical environment.

Materials and Methods: The experiment was conducted on 20-week old turkeys consisting of 20 males and 20 females. Blood was collected from all turkeys during January and May. Hemoglobin (Hb), red blood cell (RBC), packed cell volume (PCV), mean corpuscular volume (MCV), mean corpuscular hemoglobin (MCH), and mean corpuscular hemoglobin concentration (MCHC) were estimated in whole blood and glucose, protein, albumin, globulin, A/G ratio, calcium, phosphorus, alanine aminotransferase (ALT), and aspartate aminotransferase (AST) in serum.

Result: Season has significant (p<0.05) effect on Hb concentration, RBC, and PCV in both male and female. Male has significantly higher (p<0.05) Hb concentration, RBC, and PCV. There is no significant effect of sex, and season was observed on MCV, MCH, and MCHC. Glucose, protein, albumin, globulin, and A/G ratio were significantly (p<0.05) affected by season and sex. AST and ALT were significantly (p<0.05) affected by season in both sexes. There is no significant difference was recorded on calcium, phosphorus due to season and sex.

Conclusion: Under arid tropical environment, turkey hemato-biochemical parameters are influenced by both sex and season.

Keywords: alanine aminotransferase, aspartate aminotransferase, season, sex, turkey.

Introduction

Turkey (*Meleagris gallopavo*) is a prized avian species reared all over the world for their tasty and high-quality meat besides, its link with celebrations of "Christmas" and "Thanksgiving celebrations" in the western world [1]. It originates from North America and has now been introduced nearly worldwide including India. The production of this poultry species is gaining momentum as a new agricultural activity for the commercial production of meat in India as a source of animal protein due to its comparatively high percentage of protein and low percentage of fat [2-4]. In general, blood examination is considered most dependable indicator of health status. Blood biochemical profile such as glucose, calcium, total protein, aspartate aminotransferase (AST), alanine aminotransferase (ALT), urea, and chloride levels are of diagnostic values for various disease conditions and having particular reference to liver disorders, kidney diseases, diarrhea, dehydration, etc. [5]. Enzyme activity can be useful in selecting males to improve fertility and or hatchability of females in chicken.

The information on these is useful for diagnostic and management purposes which could further be incorporated into breeding programs for genetic improvement of turkeys. Values for the hematology and serum biochemical characters for turkey have been reported elsewhere [6,7], but literature is still incomplete with respect to variability of these parameters in the different climatic seasons, especially in the semi-arid region of India. Thus, to generate baseline data, the present study was planned. This will help in furtherance of research on breed improvement programs at geo-climatic conditions of this tract.

Therefore, the present study was undertaken to evaluate the effect of sex and season on the hematology and serum biochemical profile of turkey in the arid tropical environment.

Materials and Methods

Ethical approval

The prior approval from the Institutional Animal Ethics Committee (Apollo College of Veterinary Medicine, Jaipur) was obtained for use of animal in this study.

Experimental animals

The present experiment was conducted at Poultry complex, Apollo College of Veterinary Medicine,

Jaipur, from January to May 2011 on 20 weeks old Beltsville small white turkey. During the experiment, in January 2011, average temperature was 6.8°C (1.4-13.8) and mean humidity was 54.6%, and in May 2011, average temperature was 34.4° (39.6-13.9) and mean humidity was 27.4%. A total of 40 adult turkeys (20 males and 20 females) were selected for this study. The turkeys were housed in a floor pen and were fed standard chicken layer ration supplied by Godrej agrovet. Feed and water provided *ad lib*. Deworming of birds was done regularly.

Collection and analysis of blood samples

Blood samples were collected aseptically two times in summer and winter season from the superficial ulnar vein of all 40 turkeys in EDTA containing vial for hematological study. Hematological study was performed within 24 h after blood collection. Hemoglobin (Hb) was estimated using drabkin's solution (Span diagnostic, India); red blood cell (RBC) using Neubauer chamber; other erythrocytes indices such as mean corpuscular volume (MCV), mean corpuscular hemoglobin (MCH), and mean corpuscular hemoglobin concentration (MCHC) were estimated using the standard formulae. Blood samples were also collected for separation of serum and stored at −20° for further use. These serum samples were used for biochemical studies. The enzymatic estimations were done within 24 h of collection. The serum biochemical parameters including serum glucose, protein, albumin, globulin, A/G ratio, calcium, phosphorus, ALT, and AST were estimated using kits (Span diagnostic, India).

Statistical analysis

All the data were expressed as mean±standard error (SE) values. The data were subjected to statistical analysis by Paired Sample t-test using SPSS version 17 according to Snedecor and Cochran [8].

Results

The results of the hemato-biochemical parameters of turkey in different season and sex are summarized as mean±SE in Table-1.

Hematological profile

The erythrocytic profile is represented in Table-1. Hb in male was 11.97±0.25 and 10.88±0.25 during winter and summer season, respectively, whereas in the female, it was 11.43±0.36 and 10.09±0.22 in both the seasons. Hb is significantly (p<0.05) affected by the season in both the sexes. Significant (p<0.05) effect of sex and season was observed on packed cell volume (PCV) and RBC. Significantly (p<0.05) lower PCV values were observed in female (38.85±0.65 and 32.65±0.70), in both winter and summer seasons, than male (40.95±0.78 and 34.55±0.54). However, both male and female have significantly (p<0.05) higher value during the winter season than summer. Similarly, RBC is significantly (p<0.05) higher in male (2.97±0.15 and 2.64±0.07) than female

(2.55±0.10 and 2.33±0.08), in winter and summer season, respectively. MCV and MCH were marginally higher during the winter season in both sexes. Further female has higher MCV and MCH than its male counterpart. MCHC was slightly higher during the summer season in male (31.60±0.70) and female (31.16±0.89) than winter season (29.42±0.79 and 29.55±1.03), respectively.

Biochemical profile

Male has significantly (p<0.05) higher glucose level in comparison to female. In the winter season, the level of glucose was significantly (p<0.05) higher both in male (251±12.19) and female (219.49±8.45) than that of summer season (220.42±8.92 and 193.53±7.34, respectively). Total protein concentration was significantly (p<0.05) higher in female during winter and summer season (5.45±0.16 and 4.25±0.25) than their male counterpart (4.12±0.15 and 3.42±0.09). Further, both in male and female the total protein level is significantly (p<0.05) higher in the winter season. Albumin concentration in serum was significantly (p<0.05) influenced by the season both in male and female. Female had significantly (p<0.05) high concentration (1.62±0.04 and 1.45±0.04) of albumin than male (1.45±0.03 and 1.31±0.04) in winter and summer season, respectively. Significantly (p<0.05) high globulin concentration was observed in female during both the summer and winter season (3.83±0.17 and 2.79±0.25) than male (2.66±0.15 and 2.10±0.08). Furthermore, in winter season, globulin was significantly (p<0.05) higher than summer season in both sexes. The climatic season had a significant (p<0.05) effect on A/G ratio in female. Further, male (0.58±0.03) has significantly (p<0.05) high value than female (0.44±0.03) only in winter season. ALT and AST enzyme was studied in the present study, and both have the similar trend in respect to season. In the summer season, the activity of ALT and AST was significantly (p<0.05) increased. In male, ALT activity was 15.47±1.67 and 32.07±1.86 during winter and summer season, respectively, whereas in the female, it was 14.45±1.86 and 29.84±2.32. Similarly, the AST activity was 309.22±7.95 and 348.35±9.20 in male and 282.99±15.64 and 333.52±8.39 in female during winter and summer season, respectively.

The serum concentration of Ca is non-significantly higher in the summer season. Further, female has non-significantly higher concentration (7.85±0.39 and 8.46±0.22) than male (7.82±0.28 and 8.04±0.20) during winter and summer season. A reverse trend was observed for phosphorus concentration in serum. Male has non-significantly high phosphorus (5.31±0.33 and 4.82±0.28) than female (4.74±0.28 and 4.66±0.24) in their blood during winter and summer season, respectively.

Discussion

Hematological and serums' biochemical parameters can provide importance information for animal's

Table-1: Effect of season and sex on hemato-biochemical profile in Turkey (mean±SE).

Hemato-biochemical attributes	Sex	Season	
		Winter	Summer
Hemoglobin (g/dl)	Male (20)	11.97[B]±0.25	10.88[bA]±0.25
	Female (20)	11.43[B]±0.36	10.09[aA]±0.22
PCV (%)	Male (20)	40.95[bB]±0.78	34.55[bA]±0.54
	Female (20)	38.85[aB]±0.65	32.65[aA]±0.70
RBC (millions/mm³ of blood)	Male (20)	2.97[bB]±0.15	2.65[bA]±0.07
	Female (20)	2.55[aB]±0.10	2.33[aA]±0.08
MCV (fl/cell)	Male (20)	144.35±7.52	131.88±3.91
	Female (20)	157.44±7.27	141.76±4.48
MCH (pg/cell)	Male (20)	42.57±2.64	41.67±1.46
	Female (20)	45.86±2.02	43.88±1.44
MCHC (g%)	Male (20)	29.42±0.79	31.60±0.70
	Female (20)	29.55±1.03	31.16±0.89
Glucose (mg/dl)	Male (20)	251.61[bB]±12.19	220.42[bA]±8.9
	Female (20)	219.49[aB]±8.45	193.53[aA]±7.34
Total protein (g/dl)	Male (20)	4.12[aB]±0.15	3.42[aA]±0.09
	Female (20)	5.45[bB]±0.16	4.25[bA]±0.25
Albumin (g/dl)	Male (20)	1.45[aB]±0.03	1.31[aA]±0.04
	Female (20)	1.62[bB]±0.04	1.45[bA]±0.04
Globulin (g/dl)	Male (20)	2.66[aB]±0.15	2.10[aA]±0.08
	Female (20)	3.83[bB]±0.17	2.79[bA]±0.25
A/G ratio	Male (20)	0.58[b]±0.03	0.64±0.03
	Female (20)	0.44[aA]±0.03	0.59[B]±0.04
ALT (IU/L)	Male (20)	14.45[A]±1.86	32.07[B]±1.86
	Female (20)	15.47[A]±1.67	29.84[B]±2.32
AST (IU/L)	Male (20)	309.22[A]±7.95	348.35[B]±9.20
	Female (20)	282.99[A]±15.64	333.52[B]±8.39
Ca (mg/dl)	Male (20)	7.82±0.28	8.04±0.20
	Female (20)	7.85±0.39	8.46±0.22
P (mg/dl)	Male (20)	5.31±0.33	4.82±0.28
	Female (20)	4.74±0.28	4.66±0.24

Superscripts (A, B) indicate significant difference ($p<0.05$) row wise. Different superscripts (a, b) indicate significant difference ($p<0.05$) column wise. SE=Standard error, PCV=Packed cell volume, RBC=Red blood cell, MCV=Mean corpuscular volume, MCH=Mean corpuscular hemoglobin, MCHC=Mean corpuscular hemoglobin concentration, ALT=Alanine aminotransferase, AST=Aspartate aminotransferase

immune status and beside of diagnostic and management purposes, can be used for developing new strains that are genetically resistant to poultry diseases as well as for genetic improvement programs [9].

Hematological traits

The erythrocytic profile in the present study is in the range reported by other workers in different part of the globe [10,11]. Higher values of Hb, PCV, and RBC observed during winter months in both male and female turkey is in accord with finding in Nigerian ducks [12]. The variation in the environment temperature and photoperiod is considered as the most important factor that affects the erythrocyte count, Hb, and hematocrit values. A decline in environmental temperature resulted in significant alterations of the circulatory system. This might be due to low ambient temperature result in high oxygen demand by the body, low partial pressure of oxygen in the blood (hypoxemia), and higher metabolic rate (favors high feed intake), which stimulate erythropoiesis thereby producing higher hematological values in winter [13,14]. During summer, high ambient temperature increases body temperature, respiration and respiratory water loss and oxygen consumption of birds. The increased oxygen intake increases the partial pressure of oxygen

in the blood of birds [15] leading to decreased erythropoiesis and consequently, reducing the number of circulating erythrocyte [16].

MCV, MCH, and MCHC did not show any statistical differences between seasons, whereas numerically lower values were obtained during summer season might be due to in changes in blood volume and blood viscosity [17]. Female turkeys show lower Hb, PCV, and TEC in comparison to male, might be due high estrogen concentration [17-19].

Biochemical traits

The lowered blood glucose in female due to estradiol effect which decreases the expression of gluconeogenic genes in the liver [20,21]. Protein concentrations in the present study are in the reference range as reported elsewhere [20]. The higher protein concentration in females could be explained by the high level of estrogen hormones in females responsible of the high content of serum globulins [22]. The decrease in serum albumin during the summer season may be due to reduced protein consumption and consequently decreased supply of essential amino acids from feed, accompanied with reduced protein digestibility because exposure of broilers to high environmental temperature [23,24]. The mean activity of ALT and AST is in accordance with the other researchers [6,7,20]. The increased values of enzyme activity during summer season may be attributed to the greater influence of thermal stress [25].

Non-significant higher calcium level in female might be result of estrogen response [26,27]. Non-significant variation in serum phosphorus levels between sex can be attributed to hormonal influence and breeding activity [27]. Factors such as breed, dietary calcium source, housing system, and interaction between them affected the serum inorganic phosphorus values [28].

Conclusion

The hemato-biochemical values of adult turkeys were determined under arid tropical environment for studying the effect of season and sex. The result found that season had a significant effect on Hb, RBC, PCV, glucose, protein, albumin, globulin, A/G ratio, ALT, and AST. The sex and season have no significant effect on MCV, MCH, MCHC, Ca, and P. The effect of season and sex should, therefore, be considered when interpreting the parameters to ensure accuracy and to avoid undesirable sources of variation and thus misjudgment for hemato-biochemical parameters under tropical environment.

Authors' Contributions

JSB and AG designed the experiment. AG, AP, and VM conducted the experiment. AG and AK did technical writing and revision of the manuscript. All authors have read and approved the final version of the manuscript.

Acknowledgments

The authors are highly thankful to Dean of Apollo College of Veterinary Medicine, Jaipur, for providing the necessary grant to carry out the experiment.

Competing Interests

The authors declare that they have no competing interests.

References

1. Anna Anandh, M., Richard Jagatheesan, P.N., Senthil Kumar, P., Paramasivam, A. and Rajarajan, G. (2012) Effect of rearing systems on reproductive performance of Turkey. *Vet. World*, 5(4): 226-229.
2. Thornton, E.K., Emery, K.F., Steadman, D.W., Speller, C., Matheny, R. and Yang, D. (2012) Earliest Mexican Turkeys (*Meleagris gallopavo*) in the Maya region: Implications for pre-hispanic animal trade and the timing of Turkey Domestication. *PLoS ONE*, 7(8): e42630.
3. Hamza, H.M., Al-Mayali, Hind, A. and Kadhim, A. (2015) Ectoparasites of domestic Turkey (Meleagris gallopavo) in Al-Diwaniya City/Iraq. *Int. J. Curr. Microbiol. Appl. Sci.*, 4(10): 669-677.
4. Marchewka, J., Watanabe, T.T.N., Ferrante, V. and Estevez, I. (2013) Review of the social and environmental factors affecting the behavior and welfare of Turkeys (*Meleagris gallopavo*). *Poult. Sci.*, 92(6): 1467-1473.
5. Akporhuarho, P.O. (2011) Effect of crude oil polluted water on the haematology of cockerel reared under intensive system. *Int. J. Poult. Sci.*, 10(4): 287-289.
6. Patra, B., Das, S.K., Mishra, P.K., Mishra, S.K. and Panda, N. (2008) Evaluation of physio-biochemical traits of growing turkeys in hot and humid climate of Orissa. *Indian J. Anim. Sci.*, 78: 203-206.
7. Ibrahim, A.A., Aliyu, J., Abdu, M.I. and Hassan, A.M. (2012) Effects of age and sex on serum biochemistry values of Turkeys (*Meleagris gallopavo*) reared in the semi-arid environment of Nigeria. *World Appl. Sci. J.*, 16: 433-436.
8. Snedecor, G.W. and Cochran, W.G. (1980) Statistical Methods. 7th ed. Oxford and IBH Publishing Co., Calcutta.
9. Abdi-Hachesoo, B., Talebi, A., Asri-Rezaei, S. and Basaki, M. (2013) Sex related differences in biochemical and hematological parameters of adult indigenous chickens in Northwest of Iran. *J. Anim. Sci. Adv.*, 3(10): 512-516.
10. Strakova, E., Suchy, P., Kabelova, R., Vitula, F. and Herzig, I. (2010) Values of selected haematological indicators in six species of feathered game bird. *Acta Vet. Brno.*, 79: S3-S8.
11. Pandian, C., Pandiyan, M.T., Sundaresan, A. and Omprakash, A.V. (2012) Haematological profile and erythrocyte indices in different breeds of poultry. *Int. J. Livest. Res.*, 2: 89-92.
12. Olayemi, F.O. and Arowolo, R.O.A. (2000) Seasonal variation in the haematological values of the Nigerian Duck. *Int. J. Poult. Sci.*, 8: 813-815.
13. Blahová, J., Dobšíková, R., Straková, E. and Suchý, P. (2007) Effect of low environmental temperature on performance and blood system in broiler chickens (*Gallus domesticus*). *Acta Vet.*, 76: S17-S23.
14. Cetin, N., Bekyurek, T. and Cetin, E. (2009) Effects of sex, pregnancy and season on some haematological and biochemical blood values in Angora Rabbits. *Scand. J. Lab. Anim. Sci.*, 36: 155-162.
15. Brackenbury, J.H., Avery, P. and Glesson, M. (1981) Respiration in exercising Fowl. Oxygen consumption, respiratory rates and respired gases. *J. Exp. Biol.*, 93: 317-325.
16. Donkoh, A. (1989) Ambient temperature: A factor affecting performance and physiological response of broiler chickens. *Int. J. Biometeorol.*, 33: 259-265.
17. Priya, M. and Gomathy, V.S. (2008) Haematological and blood biochemicals in male and female turkeys of different age groups. *Tamil Nadu J. Vet. Anim. Sci.*, 4: 60-68.
18. Oyewale, J.O. and Ajibade, H.A. (1990) Osmotic fragility in two groups of Turkey. *Vet. Arch.*, 60: 43-48.
19. Nirmalan, G.P. and Robinson, G.A. (1972) Haematology of the japanese quail treated with exogenous stilbesterol dipropionate and testosterone propionate. *Poult. Sci.*, 51: 920-925.
20. Bounous, D.I., Wyatt, R.D., Gibbs, P.S., Kilburn, J.V. and Quist, C.F. (2000) Normal hematologic and serum biochemical reference intervals for juvenile wild Turkeys. *J. Wildl. Dis.*, 36: 393-396.
21. Kim, J.Y., Jo, K.J., Kim, O.S., Kim, B.J., Kang, D.W., Lee, K.H., Baik, H.W., Han, M.S. and Lee, S.K. (2010) Parenteral 17-beta-estradiol decreases fasting blood glucose levels in non-obese mice with short-term ovariectomy. *Life Sci.*, 87: 358-366.
22. Sturkie, P.D. and Newman, H.J. (1951) Plasma proteins of chickens as influenced by time of laying, ovulation, number of blood samples taken, and plasma volume. *Poult. Sci.*, 30: 240-243.
23. Khan, W.A., Khan, A., Anjum, A.D. and Rehman, Z. (2002) Effects of induced heat stress on some biochemical values in broiler chicks. *Int. J. Agric. Biol.*, 4: 74-75.
24. Bonnet, S., Geraert, P.A., Lessire, M., Carre, B. and Guillaumin, S. (1997) Effect of high ambient temperature on feed digestibility in broilers. *Poult. Sci.*, 76: 857-863.
25. Naqvi, S.M.K., Hooda, O.K. and Saxena, P. (1991) Some

plasma enzymes of sheep under thermal, nutritional and exercise stress. *Indian Vet. J.*, 68: 1045-1047.

26. Flora, P. and Ranjini, J. (2000) Effect of temperature and photoperiod on serum calcium, phosphorus, alkaline phosphatase and certain haematological parameters in Turkey (*Meleagris gallapovao*) during winter and summer seasons at Chennai (Tamil Nadu State). *Indian J. Poult. Sci.*, 35: 198-201.

27. Dacke, C.G., Musacchia, X.J., Volkert, W.A. and Kenny, A.D. (1973) Cyclical fluctuations in levels of blood calcium, pH and pCO_2 in japaneese quails. *Comp. Biochem. Physiol. A.*, 44: 1267-1275.

28. Radwan, A.A., El-Aggoury, S.A., Gado, M.S. and El-Gendi, G.M. (1989) In: Proceeding of 3rd Egypt Brit. Conference on Animal, Fish and Poultry Production. 7-10 October, 1989. Alexand, Egypt. p859-868.

30

Effect of extended photoperiod during winter on growth and onset of puberty in Murrah buffalo heifers

Ashwani Kumar Roy, Mahendra Singh, Parveen Kumar and B. S. Bharath Kumar

Division of Dairy Cattle Physiology, National Dairy Research Institute, Karnal, Haryana, India.
Corresponding author: Ashwani Kumar Roy, e-mail: royashwani@gmail.com,
MS: chhokar.ms@gmail.com, PK: drpk1959@gmail.com, BSBK: bharath.kumar.vet@gmail.com

Abstract

Aim: To investigate the effect of extended photoperiod on growth rate, hormonal levels, and puberty in Murrah heifers.

Materials and Methods: About 14 Murrah buffalo heifers were divided into normal day photoperiod (NDP; n=7) and extended NDP (ENDP; n=7) groups. The ENDP group was exposed to 4 h of extended photoperiod with artificial light (160 lux) after sunset for 3 months during winter.

Results: Group, age and group-by-age interaction effects on plasma glucose concentrations were non-significant (p>0.05). A significant effect of age on non-esterified fatty acids (p<0.05), cholesterol (p<0.01), and triglycerides (p<0.05) concentrations was observed. Group and group-by-age interaction effects on plasma T_3, T_4, leptin, 17 β estradiol, prolactin and melatonin concentrations were non-significant (p>0.05) while significant (p<0.05) age effect on T_4, leptin and melatonin concentrations was observed. With respect to the circadian pattern of melatonin and prolactin, the group, time and group-by-time interaction effects were non-significant (p>0.05). Average daily gain and dry matter intake of heifers were non-significant between the NDP and ENDP groups but were comparatively higher in ENDP group. By the end of the experiment, 6 out of 7 heifers attained puberty in ENDP group in comparison to 4 out of 7 in NDP group.

Conclusion: Extending the photoperiod by artificial light for 4 h during winter season resulted in better growth rate and early onset of puberty in Murrah buffalo heifers.

Keywords: buffalo, leptin, melatonin, metabolites, photoperiod, prolactin, puberty.

Introduction

Buffaloes are the major source of milk production, and they contribute significantly to the economy of many countries in Southeast Asia [1]. More than 50% of the world population of 148 million buffaloes is reared in India. Late maturity, silent heat coupled with poor expression of estrus, irregular estrous cycle, seasonality in breeding, anoestrus, low conception rate, long postpartum interval, and repeat breeding are the well-known drawbacks leading to low productivity in this species [2-4]. Pubertal development involves physical, behavioral, and hormonal changes that are linked to the activation of the hypothalamic-adenohypophyseal-gonadal axis [5].

Management of photoperiod influences the attainment of puberty and prolactin secretion in beef heifers housed in an outdoor environment [6]. Onset of puberty in cattle is largely influenced by feed intake, quality of feed, and body weight (BW) gain [7]. Recent research has demonstrated that feeding replacement heifers to traditional target BW increased development costs without improving reproduction or subsequent calf production relative to development systems in which heifers were developed to lighter target BW ranging from 50% to 57% of mature BW [8,9]. Murrah buffaloes attain puberty between the ages of 33.1 and 36.5 months [10], whereas indigenous breeds such as Haryana, Kankrej and Sahiwal, reared under same management and environmental conditions, attain puberty at 24.6 months [11]. Feed efficiency improves by 9% in crossbred beef heifers by extending the photoperiod during winter [12]. Strong and clear estrous, increased progesterone, estradiol-17 β, and declined plasma melatonin in buffalo heifers exposed to 4 h of artificial light have been reported during autumn and winter seasons after sunset [13]. No significant changes in eating behavior, daily intake or live weight gain in buffalo heifers subjected to artificial light after sunset for 6 h have been found [14].

Although exposing the heifers to extended photoperiod seemed to be beneficial and economical, there are only a few investigations available in this regard indicating contradictory results. With this perspective, the present study was designed to investigate the effect of extended photoperiod on certain plasma hormones, metabolites, growth and onset of puberty in Murrah buffalo heifers during winter.

Materials and Methods

Ethical approval

The experiment was duly approved by the Institutional Animal Ethical Committee.

Location and methodology

The experiment was conducted between the months of December and February at National Dairy Research Institute, Karnal, India, which is situated at an altitude of 250 m above mean sea level, latitude and longitude position being 29°42"N and 79°54"E, respectively. 14 Murrah buffalo heifers were selected and divided into control (n=7) and treatment (n=7) groups. A control group of heifers were exposed to natural photoperiod of 10.5 h. The treatment group heifers were exposed to 4 h of extended photoperiod with artificial light (160 Lux) after the sunset during the experimental period.

Daily feed intake and feed refusal of both the groups were recorded throughout the experiment. Dry matter intake (DMI) was calculated as the difference between feed intake and refusal. All the animals were reared under same management practices. BWs and blood samples were obtained from all the animals at fortnight intervals. To determine the circadian patterns of melatonin and prolactin hormones, blood samples were collected at an interval of 4 h over a period of 24-h. Immediately after collection, the samples were transported to the laboratory in an ice box, then centrifuged at 3000 rpm for 15 min to obtain plasma which was in different aliquots and stored at −20°C until analyzed for hormones and metabolites.

Plasma glucose was estimated by glucose oxidase-peroxidase method using commercial kits (Avecon Healthcare Pvt. Ltd.). Plasma cholesterol was estimated by cholesterol oxidase-phenol antipyrine (PAP) Trinder's method using commercial kits (Avecon Healthcare Pvt. Ltd.). Plasma triglycerides were estimated by glycerol phosphate oxidase-PAP Trinder's method using commercial kits (Avecon Healthcare Pvt. Ltd.). The copper soap solvent extraction method [15] was adopted for the estimation of plasma non-esterified fatty acids (NEFA). Progesterone (Cayman Chemical Company), estradiol-17 β, leptin, prolactin and melatonin (Cloud-clone Corp.) concentrations were estimated by enzyme immunoassays kits. The intra- and inter-assay

coefficients of variation were <10% for all the hormones. Age at puberty was determined by behavioral signs, plasma progesterone levels [13] and ultrasound examination of the ovaries.

Statistical analysis

Mixed model ANOVA (repeated measures linear model) was conducted to compare the BWs, metabolites, and hormone concentrations between normal day photoperiod (NDP) and extended NDP (ENDP) groups across the time periods. With respect to the circadian pattern of melatonin and prolactin, group, time and group-by-time interaction effects were determined by using mixed model ANOVA. The mean differences in BW, metabolites and hormone concentrations between the NDP and ENDP groups at each fortnight were analyzed by Student's t-test. GraphPad Prism (Version 5) and SPSS (Version 16) software was used to perform the statistical analysis.

Results and Discussion

BWs (Figure-1) and DMI (Figure-2) of heifers did not differ significantly ($p > 0.05$) between short day (NDP) and extended short day photoperiods (ENDP). The mean ± standard error of mean (SEM) glucose concentrations in the short day (NDP) and extended short day photoperiod (ENDP) groups were 76.4±0.98 and 78.4±1.05 mg/dl, respectively (Table-1). There were no effects of group, age and group-by-age interaction on plasma glucose concentrations. The mean NEFA concentrations in NDP and ENDP groups were 136±53.6 and 168±54.6 mM/L, respectively. A significant ($p < 0.05$) effect of age on NEFA concentrations

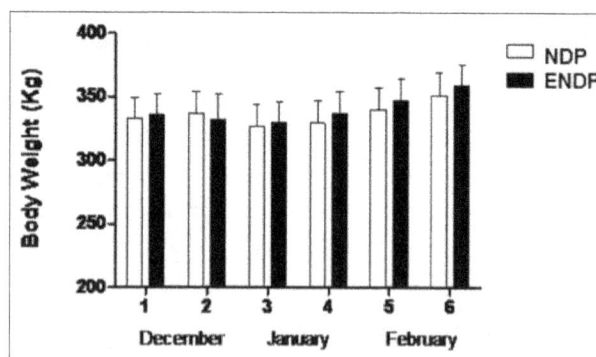

Figure-1: Mean (±standard error) body weight values in normal day photoperiod (NDP) and extended NDP groups.

Table-1: Mean±SE values of different metabolites in NDP and ENDP groups during the experimental period.

Fortnight	Glucose (mg/dl)		NEFA (μm/L)		Cholesterol (mg/dl)		Triglycerides (mg/dl)	
	NDP	ENDP	NDP	ENDP	NDP	ENDP	NDP	ENDP
1	77.2±1.54	75.8±3.21	40.0±16.2	159±128	101±7.19	98.0±5.90	91.0±4.21	74.3±5.40
2	79.41±2.61	80.67±2.97	363±144	413±111	110±13.1	108±6.97	86.3±7.52	84.7±10.1
3	77.26±2.33	81.37±4.59	158±66.7	98.9±41.1	101±5.94	102±7.24	78.6±8.77	70.0±3.90
4	76.71±2.10	76.17±2.63	190±78.3	132±47.9	77.6±3.47	88.9±5.28	87.8±8.60	97.5±5.11
5	75.39±1.60	76.35±2.10	40.3±18.84	186±139	79.7±6.25	76.9±6.10	83.8±4.67	85.0±4.57
6	72.24±1.51	80.20±2.20	24.1±4.25	18.0±8.64	82.5±5.91	87.5±12.5	92.4±4.91	81.0±3.84

NDP=Normal day photoperiod group, ENDP=Extended normal day photoperiod group, NEFA=Non-esterified fatty acids, SE=Standard error

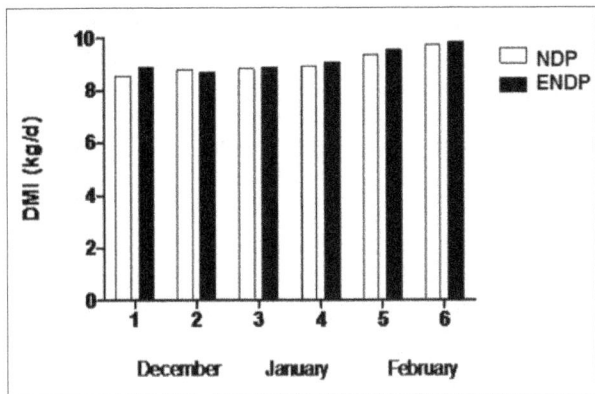

Figure-2: Mean (±standard error) dry matter intake in normal day photoperiod (NDP) and extended NDP groups.

was observed. A similar range of plasma glucose and NEFA was observed in Murrah buffaloes during winter [16]. The mean plasma cholesterol concentrations in NDP and ENDP groups were 92.3±5.75 and 93.8±4.72 mg/dl, respectively. There was significant (p<0.01) effect of age on plasma cholesterol concentrations. Plasma triglycerides concentrations in NDP and ENDP groups were 86.7±2.05 and 82.1±3.92 mg/dl, respectively. Significant (p<0.05) effect of age on triglycerides concentrations was observed.

The mean ± SEM concentrations of plasma T_3, T_4, leptin, 17 β estradiol, prolactin and melatonin in NDP group were 1.43±0.07 ng/ml, 46.0±2.05 ng/ml, 413±56.4 pg/ml, 2.68±0.35 pg/ml, 14.1±2.11 ng/ml

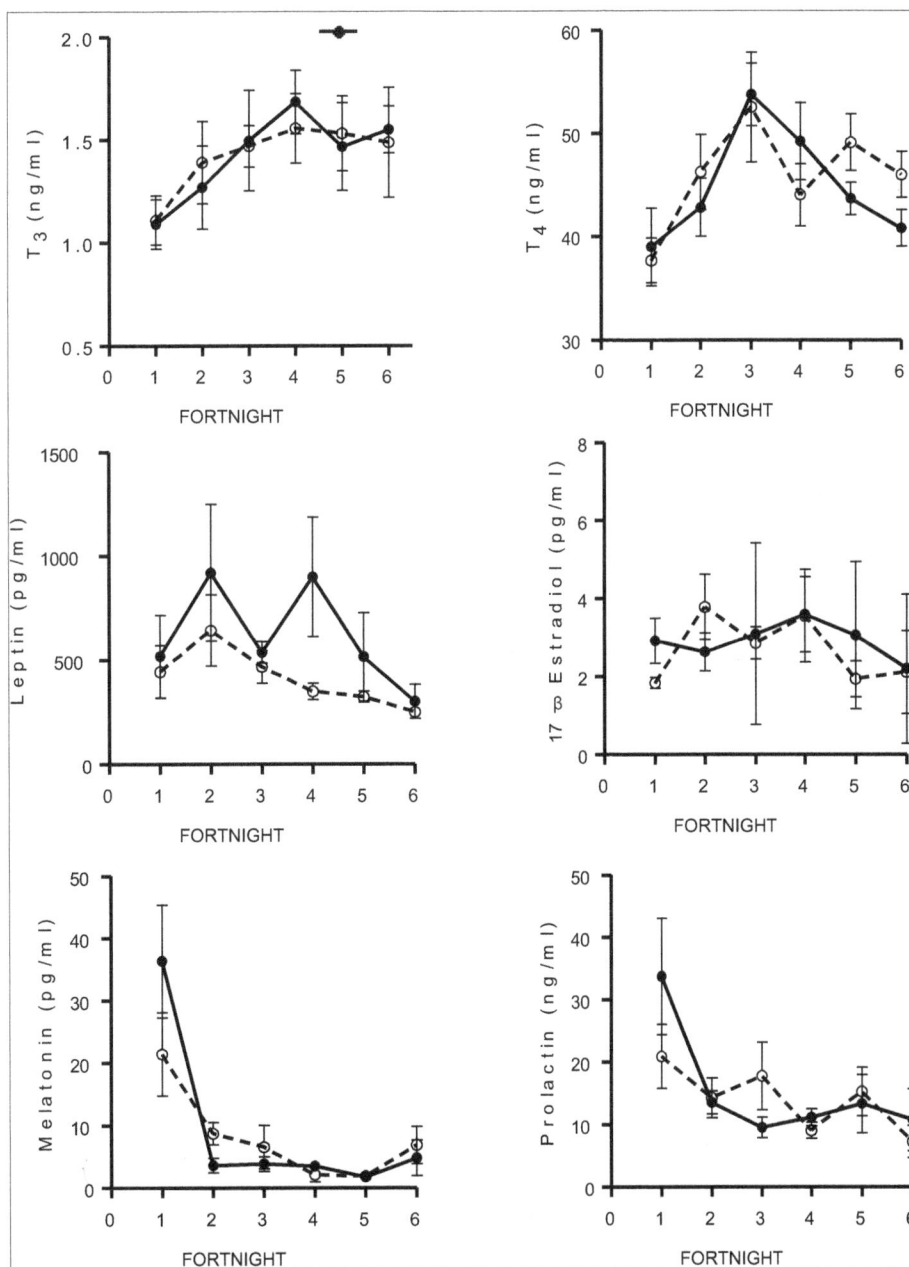

Figure-3: Mean (±standard error) plasma concentrations of T_3, T_4, leptin, 17 β estradiol, melatonin and prolactin in normal day and extended normal day photoperiod groups.

and 7.95±2.92 pg/ml, respectively (Figure-3). Plasma T_3, T_4, leptin, 17 β estradiol, prolactin and melatonin in ENDP group were 1.43±0.09 ng/ml, 44.9±2.27 ng/ml, 616±99.7 pg/ml, 2.92±0.19 pg/ml, 15.4±3.74 ng/ml, and 9.00±5.49 pg/ml, respectively. Group and group-by-age interaction effects on all the hormone concentrations were non-significant ($p>0.05$). Significant ($p<0.05$) age effect on plasma T_4, leptin and melatonin concentrations was observed. The plasma T_3 and T_4 levels observed in this experiment was in accordance with a similar study conducted on peripubertal Murrah buffaloes [17]. The lower plasma 17 β

estradiol concentrations (<5 pg/ml) observed in both the groups of this study was also in accordance with the results obtained [18]. By the end of the experiment, 6 out of 7 heifers attained puberty in ENDP group, whereas only 4 out of 7 heifers attained puberty in NDP group. Attainment of puberty was determined by behavioral signs, and confirmed by both plasma progesterone levels (>1 ng/ml) and presence of corpus luteum through ultrasound examination of ovaries.

The circadian pattern of melatonin and prolactin in both NDP and ENDP groups are depicted in Figure-4. There were no group, time and

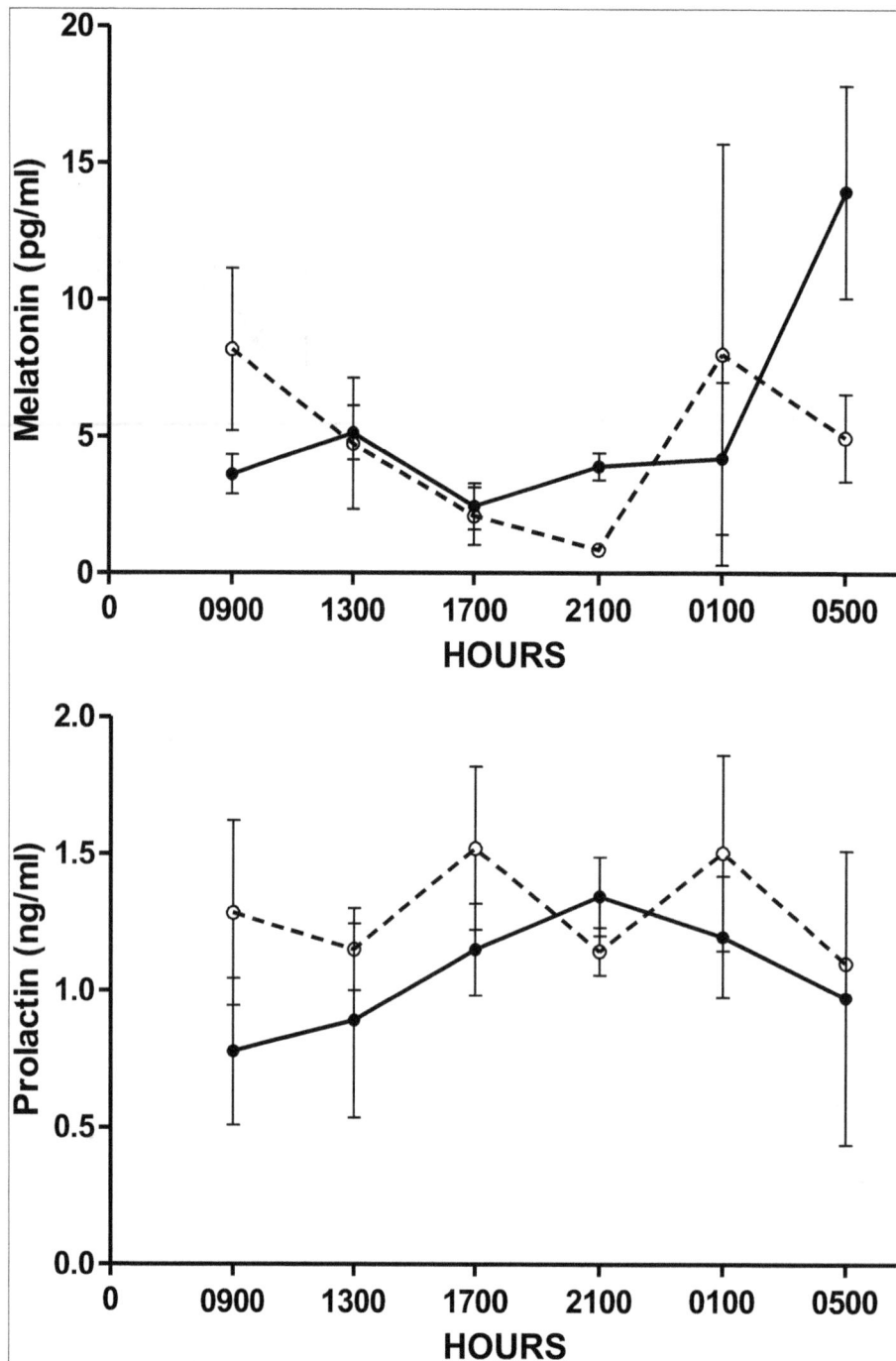

Figure-4: Circadian trend of prolactin and melatonin in   normal day and extended normal day photoperiod groups.

group-by-time interaction effects on both plasma melatonin and prolactin concentrations. Each heifer, irrespective of their group, showed different levels and pattern of melatonin and prolactin release. The plasma melatonin concentrations in NDP and ENDP groups ranged between 0.82-23.4 and 1.16-20.7 pg/ml, respectively. Plasma prolactin concentrations in NDP and ENDP groups ranged between 0.97-2.19 and 0.35-1.87 ng/ml, respectively. There was a definite circadian trend of plasma melatonin in buffaloes reared in few farms of Italy [19]. However, the buffaloes reared in a certain farm did not show a definite circadian pattern. The different trends of melatonin could be attributed to selection process practiced in the farms and targeted elimination of seasonal buffaloes [20]. The genetic selection criteria implemented to maintain the breeding herd in our farm reasons for the different pattern of melatonin release, irrespective of group.

In the present study, the DMI and BWs of NDP and ENDP groups did not differ significantly (p>0.05). However, the higher average daily gain was observed among the heifers of ENDP as compared to NDP group. Exposure of experimental group to 4 h of extended photoperiod with artificial light (160 Lux) after sunset may have increased their feed efficiency ratio and thus higher average daily gain. An increase in feed efficiency by extending photoperiod during winter in crossbred beef heifers corroborates the result of this study [21]. They also observed a non-significant difference in DMI between the natural and extended photoperiod groups, which agreed with our results. Plasma leptin appears to be an important link between metabolic status, the neuroendocrine axis and subsequent fertility in farm animals [21-23]. It also serves as a metabolic signal that acts on the hypothalamic-pituitary-ovarian axis to enhance gonadotropin-releasing hormone and luteinizing hormone secretion and ovarian function [24,25]. Proper management practices, nutrition, and optimum climatic conditions are indispensable for homeostasis and optimum productivity in cattle [26]. In the present study, the mean plasma leptin concentrations were comparatively higher in the ENDP (616±99.7 pg/ml) group than in NDP (413±56.4 pg/ml) group. An improved feed efficiency and better average daily gain in ENDP group may have influenced the plasma leptin concentrations and further attainment of puberty.

Conclusion

Extending the natural photoperiod by artificial light (160 Lux) for 4 h daily during winter season resulted in better growth rate and early onset of puberty in Murrah buffalo heifers.

Authors' Contributions

AKR: Planning and execution of experiment. Drafted and revised the manuscript; MS: Hormone assays; PK: Management of animals in the farm;

BSBK: Statistical analysis of data. All authors read and approved the final manuscript.

Acknowledgments

Financial support provided by the Director, National Dairy Research Institute, India and the National Initiative on Climate Resilience in Agriculture, India are greatly acknowledged.

Competing Interests

The authors declare that they have no competing interests.

References

1. Mirmahmoudi, R. and Prakash, B.S. (2012) The endocrine changes, the timing of ovulation and the efficacy of the doublesynch protocol in the murrah buffalo (*Bubalus bubalis*). *Gen. Comp. Endocrinol.*, 177(1): 153-159.
2. Terzano, G.M., Lucia, B.V. and Antonio, B. (2012) Overview on reproductive endocrine aspects in buffalo. *J. Buffalo Sci.*, 1: 126-138.
3. Perera, B.M.A. (2011) Reproductive cycles of buffalo. *Anim. Reprod. Sci.*, 124(3), 194-199.
4. Mirmahmoudi, R., Souri, M. and Prakash, B.S. (2014) Comparison of endocrine changes, timing of ovulations, ovarian follicular growth, and efficacy associated with estradoublesynch and heat synch protocols in Murrah buffalo cows (*Bubalus bubalis*). *Theriogenology*, 82(7): 1012-1020.
5. Sisk, C.L. and Foster, D.L. (2004) The neural basis of puberty and adolescence. *Nat. Neurosci.*, 7: 1040-1047.
6. Small, J.A., Glover, N.D., Kennedy, A.D., McCaughey, W. P. and Ward, D.R. (2003) Photoperiod effects on the development of beef heifers. *Can. J. Anim. Sci.*, 83: 721-730.
7. Brito, L.F.C., Barth, A.D., Rawlings, N.C., Wilde, R.E., Crews, D.H., Boisclair, Y.R. and Kastelic, J.P. (2007) Effect of feed restriction during calf-hood on serum concentrations of metabolic hormones, gonadotropins, testosterone, and on sexual development in bulls. *Reproduction*, 134(1): 171-181.
8. Davis Rincker, L.E., Vandehaar, M.J., Wolf, C.A., Liesman, J.S., Chapin, L.T. and Weber Nielsen, M.S. (2011) Effect of intensified feeding of heifer calves on growth, pubertal age, calving age, milk yield, and economics. *J. Dairy Sci.*, 94: 3554-3567.
9. Funston, R.N., Martin, J.L., Larson, D.M. and Roberts, A.J. (2012) Physiology and endocrinology symposium: Nutritional aspects of developing replacement heifers. *J. Anim. Sci.*, 90: 1166-1171.
10. Saini, M.S., Dhanda, O.P., Singh, N. and Georgie, G.C. (1998) The effect of improved management on the reproductive performance of pubertal buffalo heifers during the summer. *Indian J. Dairy Sci.*, 51(4): 250-253.
11. Jamara, M.S., Mehla, R.K., Singh, M., Ali, M.M. and Chouhan, N. (2014) Effect of the feed Shatavari (*Asparagus racemosus*) on body weight and puberty of Sahiwal heifers. *Int. J. Agric. Sci. Vet. Med.*, 2(1): 64-67.
12. Kennedy, A.D., Bergen, R.D., Lawson, T.J., Small, J.A. and Veira, D.M. (2004) Effects of evening feeding and extended photoperiod on growth, feed efficiency, live animal carcass traits and plasma prolactin of beef heifers housed outdoors during two Manitoba winters. *Can. J. Anim. Sci.* 84: 491-500.
13. Kassim, N.S.I., Afify, A.A. and Hassan, H.Z. (2008) Effect of photoperiod length on some reproductive traits and hormonal profiles in buffalo heifers. *Am. Euras. J. Agric. Environ. Sci.*, 3(4): 646-655.
14. Somparn, P., Gibb, M.J., Markvichitr, K., Chaiyabutr, N., Thummabood, S. and Vajrabukka, C. (2007) Effect of

supplementary lighting on eating behaviour by corralled swamp buffalo (*Bubalus bubalis*) heifers in Thailand. *Songklanakarin J. Sci. Technol.*, 29(2): 399-411.

15. Shipe, W.F., Senyk, G.F. and Fountain, K.B. (1980) Modified copper soap solvent extraction method for measuring free fatty acids in milk. *J. Dairy Sci.* 63: 193-198.

16. Khan, H.M., Mohanty, T.K., Bhakat, M., Raina, V.S. and Gupta, A.K. (2011) Relationship of blood metabolites with reproductive parameters during various seasons in Murrah buffaloes. *Asian Australas. J. Anim. Sci.*, 24(9): 1192-1198.

17. Ingole, S.D., Deshmukh, B.T., Nagvekar, A.S. and Bharucha, S.V. (2012) Serum profile of thyroid hormones from birth to puberty in buffalo calves and heifers. *J. Buffalo Sci.*, 1(1): 39-49.

18. Mondal, S., Prakash, B.S. and Palta, P. (2007) Endocrine aspects of oestrous cycle in buffaloes (*Bubalus bubalis*): An overview. A*sian-Aust. J. Anim. Sci.*, 20(1): 124-131.

19. Parmeggiani, A., Di Palo, R. and Zicarelli, L. (1994) Melatonin and reproductive seasonality of the Della Buffalo, *Agri. Res.* 16: 41-8.

20. Seren, E., Parmeggiani, A., Campanile, G. (1995) The control of ovulation in Italian buffalo. In: Enne, G., Greppi, G.F. and Lauria, A., editors. Reproduction and Animal Breeding Advances and Strategy. Elsevier, Amsterdam. p265-275.

21. Barb, C.R. and Kraeling, R.R. (2004) Role of leptin in the regulation of gonadotropin secretion in farm animals. *Anim. Reprod. Sci.*, 82: 155-167.

22. Lomniczi, A., Wright, H. and Ojeda, S.R. (2015) Epigenetic regulation of female puberty. *Front. Neuroendocrinol.*, 36: 90-107.

23. Vázquez, M.J., Romero-Ruiz, A. and Tena-Sempere, M. (2015) Roles of leptin in reproduction, pregnancy and polycystic ovary syndrome: Consensus knowledge and recent developments. *Metabolism*, 64(1): 79-91.

24. Campbell, B.K., Guitierrez, C.G., Armstrong, D.G., Webb, R. and Baird, D.T. (2000) Leptin: *In vitro* and *in vivo* evidence for direct effects on the ovary in monovulatory ruminants. *Hum. Reprod.*, 14: 15-16.

25. Takumi, K., Shimada, K., Iijima, N. and Ozawa, H. (2015) Maternal high-fat diet during lactation increases Kiss1 mRNA expression in the arcuate nucleus at weaning and advances puberty onset in female rats. *Neurosci. Res.*, 100: 21-28.

26. Bova, T.L., Chiavaccini, L., Cline, G.F., Hart, C.G., Matheny, K., Muth, A.M., Voelz, B.E., Kesler, D. and Memili, E. (2014) Environmental stressors influencing hormones and systems physiology in cattle. *Reprod. Biol. Endocrinol.*, 12: 58.

31

Occurrence of pathogenic *Vibrio parahaemolyticus* in crustacean shellfishes in coastal parts of Eastern India

S. Parthasarathy[1], Suresh Chandra Das[2] and Ashok Kumar[3]

1. Division of Veterinary Public Health, Indian Veterinary Research Institute, Izatnagar, Bareilly - 243 122, Uttar Pradesh, India; 2. Veterinary Public Health Laboratory, Indian Veterinary Research Institute, Eastern Regional Station, Kolkata - 700 037, West Bengal, India; 3. Assistant Director General (Animal Health), Indian Council of Agricultural Research, Krishi Bhawan, New Delhi, India.
Corresponding author: Suresh Chandra Das, e-mail: dasivriers@gmail.com,
SP: parthasarathyvet@gmail.com, AK: ashokakt@rediffmail.com

Abstract

Aim: The objective of the study was to isolate and characterize pathogenic *Vibrio parahaemolyticus* from crustacean shellfishes (crab and shrimp) commonly retailed in coastal parts of eastern India.

Materials and Methods: Samples were processed by bacteriological isolation followed by biochemical characterization in Kaper's medium. Presumptively identified isolates were confirmed by species-specific Vp-*toxR* polymerase chain reaction (PCR) assay. Virulence and pandemic property of the confirmed *V. parahaemolyticus* isolates were determined by specific PCR assays.

Results: On screening of 167 samples comprising crabs (n=82) and shrimps (n=85) by the standard bacteriological cultural method, *V. parahaemolyticus* was presumptively identified in 86.6% (71/82) and 82.3% (70/85) of respective samples. Of these, 46 (56%) and 66 (77.6%) isolates from crab and shrimp, respectively, were confirmed as *V. parahaemolyticus* by biochemical characterization (Kaper's reaction) followed by specific Vp-*toxR* PCR assay. About 10 isolates each from crab and shrimp was found to carry the virulence gene (*tdh*). It denotes that 12.2% of crab and 11.7% of shrimp in the study area are harboring the pathogenic *V. parahaemolyticus*. Such *tdh*+ isolates (n=20) were subjected for screening of pandemic genotype by pandemic group specific (PGS) - PCR (PGS-PCR) and GS-PCR (*toxRS* gene) where 11 (6.5%) isolates revealed the pandemic determining amplicon (235 bp) in PGS-PCR and belonged to crab (7.3%) and shrimp (6%) samples; however, 2 (2.4%) isolates were positive in GS-PCR and belonged to crab samples only. These two GS-PCR+ isolates from crab were also positive in PGS-PCR.

Conclusion: The findings of the study conclusively indicated that a considerable percentage of crab and shrimp in these areas were harboring pathogenic and pandemic *V. parahaemolyticus* posing a public health risk in consumption of improperly processed such shellfishes. Cross contamination of other marine and fresh water market fishes by such shellfishes in these areas may provide scope for spreading this pathogen in community food chain.

Keywords: crustaceans, pandemic, pathogenic, *toxR*-gene, *Vibrio parahaemolyticus*.

Introduction

Globalization of the food supply and increased international travel has enhanced the risk of occurrence of different diseases in many parts of the world. Moreover, changes in nutritional habits brought about an increase in consumption of undercooked or raw foods, especially sea foods such as marine fish and shellfish implicated with *Vibrio parahaemolyticus* exposing consumers to different diseases more specifically gastroenteritis and diarrhea [1]. Occupying a variety of niches, *V. parahaemolyticus* is a common bacterium in marine and estuarine environments [2]. It can exist planktonically or attached to submerged inert and animate surfaces, including suspended particulate matter, zooplankton, fish and shellfish [3]. It belongs to genus *Vibrio* and commonly isolated from various seafoods including oyster, mussel, scallop, octopus, shrimp, clam, crab, mackerel, sardines, codfish, etc., worldwide [4]. This organism is recognized globally as one of the leading causes of food poisoning (toxi-infection), diarrhea and gastroenteritis in human resulting from the consumption of raw or insufficiently cooked seafood [1,5]. Thermostable direct hemolysin (TDH) and TDH-related hemolysin (TRH), encoded by the *tdh* and *trh* genes, respectively, have been recognized as the major virulence factors of this organism [6,7]. TDH causes β-hemolysis of human erythrocytes in Wagatsuma agar medium, popularly known as the Kanagawa phenomenon [8].

West Bengal and Odisha, the two eastern coastal states of India are important hub for the harvesting of marine fish and shellfishes. The average brackish water fish production was around 30,000 MT which includes 5000 MT of shrimp and 350 MT of crab harvested from the Chilika Lake, the important saltwater fishing harbor in Odisha (Directorate of Fisheries, Government of Odisha; website link: http://www.odishafisheries.com). The export of marine products to foreign countries, such as Japan, Thailand, and Indonesia, is about 30,900 MT which costs around 1800 crores annually (Directorate of Fisheries, Government of Odisha). West Bengal is the only state in India, where fishes have been cultivated in all types of water bodies', i.e., sweet water, brackish water, sewage water, and marine water, etc. The total productions of inland fish and marine fish in WB are 15.30 Lac ton and 2 Lac ton, respectively. These are mainly consumed in the state and rest spare for Delhi, Uttar Pradesh, Madhya Pradesh, Bihar, and other adjoining states. Export of marine fish earned handsome revenue of Rs.700 crore in the year 2009-2010. West Bengal occupies the 4th position in the country regarding export of seafood products. Fishes are exported primarily to Japan, Vietnam, and China. Out of the total exports, 90% are shrimps and the rest includes ornamental fish, crab, fresh water prawns (Food Processing Industries Survey, West Bengal, 2012-13; website link: http://www.wbfpihgov.in).

Ingestion of raw or improperly cooked seafoods, mainly crustacean and molluscan shellfishes have been identified the main sources of *V. parahaemolyticus* infections, and this has emerged as a growing concern in the production and trade of seafoods [1,2]. Kolkata, an inland metropolis is an endemic area for diarrheal diseases and *V. parahaemolyticus* was detected from 3.5% to 23.9% of acute human diarrheal cases [9]. Since 1996, the incidence of *V. parahaemolyticus* associated infections has increased with an emergence of highly virulent pandemic O3: K6 clone [10]. On the other hand, magnitude of occurrence of this organism has not been properly addressed in coastal Odisha, i.e. in and around Bhubaneswar, India. These marine shellfishes, such as crab and shrimps, provide an affordable protein dishes in this geographical region that replaces more than 30% of the local fish consumption and are suspected as a potential source of diarrheal diseases. Further, in Indian context, the past studies, so far, reported the incidence of this organism mostly from clinical diarrhea [11-13] and a few studies from marine fishes [14-16] but not from the different shellfishes retailed in suburban and proper Kolkata and Bhubaneswar areas. Keeping this in view, the present investigation was undertaken to determine the occurrence of pathogenic *V. parahaemolyticus* in shellfishes namely crabs and shrimp in these areas as well as to identify their pandemic population.

Materials and Methods

Ethical approval

In this study, samples from saline water shellfishes viz, crab and shrimp were collected from retail market and examined for presence of the organism by cultural isolation and thereafter, characterized for

their virulence traits in the laboratory adopting the recommended assays where no animal experiment was involved.

Design of study

The study was designed for isolation and identification of *V. parahaemolyticus* from saline water origin shellfishes such as crab and shrimp by bacteriological isolation and biochemical characterization followed by confirmation in species-specific Vp-*toxR* polymerase chain reaction (PCR) assay. The confirmed isolates were further characterized for their pathogenic and pandemic property by molecular characterization employing specific PCR methods.

Study area

A total of 167 samples of crab (n=82) and shrimp (n=85) collected aseptically in sterile sample container from different retail fish markets in and around the city of Kolkata and Bhubaneswar, India (Figure-1) and transported in ice packs to the laboratory for further processing.

Sample processing

Intestinal mass of crab and head portions of shrimp were considered for processing. About 10-20 g of sample was aseptically grinded using pestle and mortar. The masses were inoculated in 50 ml of alkaline peptone water containing 3% NaCl at pH 8.5 (pre-enrichment) and incubated aerobically for 24 h at 37°C. During processing, all necessary precautions were taken to avoid cross-contamination of the samples.

Cultural isolation

Isolation and identification of *V. parahaemolyticus* were carried out by adopting standard bacteriological methods [17] with minor modifications. Briefly, a loop full of overnight broth was streaked on thiosulfate citrate bile salts sucrose agar and the plates were incubated at 37°C for 24 h. Presumptive identification of *V. parahaemolyticus* was carried out based on typical colony characteristics, i.e., round, 2-3 mm in diameter with green or blue center. Five typical colonies from each plate (each sample) were selected for

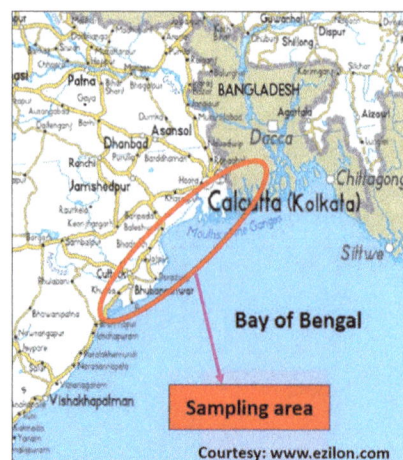

Figure-1: Location of sampling areas.

biochemical characterization in the Kaper's multi test medium where characteristic colonies of the *V. parahaemolyticus* revealed acidic (yellow) butt and alkali (purple) slant (K/A) reaction. Such characteristic colonies (n=112; Table-1) were subjected to screen for species-specific *toxR* gene by Vp-*toxR* PCR assay.

Confirmation of isolate by species-specific Vp-*toxR* PCR assay

The Vp-*toxR* PCR assay was standardized for detection of species-specific *toxR* gene of *V. parahaemolyticus* adopting the described method [18] with some modification using the bacterial lysate as template DNA prepared from the lawn culture on LB agar plates by snap chill method. Briefly, a loopful of fresh bacterial culture was mixed with 100 µl Mlli Q water in a microcentrifuge tube and centrifuged at 10,000 rpm for 5 min. The tube was kept in a boiling water bath for 10 min. After heat treatment, the cell lysate was immediately kept in ice cubes. After 10 min, it was centrifuged at 6000 rpm for 5 min and supernatant was used as template DNA. The primers as mentioned in Table-2 were used in this assay. Amplification reaction was performed in 25 µl reaction volume containing 2.5 µl 10× PCR amplification buffer (500 mM KCl, 100 mM Tris-HCl, pH-8.3; 15 mM MgCl$_2$), 0.5 µl dNTP mix (10 mM each), 1 µl (10 pmol/µl) each of forward and reverse primers, 0.2 µl (1 unit) Taq DNA polymerase, 5.3 µl of 1:10 diluted bacterial lysate and sterile deionized water to make volume up to 25 µl. Cycling conditions include initial denaturation at 95°C for 5 min followed by 20 cycles of denaturation (94°C for 1 min), annealing (63°C for 1.30 min) and extension (72°C for 1.30 min) and final extension was carried out at 72°C for 7 min. The amplified product (368 bp) was electrophoresed on 1.5% agarose gel, visualized under ultraviolet (UV) light after staining with ethidium bromide (0.5 µg/ml), and the result was recorded comparing with reference strain Vp-Kx-V138 (Figure-2).

Detection of virulence gene (*tdh*)

Virulence of the confirmed isolates was determined by defining the presence of cardinal virulence gene, i.e., *tdh* gene for hemolysin production. The *tdh* PCR assay was accomplished following the method [19] using the primers as mentioned in Table-2. The assay involved 2.5 µl of 10× PCR amplification buffer (500 mM KCl, 100 mM Tris-HCl, pH-8.3; 15 mM MgCl$_2$), 0.5 µl of dNTP mix (10 mM each), 1 µl (10 pmol/µl) each of forward and reverse primers, 0.2 µl (1 unit) of Taq DNA polymerase, 5.3 µl of bacterial lysate (1:10 dilution) and sterile deionized water to make final reaction volume up to 25 µl. The reaction mixture was cycled at 94°C for 5 min for initial denaturation, then 30 cycles of

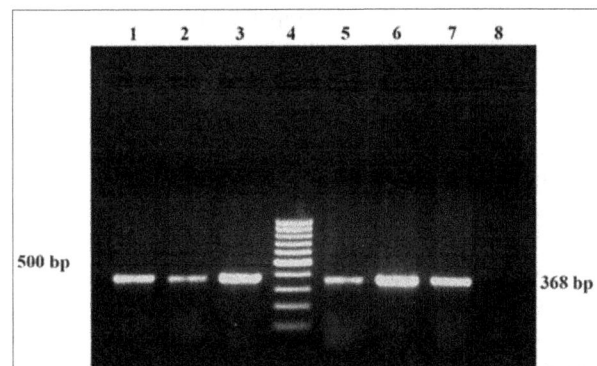

Figure-2: Polymerase chain reaction amplification of *toxR* gene of *Vibrio parahaemolyticus*, Lane 1, 2, 3, 5, 6: Sample DNA (C2, C25, C57, S8, S38) with positive amplicon (368 bp), Lane 4: DNA ladder of molecular weight 100 bp, Lane 7: Positive control (*V. parahaemolyticus* Vp-Kx-V$_{138}$ strain), Lane 8: Negative control, C - Crab, S – Shrimp.

Table-1: Occurrence of *V. parahaemolyticus* in shellfishes.

Samples screened (n)	Cultural isolation in TCBS (%)	Biochemical characterization (Kaper's Reaction) (%)	PCR assay			
			Species confirmation (Vp-*toxR*) (%)	Virulence characterization (%)		
				tdh	GS-PCR	PGS-PCR
Crab (82)	71 (86.6)	46 (56)	46 (56)	10 (12.2)	2 (2.4)	6 (7.3)
Shrimp (85)	70 (82.3)	66 (77.6)	66 (77.6)	10 (11.7)	0	5 (6)
Total (167)	141 (84.4)	112 (67)	112 (67)	20 (11.9)	2 (1.2)	11 (6.5)

TCBS=Thiosulfate citrate bile salts sucrose, PGS=Pandemic group specific, PCR=Polymerase chain reaction, *V. parahaemolyticus*=*Vibrio parahaemolyticus*

Table-2: Oligonucleotide primers used in different PCR assays.

PCR assay	Target gene	Primer sequences (5`-3`)	Amplicon	References
Vp-toxR PCR	*tox*R	F: GTC TTC TGA CGC AAT CGT TG R: ATA CGA GTG GTT GCT GTC ATG	368 bp	[18]
tdh PCR	*tdh*	F: CCA AAT ACA TTT TAC TTG G R: GGT ACT AAA TGG CTG ACA TC	199 bp	[19]
GS-PCR	*toxRS*/new sequence	F: TAA TGA GGT AGA AAC A R: ACG TAA CGG GCC TAC A	651 bp	[20]
PGS-PCR	PGS sequence	F: TTC GTT TCG CGC CAC AAC T R: TGC GGT GAT TAT TCG CGT CT	235 bp	[21]

PGS=Pandemic group specific, PCR=Polymerase chain reaction

denaturation at 94°C for 1.30 min, annealing at 50°C for 1.30 min and elongation at 72°C for 1.30 min followed by final extension for 7 min at 72°C. At the end of reaction, the amplified product (199 bp) was electrophoresed on 1.5% agarose gel, visualized under UV light after staining with ethidium bromide (0.5 µg/ml), and the result was recorded comparing with reference strain Vp-Kx-V$_{138}$ (Figure-3).

Detection of pandemic marker (*toxRS* new/GS-PCR and pandemic group specific-PCR [PGS-PCR])

All the 20 *tdh*$^+$ isolates obtained from crab and shrimp were further subjected to GS-PCR and PGS-PCR assay to determine the presence of pandemic gene by employing the published methods [20,21] using primers as mentioned in Table-2. The reaction mixture was optimized to contain 2.5 µl of 10× PCR buffer (500 mM KCl, 100 mM Tris-HCl, pH-8.3; 15 mM MgCl$_2$), 0.5 µl of dNTP mix (10 mM each), 1.0 µl (10 pmol/µl) each of forward and reverse primers, 0.2 µl (1 unit) of Taq DNA polymerase, 5.3 µl of bacterial lysate (1:50 dilution for GS-PCR and 1:10 for PGS-PCR) prepared by boiling and snap chilling method and sterile deionized water to make final volume 25 µl. The reaction was performed in a thermal cycler with preheated lid (lid temp 105°C). The cycling condition for GS-PCR was an initial denaturation at 96°C for 5 min, followed by 25 cycles each of denaturation at 96°C for 1 min, annealing at 45°C for 2 min, elongation at 72°C for 3 min and final extension step at 72°C for 7 min. Similarly, for PGS-PCR assay, the initial denaturation was at 94°C for 5 min followed by 25 cycles each of denaturation at 94°C for 1 min, annealing at 59°C for 1 min, elongation at 72°C for 1 min and final extension step at 72°C for 7 min. On completion of the reaction, the amplified products (651 bp and 235 bp) were held briefly at 4°C, and then, analyzed by agarose (1.2%) gel electrophoresis

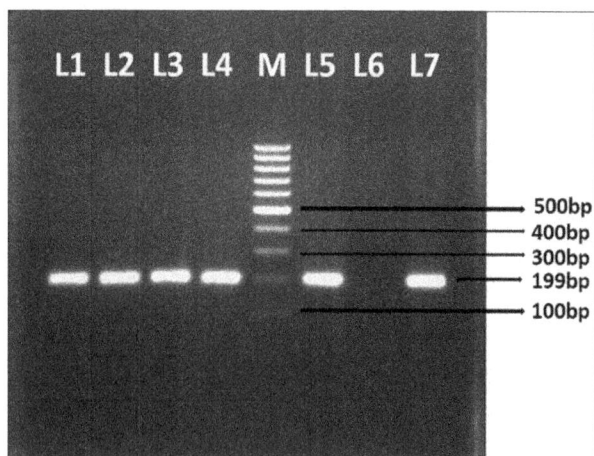

Figure-3: Polymerase chain reaction amplification of *tdh* gene of *Vibrio parahaemolyticus*, Lane 1, 2, 3, 4, 6: Sample DNA (C2, C25, C57, S8, S38) with positive amplicon (199 bp), Lane 5: DNA ladder of molecular weight 100 bp, Lane 7: Negative control, Lane 8: Positive control (*V. parahaemolyticus* Vp-Kx-V$_{138}$ Strain), C - Crab, S – Shrimp.

stained with ethidium bromide (0.5 µg/ml) and visualized under UV transilluminator. DNA ladder of 100 bp (Thermo Fischer Scientific, USA) was used as molecular weight marker. The lysate DNA of reference culture Vp-Kx-V$_{138}$ and *E. coli* K12 were used as positive and negative control, respectively.

Results

A total of 167 samples from crab (n=82) and shrimp (n=85) were examined for the presence of *V. parahaemolyticus* by cultural isolation and biochemical characterization followed by confirmation of the species by species-specific Vp-*toxR* PCR assay. Of the total 167 samples screened by standard bacteriological cultural method, *V. parahaemolyticus* was presumptively identified in 86.6% (71/82) crab and 82.3% (70/85) shrimp samples, respectively (Table-1). On biochemical characterization in Kaper's multi test medium with such presumptively identified 71 and 70 isolates from crab and shrimp, 46 (56%) and 66 (77.6%) were produced positive K/A reaction, respectively. All the Kaper's positive isolates were confirmed as *V. parahaemolyticus* in species-specific Vp-*toxR* PCR assay (Table-1). The identified isolates were characterized by *tdh* PCR assay for the presence of cardinal virulence gene, i.e., *tdh* gene responsible for hemolysin production. Of the total 112 confirmed isolates, 10 isolates each from crab (12.2%) and shrimp (11.7%) was found to carry the virulence gene (*tdh*) (Table-1). Subsequently, such *tdh*$^+$ isolates (n=20) were subjected for screening of pandemic genotype by PGS-PCR (235 bp amplicon of the AP-PCR fragment for 930 bp) and GS-PCR (*toxRS*/new sequence) where 11 (6.5%) isolates revealed the pandemic determining amplicon (235 bp) in PGS-PCR and belonged to crab (7.3%) and shrimp (6%) samples; however, 2 (2.4%) isolates were positive in GS-PCR and belonged to crab samples only. These two (2) GS-PCR$^+$ isolates from crab were also positive in PGS-PCR.

Discussion

With the increase in human population and growing demand of more food, the aquatic foods including seafoods has been considered as an alternative source of dietetic protein to meet up the growing need of the community. This situation considered as an important cause for a large number of foodborne diseases including of *V. parahaemolyticus* in food chain [22] that causes gastroenteritis (toxi-infection) associated with the ingestion of contaminated raw or improperly cooked saline water origin fish and shellfishes [1,2]. In spite of the large infective dose (10^7 to 10^8), the short generation time (8-9 min) enables the organisms to multiply rapidly at ambient temperatures in foods and facilitate to cause disease. Shellfishes including crab and small shrimps serve a staple dietary protein for non-veg fish eaters in Eastern India coastal areas including suburban and proper Kolkata and Bhubaneswar. In 1996, an abrupt increase in diarrheal cases and isolation of *V. parahaemolyticus* was reported in Infectious Disease Hospital, Kolkata with the emergence of highly virulent pandemic strain O3:K6 [10]. Moreover, the first outbreak of *V. parahaemolyticus* mediated diarrhea was reported in Vellore, Tamil Nadu [10]. Further, in India, the incidence of *V. parahaemolyticus* is reported to have doubled during 1996-2000 [11] fetch its clinical and public health importance. Primarily this organism was considered for study because, since 1996, it has been frequently associated in human diarrheal cases in eastern coastal areas and has gained a new global dimension in its pathogenicity by virtue of its emerging the virulence and pandemic characters. Moreover, this is capable of infecting wide host range of marine animals including marine shellfishes which still remains to be the main source of food borne infection in these areas. The perusal of literature suggested that past studies on occurrence of this pathogen were mainly centered on the clinical cases and very few studies with saline water fishes. However, the occurrence of this pathogen in shellfishes available in coastal areas particularly in Odisha has not been addressed where seafood especially crabs and shrimps are included in the daily dishes by a considerable size of population.

Among all the 167 shellfish samples, 141 (84.4%) yielded characteristic *V. parahaemolyticus* in cultural isolation; however, isolates from 112 (67%) such samples revealed positivity in biochemical characteristics and the species-specific *toxR* gene amplicon (368 bp) in Vp-*toxR* PCR assay thereby confirmed the occurrence of *V. parahaemolyticus*. Further, this organism was recorded in little higher frequency (77.6%) in shrimp than crab (56%) (Table-1). The result recorded the sizeable difference in identification of *V. parahaemolyticus* from samples by traditional cultural isolation and the PCR assay. Incidence (67%) of this pathogen in common shellfishes in these areas revealed its potentials as a food borne problem. The observation for the isolation in this study is in accordance with the earlier published works [15] where marine fishes were sampled. The present findings deferred with the observation of Deepanjali *et al*. [23] who reported *V. parahaemolyticus* in 93.87% of oysters. This difference in occurrence may be attributed to variation in factors for geographical areas and type of sample studied. The study findings were also in concordance with earlier studies that reported the presence of this organism in about 50-70% of seafood [24].

PCR was used to detect *tdh* gene using DNA primers that are specific for encoding TDH to determine the pathogenic population among the confirmed *V. parahaemolyticus*. Out of 167 samples, 20 (11.9%) were identified to be virulent by producing specific amplicon for *tdh* gene recognized for production of β-hemolysis evident on Wagatsuma agar referred as Kanagawa phenomena [25]. Moreover, there was no significant difference in occurrence of *tdh*+ isolates in the two sample sources, i.e. crab (12.2%) and shrimp

(11.7%). In this study, population of *tdh*+ *V. parahaemolyticus* was comparatively high than the works of Deepanjali *et al.,* [23] where *tdh*+ was recorded in 6.1% isolates in South West coast of India and also to the observation of Sakazaki *et al.,* [8] who reported that 1-2% of environmental samples contain virulent (*tdh*+) isolates. The study findings were also in agreement with previous studies [26,27] where *tdh*-positive *V. parahaemolyticus* was recovered in 10%, 11% and 15% of shellfishes such as oyster and shrimps. The high frequency of occurrence of pathogenic (*tdh*+) *V. parahaemolyticus* in shellfishes (crab and shrimp) in these areas indicates the potentials of common market shellfishes for causing food-borne gastroenteritis linked to food chain. The present study also highlighted the real magnitude of public health risk in terms of gastroenteritis attributed to routine intake of such improperly processed shellfishes that carry pathogenic *V. parahaemolyticus* in their considerable population (11.9%).

In reality, in Indian context, gastroenteritis to the consumers are not reported so frequently; hopefully, it is the boon of the Indian cuisine that attained much higher temperature than the thermal death point of this pathogen. Since 1996, occurrence of *V. parahaemolyticus* in endemic and epidemic situations has been increasingly reported in many Asian countries including India [28]. Regular rise of ambient and aquatic environment temperature as well as acquiring virulent gene(s) may be associated in abetting such increasing incidences of pathogenic *V. parahaemolyticus* [29]. Warmer sea temperatures (the El Nino effect) have resulted in the emergence of more virulent *V. parahaemolyticus* in USA [30]. Increasing environmental temperature in these areas may facilitate to cope up and propagate the pathogenic strains of this organism.

Epidemiological study revealed that most of the reported outbreaks of *V. parahaemolyticus* infection were due to consumption of raw or insufficiently cooked sea foods especially crustacean and molluscs [4]. The linkage in the transmission of this pathogen through food chain among the consumers of shellfishes in eastern India and probability for incidence of gastroenteritis are seems to be almost similar with the earlier studies because lower income group people of these areas prefer these shellfishes in their daily with dishes that serves the low-cost common dietary affordable protein sources. In modern era of fast food practice, some group of Indian people skip the recommended cooking temperature and time protocol that may accidentally allow entry of this pathogen in food chain. In Indian circumstances, contamination of freshwater fishes at the market level through shellfishes implicated with *V. parahaemolyticus* and subsequently, contamination of other foods in the kitchen by contaminated shellfish brought from markets are believed to be the possible sources of entry of this organism in food chain [31,32]. Factors like improper handling and processing of fish and shellfish at fishing harbors as well as in market are major contributors to contamination by *V. parahaemolyticus* [31]. In Indian context, the physical facilities and infrastructure in all types of fish markets are far from satisfactory. Most fish landing centers and fish markets are old, crowded and have an excess number of traders, even in the passages and without proper infrastructure facilities, thereby resulting in poor fish handling. Most retailers were found selling fish by the roadside without considering either quality or hygiene.

In this investigation, the *tdh*⁺ isolates were screened for the presence of pandemic potential GS gene sequence by employing the GS-PCR and PGS-PCR assay. The GS-PCR elucidates the GS sequence (*toxRS* operon) of *V. parahaemolyticus* that encodes the transmembrane protein involved in the regulation of virulence-associated genes. On comparison sequence in this *toxRS* coding region (1364 bp) between two sets of *V. parahaemolyticus* isolates of O3:K6 serotype (pandemic strain) that was isolated before and after 1995 in different parts of the world, difference was recorded in 7 bases. Moreover, these 7 bases were found conserved in the isolates of such *V. parahaemolyticus* O3:K6 serotype that was isolated after 1995 and termed as *toxRS*/new sequence [20]. With this concept, the sense and antisense primer were designed to amplify the *toxRS*/new sequence by GS-PCR. Similarly, the PGS-PCR yields an amplicon of 235-bp GS sequence of an arbitrarily primed-PCR fragment for 930 bp carried by the pandemic strains of this organism. Accordingly, all the pathogenic (*tdh*⁺) isolates (n=20) were subjected for both PGS-PCR and GS-PCR to determine their pandemic potentials and 11 (6.5%) were found positive in PGS-PCR assay that belonged to crab 6 (7.3%) and shrimp 5 (6%) (Table-1). However, two isolates were found positive in GS-PCR assay and belonged to crab. These two GS-PCR⁺ isolates from crab were also positive in PGS-PCR. The findings indicate that a considerable percentage of shellfishes in these areas were carrying pathogenic *V. parahaemolyticus* that was having well-recognized pandemic potentials in their genotype. The findings also highlight the alarm of public health risk on consumption of improperly processed and cooked shellfishes from such sources. The result also revealed that the PGS-PCR could identify the pandemic potential GS sequence in 6.5% of *tdh*⁺ *V. parahaemolyticus* isolates whereas GS-PCR could do in 1.2% of such isolates. The findings support the preference of PGS-PCR on GS-PCR in detecting the pandemic strains of *V. parahaemolyticus* of saline water origin. The present findings were in accord to the observation of earlier study [21] where a group of pandemic and non-pandemic *V. parahaemolyticus* isolates were extensively examined for identifying the GS pandemic potential gene sequence and concluded that the PGS-PCR assay can be a useful molecular tool not only for identification of pandemic *V. parahaemolyticus* strains but also for direct detection of this organism contaminating food and environmental samples.

Altogether, a constant surveillance on the occurrence of this pathogen in index clinical cases and thereafter, identifying the suspected foods may be beneficial to a large extent to combat the public health problems caused by this pathogen. Further, inculcation of the utmost effective measures, i.e., to educate the people routinely about fundamentals of public health and hygiene will certainly be contributory to reduce the occurrence of health problem with this pathogen and to project a healthy community life.

Conclusion

This study was envisaged to proximate the occurrence of pathogenic and pandemic *V. parahaemolyticus* in saline water origin shellfishes retailed in coastal parts of Eastern India mainly in and around Kolkata and Bhubaneswar by characterizing their virulence and pandemic genotypes. From the present study, it was concluded that a considerable percentage of shellfishes in these areas are inflicted with pathogenic (*tdh*⁺) (11.9%) and pandemic (6.5%) *V. parahaemolyticus*. This poses public health risk in consumption of improperly processed shellfishes. The health risk arising with cross contamination by such shellfishes to other marine and fresh water market fishes in these areas may be an additional point of risk.

Authors' Contributions

This work is the part of M. V. Sc. dissertation work of SP. SP and SCD designed the experiment. SP conducted the experimental work. SCD and AK were involved in scientific discussion and analysis of the data. SCD and AK drafted and revised the manuscript. All authors read and approved the final manuscript.

Acknowledgments

The authors are thankful to the Director, ICAR-IVRI, Deemed University, Bareilly, Uttar Pradesh for providing the necessary funds and facilities for the current study. The authors are also thankful to Dr. T. Ramamurthy, Senior Deputy Director, National Institute of Cholera and Enteric diseases, Kolkata for providing reference *V. parahaemolyticus* strains Vp-Kx-V₁₃₈ and technical advises.

Competing Interests

The authors declare that they have no competing interests.

References

1. Newton, A., Kendall, M., Vugia, D.J., Henao, O.L. and Mahon, B.E. (2012) Increasing rates of Vibriosis in the United States, 1996-2010: Review of surveillance data from 2 systems. *Clin. Infect. Dis.*, 54(5): 391-395.

2. Nelapati, S., Nelapati, K. and Chinnam, B.K. (2012) *Vibrio parahaemolyticus*: An emerging foodborne pathogen - A review. *Vet. World*, 5(1): 48-62.

3. Kaneko, T. and Colwell, R.R. (1973) Ecology of *Vibrio parahaemolyticus* in Chesapeake bay. *J. Bacteriol.*, 113: 24-32.

4. Su, Y.C. and Liu, C. (2007) *Vibrio parahaemolyticus*: A concern of seafood safety. *Food Microbiol.*, 24: 549-558.

5. Charles-Hernandez, G.L., Cifuentes, E. and Rothenberg, S.J. (2006) Environmental factors associated with the presence of *Vibrio parahaemolyticus* in sea products and the risk of food poisoning in communities bordering the Gulf of Mexico. *J. Environ. Health* Res., 5: 75-80.

6. Ray, B. and Bhunia, A. (2008) Fundamental Food Microbiology. 4th ed. CRC Press, New Delhi.

7. Jones, J.L., Ludeke, C.H.M., Bowers, J.C., Garrett, N., Fischer, M., Parsons, M.B., Bopp, C.A. and DePaola, A. (2012) Biochemical, serological, and virulence characterization of clinical and oyster *Vibrio parahaemolyticus* Isolates. *J. Clin. Microbiol.*, 50(7): 2343-2352.

8. Sakazaki, R., Tamura, K., Kato, T., Obara, Y., Yamai, S. and Hobo, K. (1968) Studies of enteropathogenic facultative halophilic bacteria *Vibrio parahaemolyticus* III. Enteropathogenicity. *Jpn. J. Med. Sci. Biol.*, 21: 325-331.

9. Pal, S.C., Sircar, B.K., Nair, G.B. and Deb, B.C. (1985) Epidemiology of bacterial diarrheal diseases in India with special reference to *Vibrio parahaemolyticus* infections. In: Takeda, Y. and Miwatani, T. editors. Bacterial Diarrheal Diseases. KTK Scientific Publishers, Tokyo, Japan. p65-73.

10. Okuda, J., Ishibashi, M., Hayakawa, E., Nishino, T., Takeda, Y., Mukhopadhyay, A.K., Garg, S., Bhattacharya, S.K., Nair, G.B. and Nishibuchi, M. (1997) Emergence of a unique O3:K6 clone of *Vibrio parahaemolyticus* in Calcutta, India and isolation of strains from the same clonal group from Southeast Asian travelers arriving in Japan. *J. Clin. Microbiol.*, 35(12): 3150-3155.

11. Chowdhury, N.R., Chakraborty, S., Ramamurthy, T., Nishibuchi, M., Yamasaki, S., Takeda, Y. and Nair, G.B. (2000) Molecular evidence of clonal *Vibrio parahaemolyticus* pandemic strains. *Emerg. Infect. Dis.*, 6: 631-636.

12. Kanungo, S., Sur, D., Ali, M., You, Y.A., Pal, D., Manna, B., Niyogi, S.K., Sarkar, B., Bhattacharya, S.K., Clemens, J.D. and Nair, G.B. (2012) Clinical, epidemiological, and spatial characteristics of *Vibrio parahaemolyticus* diarrhea and cholera in the urban slums of Kolkata, India. *BMC Public Health*, 12: 830-838.

13. Pazhani, G.P., Bhowmik, S.K., Ghosh, S., Guin, S., Dutta, S., Rajendran, K., Saha, D.R., Nandy, R.K., Bhattacharya, M.K., Mukhopadhyay, A.K. and Ramamurthy, T. (2014) Trends in the epidemiology of pandemic and non pandemic strains of *Vibrio parahaemolyticus* isolated from Diarrheal Patients in Kolkata, India. *PLoS Negl. Trop. Dis.*, 8(5): e2815.

14. Pal, D. and Das, N. (2010) Isolation, identification and molecular characterization of *Vibrio parahaemolyticus* from fish samples in Kolkata. *Eur. Rev. Med. Pharmacol. Sci.*, 14: 545-549.

15. Anjay, Das, S.C., Kumar, A., Kaushik, P. and Kurmi, B. (2013) Detection of *Vibrio parahaemolyticus* from saltwater fish samples by Vp-*toxR* PCR. *Indian J. Fish.*, 60(1): 141-143.

16. Anjay, Das, S.C., Kumar, A., Kaushik, P. and Kurmi, B. (2014) Occurrence of *Vibrio sswparahaemolyticus* in marine fish and shellfish. *Indian J. Geo-Marine Sci.*, 43(5): 887-990.

17. Food and Drug Administration (FDA). (2004) Bacteriological Analytical Manual on Line. 8th ed., Ch. 9. Revision A. 1998. AOAC International, Arlington, VA.

18. Kim, Y.B., Okuda, J., Matsumoto, C., Takahasi, N., Hashimoto, S. and Nishibuichi, M. (1999) Identification of *Vibrio parahaemolyticus* strains at species level by PCR targeted to *toxR* gene. *J. Clin. Microbiol.*, 37: 1173-1177.

19. Tada, J., Ohashi, T., Nishimura, N., Shirasaki, Y., Ozaki, H., Fukushima, S., Takano, J., Nishibuchi, M. and Takeda, Y. (1992) Detection of the thermostable direct hemolysin gene (tdh) and the thermostable direct hemolysin-related hemolysin gene (trh) of *Vibrio parahaemolyticus* by polymerase chain reaction. *Mol. Cell. Probes*, 6(6): 477-487.

20. Matsumoto, C., Okuda, J., Ishibashi, M., Iwanaga, M., Garg, P., Ramamurthy, T., Wong, H., Depaola, A., Kim, Y.B., Albert, M.J.M. and Nishibushi, M. (2000) Pandemic spread of an O3:K6 clone of *Vibrio parahaemolyticus* and emergence of related strains evidenced by arbitrarily primed PCR and toxRS sequence analysis. *J. Clin. Microbiol.*, 38: 578-585.

21. Okura, M., Osawa, R., Iguchi, A., Takagi, M., Arakawa, E., Terajima, J. and Watanabe, H. (2004) PCR-based identification of pandemic group *Vibrio parahaemolyticus* with a novel group-specific primer pair. *Microbiol. Immunol.*, 48: 787-790.

22. Austin, B. (2010) Vibrios as causal agents of zoonoses. *Vet. Microbiol.*, 140: 310-317.

23. Deepanjali, A., Kumar, H.S. and Karunasagar, I. (2005) Seasonal variation in abundance of total and pathogenic *Vibrio parahaemolyticus* bacteria in oysters along the Southwest coast of India. *Appl. Environ. Microbiol.*, 71: 3575-3580.

24. Ward, L.N. and Bej, A.K. (2006) Detection of *Vibrio parahaemolyticus* in shellfish by use of multiplexed real-time PCR with *Taq*Man fluorescent probes. *Appl. Environ. Microbiol.*, 72(3): 2031-2042.

25. Broberg, C.A., Calder, T.J. and Orth, K. (2011) *Vibrio parahaemolyticus* cell biology and pathogenicity determinants. *Microbes Infect.*, 13: 992-1001.

26. Hara-Kudo, Y., Sugiyama, K., Nishibuchi, M., Chowdhury, A., Yatsuyanagi, J., Ohtomo, Y., Saito, A., Nagano, H., Nishina, T., Nakagawa, H., Konuma, H., Miyahara, M. and Kumagai, S. (2003) Prevalence of thermostable direct haemolysin-producing *Vibrio parahaemolyticus* O3:K6 in seafood and coastal environment in Japan. *Appl. Environ. Microbiol.*, 69(7): 3883-3891.

27. Sujeewa, A.K., Norrakiah, A.S. and Laina, M. (2009) Prevalence of toxic genes of *Vibrio parahaemolyticus* in shrimps (*Penaeus monodon*) and culture environment. *Int. Food Res. J.*, 16: 89-95.

28. Koralage, M., Alter, T., Pichpol, D., Strauch, E., Zessin, K. and Huehn, S. (2012) Prevalence and molecular characteristics of *Vibrio* spp. Isolated from pre-harvest shrimp of the North Western Province of Sri Lanka. *J. Food Prot.*, 75: 1846-1850.

29. Martinez-Urtaza, J., Simental, L., Velasco, D., DePaola, A., Ishibashi, M., Nakaguchi, Y., Nishibuchi, M., Carrera-Flores, D., Rey-Alvarez, C. and Pousa, A. (2005) Pandemic *Vibrio parahaemolyticus* O3:K6, Europe. *Emerg. Infect. Dis.*, 11(8): 1319-1320.

30. Daniels, N.A., MacKinnon, L., Bishop, R., Altekruse, S., Ray, B., Hammond, R.M., Thompson, S., Wilson, S., Bean, N.H., Graffin, P.M. and Slutsker, L. (2000) *Vibrio parahaemolyticus* infections in the United States, 1973-1998. *J. Infect. Dis.*, 181: 1661-1666.

31. Sudha, S., Divya, P.S., Francis, B. and Hatha, A.A.M. (2012) Prevalence and distribution of *Vibrio parahaemolyticus* in finfish from Cochin (south India). *Vet. Ital.*, 48(3): 269-281.

32. Sudha, S., Mridula, C., Selvester, R. and Hatha, A.A.M. (2014) Prevalence and antibiotic resistance of pathogenic Vibrios in shellfish from Cochin market. *Indian J. Geo-Marine Sci.*, 43(5): 815-824.

32

Effect of supplemental heat on mortality rate, growth performance, and blood biochemical profiles of Ghungroo piglets in Indian sub-tropical climate

Hemanta Nath[1], Mousumi Hazorika[1], Dipjyoti Rajkhowa[2], Mrinmoy Datta[1] and Avijit Haldar[1]

1. Animal Reproduction Division, ICAR Research Complex for North Eastern Hill Region, Tripura Centre, Agartala, Lembucherra, West Tripura, India; 2. ICAR Research Complex for NEH Region, Barapani, Umiam, Meghalaya, India.
Corresponding author: Avijit Haldar, e-mail: avijit_vet@rediffmail.com,
HN: johnnath2000@gmail.com, MH: mausumihazorika5@gmail.com,
DR: djrajkhowa@gmail.com, MD: mdatta2@rediffmail.com

Abstract

Aim: The present study was conducted to explore the effect of supplemental heat on mortality rate, growth performance, and blood biochemical profiles of indigenous Ghungroo piglets in sub-tropical cold and humid climatic conditions of Tripura, a state of the north eastern hill (NEH) region of India.

Materials and Methods: The experiment was conducted on 38 indigenous Ghungroo piglets from birth up to 60 days of age. Among the 38 piglets, 19 piglets were provided with supplemental heat ranging between 17.0°C and 21.1°C for the period of the first 30 days and thereafter between 24.1°C and 29.9°C for the next 30 days. The other 19 piglets were exposed to natural environmental minimum temperatures ranging between 7.2°C and 15.0°C during the first 30 days and then between 18.5°C and 25.5°C for the next 30 days.

Results: The supplemental heat resulted in 10.6% reduction of piglet mortality from the 2nd till the 7th day of age. These beneficial effects could be related with the lower ($p<0.05$) plasma glutamate pyruvate transaminase (GPT) and cortisol levels and higher ($p<0.05$) plasma alkaline phosphatase (AP) concentrations in heat supplemented group compared to control group. Plasma AP, GPT, glucose, triiodothyronine, and luteinizing hormone concentrations decreased ($p<0.05$) gradually with the advancement of age in both control and supplemental heat treated piglets.

Conclusion: Supplemental heat could be beneficial since it is related to a reduction of piglet mortality during the first week of life under farm management system in the sub-tropical climate of NEH region of India.

Keywords: biochemical profiles, Ghungroo piglets, growth, mortality rate, neonatal, supplemental heat.

Introduction

The survivability and growth of piglets are very important economic aspects for the success of pig farming. Piglet mortality during the perinatal and lactational period is one of the most crucial factors leading to reduced production efficiency in pig farming [1,2]. Besides, the economic losses, piglet mortality also represent a livestock welfare issue. The primary causes of live born piglet mortality are hypothermia, starvation, and crushing [3]. Newborn piglets are poorly insulated and lack of brown adipose tissue, and thus rely exclusively on shivering as the main mechanism for thermogenesis in the cold environment [4]. At birth, they usually experience a sudden drop of 2-4°C in the body temperature, and recovery of a normothermic temperature of 39°C is achieved after 24-48 h of life in adequate environmental condition [5]. However, excessive hypothermia due to severe environmental conditions, low body weight, or reduced vitality at birth could significantly reduce piglet vigor leading to the death of the animal [6]. Impairment of cellular immunity, another factor strongly related to piglet survival, is associated with overexpression of heat shock protein 70 in neonatal pigs [7].

Floor heating has favorable effects on the early recovery of piglet body temperature, latency to first suckle, and survival of piglets [8]. Straw can be used on the floor to provide warmth to the piglets during winter months. However, proximity to the straw is a concern with regard to increasing the risk of piglets crushing and enteritis [9]. Recent studies indicate that the maternal diet modulates the epigenetic regulation of hepatic gluconeogenic genes in neonatal piglets [10]. Limited studies concerning the provision of the warm environment to the newborn piglets and its beneficial effects on piglet's survivability and performance have previously been performed with exotic pure or crossbred piglets in temperate climate [11]. However, there is no information on the effect of supplemental heat on the performance of indigenous piglets during winter in the Indian sub-tropical climate.

The aim of the present study was to explore the effect of supplemental heat on mortality rate, growth performance, and blood biochemical profiles of indigenous Ghungroo piglets during cold and humid weather in the north eastern sub-tropical region of India.

Materials and Methods

Ethical approval

The experimental protocol and animal care were in accordance with the National Guidelines for care and use of Agricultural Animals in Agricultural Research and Teaching.

Study area

The present study was conducted at pig farm of the Indian Council of Agricultural Research (ICAR) Complex, Tripura Centre, Lembucherra, West Tripura, India located at 22°56/N latitude and 90°09/E longitude. During the 60 days experimental period, meteorological data were daily recorded. The climate was cold and humid with environmental minimum temperature ranging between 7.2°C and 15°C and 18.5°C and 25.5°C during the periods of 1st-30th and 31st-60th day, respectively. The temperature humidity index per day was calculated according to Johnson et al. [12] and presented in Figure-1.

Animals and management

About 38 indigenous Ghungroo piglets were randomly selected from 4 lactating sows one day after their birth. Each sow with its litter was housed in well-ventilated individual pens with brick flooring and asbestos roofing. The supplemental heat was provided to 19 piglets (10 piglets from sow no. 2549 and 9 piglets from sow no. 2531) by placing three 100 W bulbs 3 ft high from the floor for each pen. Temperature values of the heat supplemented pens ranged from 17.0°C to 21.1°C for the first 30 days period and between 24.1°C and 29.9°C for the next 30 days. These piglets were considered as the treatment group. Another 19 piglets (11 piglets from sow no. 2541 and 8 piglets from sow no. 2546) were housed in separate two pens under natural environmental conditions and considered as the control group. The environmental minimum and maximum temperature along with room temperature after supplemental heat are shown in Figure-2.

Fresh and clean water was offered *ad libitum* by a water trough and piglets had also free access to suckle. They were treated with iron dextran (Imferon®, M/s. Shreya, India) intramuscularly at 3, 7, and 14 days of age and vaccinated with swine fever vaccine at 45 days of age. Piglet mortality rates were daily recorded during the experimental period.

Body weight and rectal temperature recording

Body weight of each piglet was recorded on the day of birth and then on a weekly basis up to 56 days of age. Rectal temperature was also recorded on the day of birth and then at 3 days interval for 60 days.

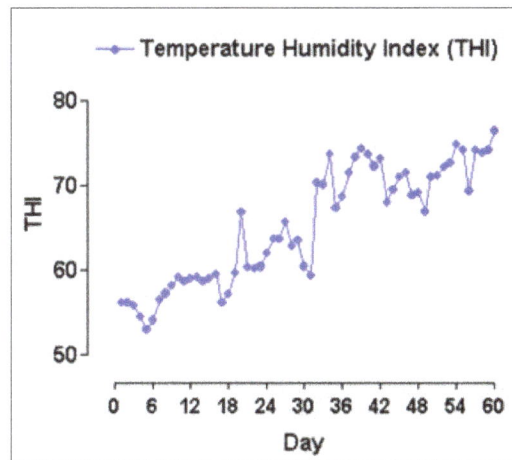

Figure-1: Daily temperature humidity index during the 60 days experimental periods (values ranged between 52.98 and 76.45).

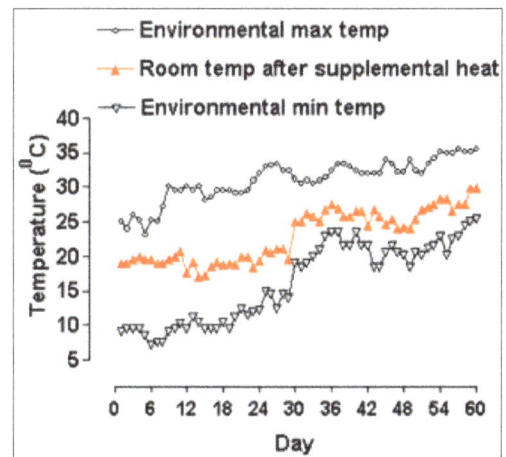

Figure-2: Daily temperature values during the 60 days experimental periods (ambient temperature ranged between 7.2°C and 15.0°C and 18.5°C and 25.5°C for the period of 1st-30th and 31st-60th day of age, respectively. In case of supplemental heat, values ranged between 17.0°C and 21.1°C and 24.1°C and 29.9°C for the period of 1st-30th and 31st-60th day of age, respectively).

Blood sampling

Each piglet was restrained in dorsoventral position and blood sample was collected into heparinized 5 ml polypropylene tubes (20 IU heparin/ml of blood) from anterior vena cava under aseptic condition using 18 gauge needle between 09:30 and 10.30 h on day 7, 15, 30, 45, and 60 of age. A fraction of blood sample was used for hemoglobin estimation using standard Sahli's acid hematin method [13]. Plasma samples were collected after centrifugation at 2500 × g for 10 min at 4°C and stored at −20°C until the implementation of plasma biochemical analyzes.

Biochemical profiling

Plasma glucose, alkaline phosphatase (AP), glutamate pyruvate transaminase (GPT), and glutamate oxaloacetate transaminase (GOT) activities were estimated colorimetrically using commercially available kits (M/s. Span Diagnostic Ltd., Surat, India).

Plasma cortisol, triiodothyronine (T3), thyroxine (T4), follicle-stimulating hormone (FSH), and luteinizing hormone (LH) were quantified by an enzyme-linked immunosorbent assay technique using the commercially available kit for swine (M/s. Endocrine Technologies, Inc., Newark, CA, USA).

Statistical analysis

Data are presented as the mean±standard error of the mean. The mean±standard error of the mean of different parameters studied were graphically presented using graph pad PRISM 2.01 Software Package (1995). The effect of treatment and period (week/day) on body weight and biochemical parameters was determined by performing an ANOVA analysis appropriate for repeated measures using the SPSS Statistical Software Package (1999), SPSS, Inc., USA.

Results and Discussion

Mortality rate

The rates of piglet mortality in control and supplementary heat treated piglet groups are presented in Figure-3. In the present experiment, mortality rates of 17.3% and 20.9% were observed at the day of birth in control and treatment groups, respectively, due to stillbirth, asphyxia, low birth weight, crushing, etc. The period between the 2nd and 7th day of age, mortality rates were 31.6% and 21.0% in control and heat supplemented groups, respectively.

This finding may be comparable to earlier observations [14]. Piglet mortality was invariably high in the first few days after birth, reflecting the problems of transition from the totally protected intrauterine life to an unpredictable extrauterine existence.

Rectal temperature

Figure-4 shows that the mean rectal temperature in both control and supplemental heat treated piglets remain between 37.31°C and 38.83°C indicating the maintenance of a normothermic temperature of 38-39°C [5].

Body weight

The mean±standard error of the mean (SEM) body weight values is presented in Figure-5. No effect (p>0.05) of supplemental heat on body weight was shown, and the daily weight gain for both groups was approximately 130 g/day. This finding is in agreement with the data of exotic piglets, which were reared under an artificial temperature between 18.5°C and 22.5°C [14]. In contrast, Adams *et al.* [15] reported that supplemental heat improved weight gain, while pigs were housed in farrowing crates with 250-watt lamp and the ambient temperature of the farrowing house was approximately 21°C at sow's level. Weight is considered as the most important factor in successful recovery from postnatal hypothermia [16].

Plasma biochemical profiles

The mean±SEM blood hemoglobin and glucose concentrations of the supplemental heat treated and the control piglets recorded at 7, 15, 30, 45, and

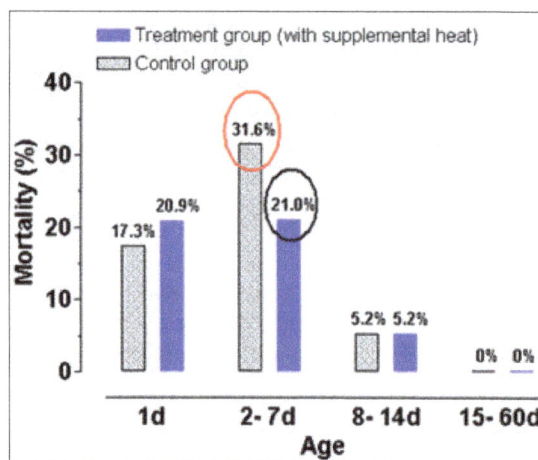

Figure-3: Piglet mortality (%) of control and supplemental heat treated piglets during the experimental period.

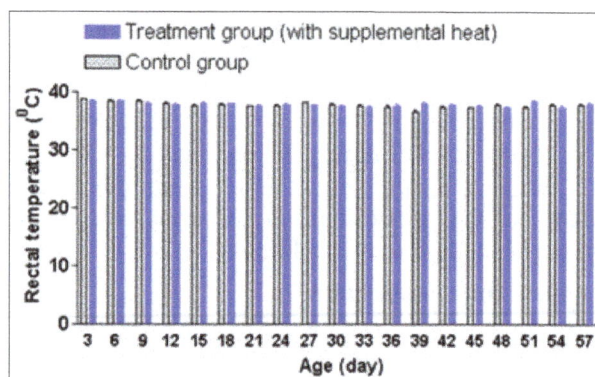

Figure-4: Mean±standard error of mean rectal temperature of control and supplemental heat treated piglets during the experimental period.

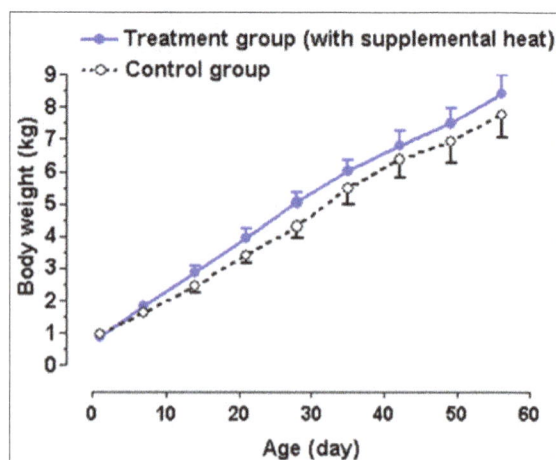

Figure-5: Mean±standard error of mean body weight of control and supplemental heat treated piglets during the experimental period.

60 days of age are presented in Figures-6 and 7, respectively. There was no significant effect (p>0.05) of the supplemental heat on the levels of these blood parameters. The mean blood hemoglobin and glucose concentrations in both groups were comparable with the values reported in 6-8 months old indigenous Assam pigs [17] and weaned Burmese pigs [18].

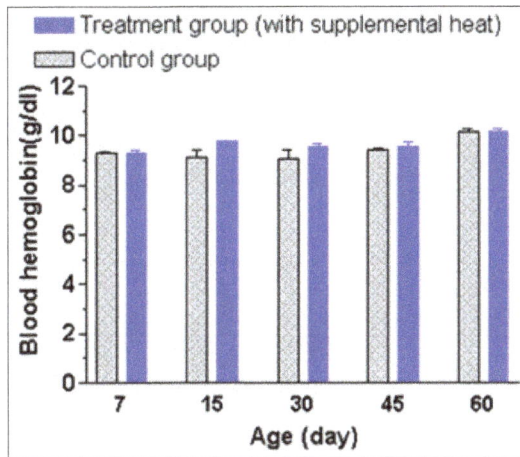

Figure-6: Mean±standard error of mean blood hemoglobin levels (g/dl) of control and supplemental heat treated piglets during the experimental period.

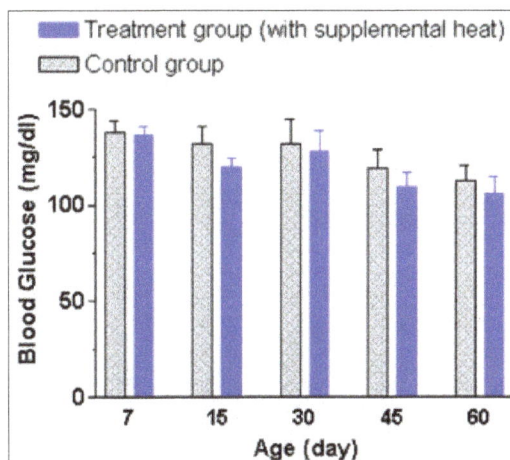

Figure-8: Mean±standard error of mean plasma alkaline phosphatase levels (U/L) of control and supplemental heat treated piglets during the experimental period (*p<0.05).

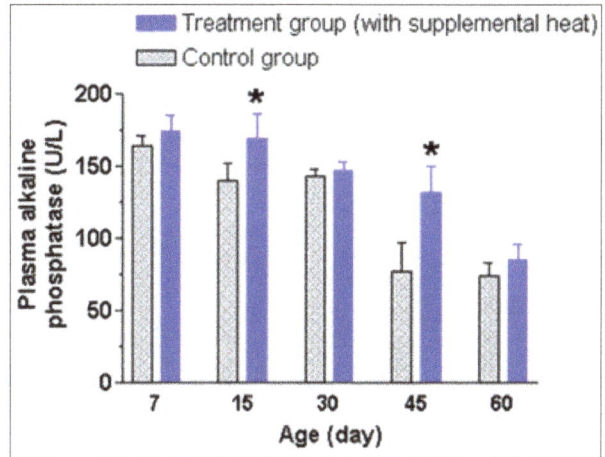

Figure-7: Mean±standard error of mean plasma glucose levels (mg/dl) of control and supplemental heat treated piglets during the experimental period.

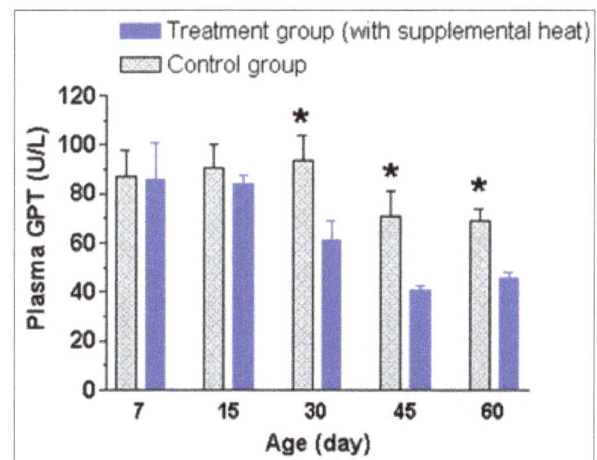

Figure-9: Mean±standard error of mean plasma glutamate pyruvate transaminase levels (U/L) of control and supplemental heat treated piglets during the experimental period (*p<0.05).

Recent reports indicated that maternal dietary protein level induced changes in the epigenetic regulation of the glucose metabolism [19] and microRNA involved lipid metabolism [20] in newborn piglet liver. Other reports indicated that plasma glucose level increased linearly when newborn piglets were exposed to the temperature of 14°C for 2-2.5 h [5]. The gradual decrease in plasma glucose concentration with the advancement of age in both experimental groups could be a result of the increase in environmental temperature as the experiment continued.

The mean±SEM plasma AP, GPT, GOT, and cortisol levels of the supplemental heat treated and the control piglets at 7, 15, 30, 45, and 60 days of age presented in Figures-8-11, respectively. Plasma AP and GPT concentration gradually decreased (p<0.05) with age in both groups (Figures-8 and 9). This decrease of plasma AP with the advancement of age in both groups indicated that the higher activity of AP possibly had a positive effect on mineralization process, osteoblastic activity, and rapid growth process of bone at the early age. In addition, the supplemental heat

possibly improved bone growth process in the heat supplemented group as plasma AP concentration was significantly higher (p<0.05) compared to that of the control group at the age of 15 and 45 days (Figure-8). The supplemental heat might also have some beneficial effects on reducing protein metabolism leading to lower (p<0.05) plasma GPT concentration in the treatment compared to the control group at the age of 30, 45, and 60 days (Figure-9). Plasma GOT levels did not vary (p>0.05) between the control and treatment groups during the experimental period (Figure-10). The mean plasma GPT and GOT levels in control and treatment groups are within the range of previously reported values [21]. The increased levels of plasma GPT during the first 2 weeks of life might be an effect of the interaction of early age with the environmental low temperature [22]. On the other hand, the gradual decrease (p<0.05) in plasma GPT at the age of 45 and 60 days in both groups possibly indicated a gradual physiological adjustment to the environmental conditions. As it is presented in Figure-11, there was a

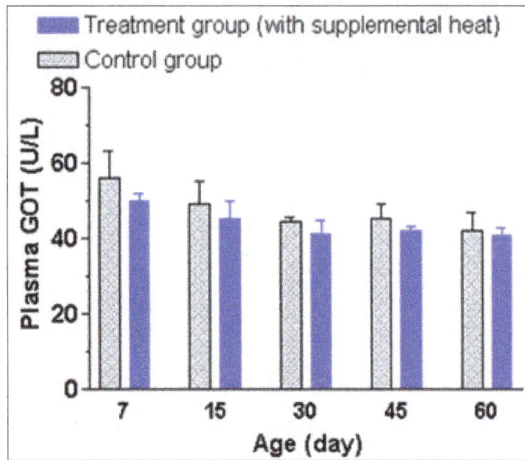

Figure-10: Mean±standard error of mean plasma glutamate oxaloacetate transaminase levels (U/L) of control and supplemental heat treated piglets during the experimental period.

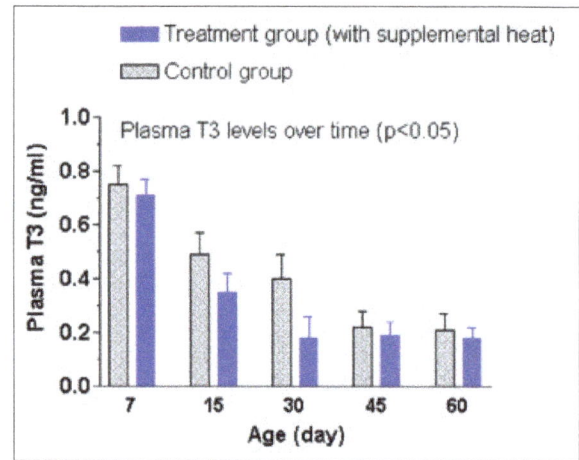

Figure-12: Mean±standard error of mean plasma triiodothyronine concentrations (ng/ml) of control and supplemental heat treated piglets during the experimental period.

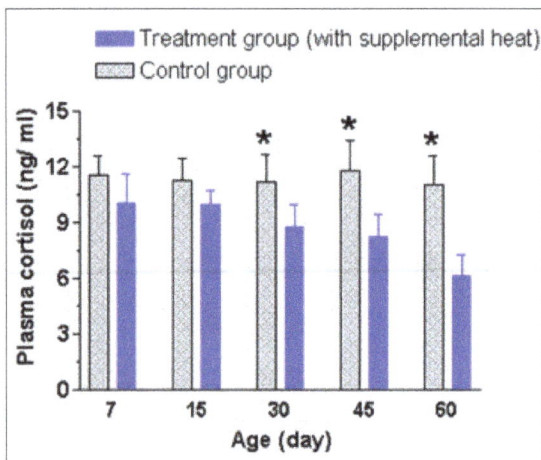

Figure-11: Mean±standard error of mean plasma cortisol concentrations (ng/ml) of control and supplemental heat treated piglets during the experimental period (*$p<0.05$).

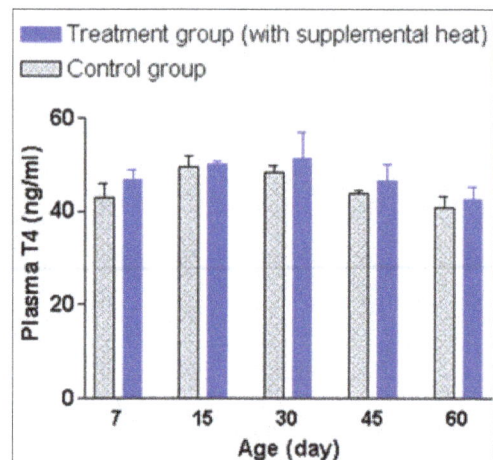

Figure-13: Mean±standard error of mean plasma thyroxine concentrations (ng/ml) of control and supplemental heat treated piglets during the experimental period.

gradual decrease of plasma cortisol concentration only in supplemental heat treated piglets. The supplemental heat resulted in lower ($p<0.05$) plasma cortisol levels on day 30, 45, and 60, as previously observed in newborn pigs on day 2 of age [14]. Possible explanation is that the supplemental heat reduced the stress of young piglets that already possess a functional hypothalamic-pituitary-adrenocortical axis.

The mean±SEM plasma T3, T4, FSH, and LH concentrations of the supplemental heat treated and the control piglets recorded at 7, 15, 30, 45, and 60 days of age are shown in Figures-12-15, respectively. No significant effect ($p>0.05$) of the supplemental heat on plasma T3, T4, FSH, and LH concentrations was demonstrated in the present study. However, plasma T3 and LH concentrations decreased ($p<0.05$) gradually with the advancement of age in both groups.

The present findings on plasma T3 and T4 concentrations in experimental piglets support the observations recorded earlier in neonatal pigs exposed to cold temperatures [23]. Evidence of an increase in the

release of thyroid-stimulating hormone (TSH) from the pituitary gland and thereby increase in secretion of the thyroid hormones from the thyroid gland in animals exposed to cold have well been documented [24]. No significant difference ($p>0.05$) of plasma T4 concentrations between the experimental groups or the gradual decrease ($p<0.05$) in plasma T3 concentrations with the advancement of age could be explained in the light of adjustments in metabolism and energy expenditure [25]. The mean plasma FSH and LH concentration in control and treatment groups were quite similar with the concentrations recorded in Landrace x Yorkshire crossbred neonatal pigs [26]. The gradual decrease ($p<0.05$) in plasma LH concentration with the advancement of age in both groups might be due to the ovarian steroid negative feedback mechanism on gonadotropin secretion in neonatal piglets [27].

Conclusions

To the best of the authors' knowledge, the present study is the first that describes the effect of

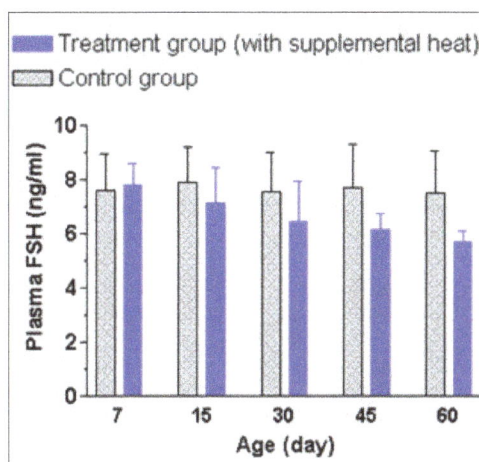

Figure-14: Mean±standard error of mean plasma follicle-stimulating hormone concentrations (ng/ml) of control and supplemental heat treated piglets during the experimental period.

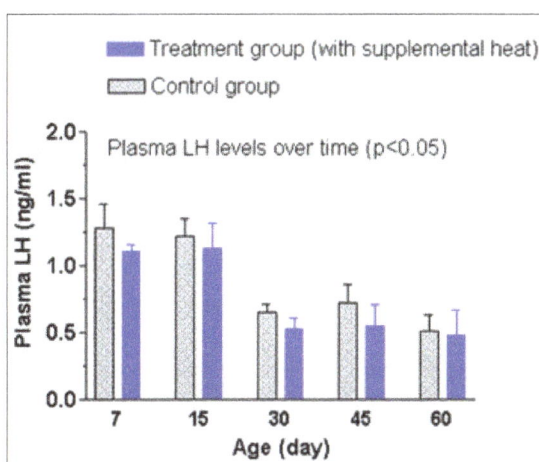

Figure-15: Mean±standard error of mean plasma luteinizing hormone concentrations (ng/ml) of control and supplemental heat treated piglets during the experimental period.

supplemental heat on mortality rate, growth performance, and blood biochemical profiles of indigenous Ghungroo piglets during cold and humid weather in north eastern hill of India. The supplemental heat resulted in approximately 10% reduction of piglet mortality during the first week of life under farm management system in the sub-tropical cold and humid climatic conditions of north eastern region of India. However, the observations on the effect of supplemental heat on piglet performance warrant validation on different breeds of piglets. The effect of supplemental heat at higher temperatures on piglet performances also needs to be examined.

Authors' Contributions

All authors contributed to conception and design of the study. HN and MH worked together at the farm as well as research laboratory to collect data. MD analyzed data. DR monitored the whole research program. AH interpreted the results and drafted the article critically for important intellectual content. All authors read and approved the final manuscript.

Acknowledgments

The necessary fund provided by National Initiative on Climate Resilient Agriculture (NICRA) of Indian Council of Agricultural Research (ICAR), New Delhi, India is duly acknowledged. The authors are thankful to the Director of ICAR Research Complex for NEH Region, Barapani, Umiam, Meghalaya - 793 103, India for his constant support to carry out the study. The authors wish to express their sincere thanks to all the technical staff of Livestock Division of ICAR Research Complex for North Eastern Hill Region, Tripura Centre, Agartala, Lembucherra - 799 210, West Tripura, India for their regular help and cooperation during the investigation.

Competing Interests

The authors declare that they have no competing interests.

References

1. Kirkden, R.D., Broom, D.M. and Andersen, I.L. (2013) Invited review: Piglet mortality: Management solutions. *J. Anim. Sci.*, 91(7): 3361-3389.
2. Strange, T., Ask, B. and Nielsen, B. (2013) Genetic parameters of the piglet mortality traits stillbirth, weak at birth, starvation, crushing and miscellaneous in crossbred pigs. *J. Anim. Sci.,* 91(4): 1562-1569.
3. Herpin, P., Damon, M. and Le Dividich, J. (2002) Development of thermoregulation and neonatal survival in pigs. *Livest. Prod. Sci.*, 78: 25-45.
4. Berthon, D., Herpin, P., Bertin, R., De Marco, F. and le Dividich, J. (1996) Metabolic changes associated with sustained 48-hr shivering thermogenesis in the newborn pig. *Comp. Biochem. Physiol. B Biochem. Mol. Biol.*, 114: 327-335.
5. Lossec, G., Herpin, P. and Le Dividich, J. (1998) Thermoregulatory responses of the newborn pig during experimentally induced hypothermia and rewarming. *J. Exp. Physiol.*, 83: 667-678.
6. Alonso-Spilsbury, M., Mota-Rojas, D., Villanueva-Garcia, D., Martines-Burnes, J., Orozco, H., Ramirez-Necoechea, R., Lopez, M.A. and Truijillo, M.E. (2005) Perinatal asphyxia pathophysiology and human: A review. *Anim. Reprod. Sci.*, 90: 1-30.
7. Zhong, X., Li, W., Huang, X., Zhang, L., Yimamu, M., Raiput, N., Zhou, Y. and Wang, T. (2012) Impairment of cellular immunity is associated with overexpression of heat shock protein 70 in neonatal pigs with intrauterine growth retardation. *Cell Stress Chaperones.*, 17(4): 495-505.
8. Pedersen, L.J., Malmkvist, J., Kammersgaard, T. and Jørgensen, E. (2013) Avoiding hypothermia in neonatal pigs: Effect of duration of floor heating at different room temperatures. *J. Anim. Sci.,* 91(1): 425-432.
9. Westin, R., Holmgren, N., Hultgren, J., Ortman, K., Linder, A. and Algers, B. (2015) Post-mortem findings and piglet mortality in relation to strategic use of straw at farrowing. *Prev. Vet. Med.,* 119(3-4): 141-152.
10. Cai, D., Jia, Y., Song, H., Sui, S., Lu, J., Jiang, Z. and Zhao, R. (2014) Betaine supplementation in maternal diet modulates the epigenetic regulation of hepatic gluconeogenic genes in neonatal piglets. *PLoS One,* 9(8): e105504.
11. Kenneth, B. (1986) Bioenergetics and growth: The whole and the parts. *J. Anim. Sci.,* 63: 1-10.
12. Johnson, H.D., Ragsdale, A.C., Berry, I.L. and

Shanklin, M.D. (1963) Temperature humidity effects including influence of acclimation feed and water consumption of Holstein cattle. Missouri University, Agricultural Experiment Station Research, Bullet No. 846. Columbia.

13. Sahli, H. (1909) Untersuchungen Methode. 5th ed. Lehrbuch d klin, Leipzig. p846.

14. McGinnis, R.M., Marple, D.N., Ganjam, V.K., Prince, T.J. and Pritchett, J.F. (1981) The effect of floor temperature, supplemental heat and drying at birth on neonatal swine. *J. Anim. Sci.*, 53: 1424-1431.

15. Adams, K.L., Baker, T.H. and Jensen, A.H. (1980) Effect of supplemental heat for nursing piglets. *J. Anim. Sci.*, 50: 779-782.

16. Kammersgaard, T.S., Pedersen, L.J. and Jørgensen, E. (2011) Hypothermia in neonatal piglets: Interactions and causes of individual differences. *J. Anim. Sci.*, 89(7): 2073-2085.

17. Phookan, A., Laskar, S., Goswami, R.N. and Deori, S. (2011) Hemoglobin type, hemoglobin concentration and serum alkaline phosphatase level in indigenous pigs of Assam. *Tamilnadu J. Vet. Anim. Sci.*, 7: 110-111.

18. Sarma, K., Konwar, B. and Ali, A. (2011) Hemato-biochemical parameters of Burmese pig of subtropical hill agro ecosystem. *Indian J. Anim. Sci.*, 81: 819-821.

19. Jia, Y., Cong, R., Li, R., Yang, X., Sun, Q., Parvizi, N. and Zhao, R. (2012) Maternal low-protein diet induces gender-dependent changes in epigenetic regulation of the glucose-6-phosphatase gene in newborn piglet liver. *J. Nutr.,* 142(9): 1659-1665.

20. Pan, S., Zheng, Y., Zhao, R. and Yang, X. (2013) MicroRNA-130b and microRNA-374b mediate the effect of maternal dietary protein on offspring lipid metabolism in Meishan pigs. *Br. J. Nutr.*, 109(10): 1731-1738.

21. Dhanotiya, R.S. (2006) Textbook of Veterinary Biochemistry. 2nd ed. Jaypee Brothers Medical Publishers, (P) Ltd., New Delhi.

22. Nirupama, R., Devaki, M. and Yajurvedi, H.N. (2010) Repeated acute stress induced alternations in carbohydrate metabolism in rats. *J. Stress Physiol. Biochem.*, 6: 44-55.

23. Macari, M., Dauncey, M.J., Ramsden, D.B. and Ingram, D.Z. (1983) Thyroid hormone metabolism after acclimatization to a warm or cold temperature under the condition of high or low energy intake. *J. Exp. Physiol.*, 68: 709-718.

24. Macari, M., Zuim, S.M., Secato, E.R. and Guerreiro, J.R. (1986) Effect of ambient temperature and thyroid hormone on food intake by pigs. *J. Physiol. Behav.*, 36: 1035-1090.

25. Laurberg, P., Anderson, S. and Kermisolt, J. (2005) Cold adaptation and thyroid hormone metabolism: Review. *Horm. Metab. Res.*, 37: 545-549.

26. Colenbrander, B., Meijer, J.C., Macdonald, A.A., Van De Wiel, D.F.M., Engel, B. and De Jong, F.H. (1987) Feedback regulation of gonadotropic hormone secretion in neonatal pigs. *Biol. Reprod.*, 36: 871-877.

27. Campbell, C.S. and Schwartz, M.B. (1977) Steroid feedback regulation of luteinizing hormone and follicle - Stimulating hormone secretion rates in male and females rats. *J. Toxicol. Environ. Health.*, 3: 61-95.

33

Immunotoxicological, biochemical, and histopathological studies on Roundup and Stomp herbicides in Nile catfish (*Clarias gariepinus*)

Gihan G. Moustafa, F. E. Shaaban, A. H. Abo Hadeed, and Walaa M. Elhady

Department of Forensic Medicine and Toxicology, Faculty of Veterinary Medicine, Zagazig University, Alzeraa Street Postal Code 44511, Zagazig City, Sharkia Province, Egypt.
Corresponding author: Gihan G. Moustafa, e-mail: gihan292@hotmail.com,
FES: mahmoudnasr292@hotmail.com, AHAH: alidido@hotmail.com, WME: drwalaaelhady@yahoo.com

Abstract

Aim: The current study was directed to investigate the immunotoxic and oxidative stress effects of Roundup and Stomp herbicides and their combination on Nile catfish (*Clarias gariepinus*).

Materials and Methods: The experiment was carried out on 120 fish that randomly divided into four equal groups with three replicates: The first group kept as control, the second group exposed to 1/2 96 h lethal concentration 50 (LC_{50}) of Roundup, the third group exposed to 1/2 96 h LC_{50} of Stomp, and the fourth one exposed to a combination of Roundup and Stomp at previously-mentioned doses. The experiment was terminated after 15 days; blood samples were obtained at 1st, 8th, and 15th days of treatment where the sera were separated for estimation of antioxidant enzymes. Meanwhile, at 15th day of exposure part of blood was collected from all groups with an anticoagulant for evaluation of phagocytic activity, then the fish were sacrificed, and specimens from the liver of all groups were obtained for histopathological examination.

Results: Our results indicated that both herbicides either individually or in combination elucidated significant decrease in phagocytic activity that was highly marked in group exposed to both herbicides. Furthermore, our data elicited an obvious elevation in the levels of superoxide dismutase (SOD), catalase (CAT), and glutathione peroxidase (GPx). Meanwhile, the data depicted reduction in levels of reduced glutathione (GSH) and glutathione-S-transferase (GST). Histopathological investigation of liver proved the aforementioned results.

Conclusion: It could be concluded that either Roundup or Stomp alone cause significant deleterious effects on aquatic vertebrates. However, the use of their combination enhanced their toxic effects. Toxicity can end up in humans through the food chain.

Keywords: antioxidant enzymes, fish, phagocytosis, Roundup, Stomp.

Introduction

Worldwide, pesticide use has increased dramatically over the past two decades [1]. Pesticides have become some of the most frequently occurring organic pollutants of agricultural soils, ground and surface water, causing ecological imbalances [2] that may have toxicological effects on natural ecosystems, especially aquatic systems [3]. They cause damage to non-target organisms including fish [4]. The runoff of pesticides (insecticides, herbicides, and fungicides) from agricultural lands is a key concern for the health of aquatic organisms [5].

Herbicides are actively used in terrestrial and aquatic ecosystems to control unwanted weeds, and their use has generated serious concerns about the potential adverse effects of these chemicals on the environment and human health [6]. They are the most widely used chemicals in agriculture as they are account for about 40% of the pesticides volume used worldwide. Roundup is one of the most common herbicides used in agriculture and also used in forestry and horticulture including home use [7]. Moreover, it is being the most popular and widely used herbicide in most parts of the world [8]. The indiscriminate use of Roundup associated with careless handling, accidental spillage, or discharge of untreated effluents into natural waterways has caused harmful effects on aquatic life and may have contributed to long-term biological effects [9].

Stomp is liquid emulsive herbicide of the dinitroaniline type; its active ingredient is pendimethalin [10]. Pendimethalin is highly toxic to fish and aquatic invertebrates [11].

Reactive oxygen species (ROS) generation is continuously produced in biological systems either as side products of aerobic metabolism or products of specialized systems designed to produce ROS [12]. Perez *et al.* [13] examined the effects of three widely used pesticides that have been widely detected in aquatic systems, in which they found that binary mixtures elicited synergistic responses; however, aquatic organisms are rarely exposed to only one single contaminant but typically to mixtures of numerous pesticides with varying constituents in varying concentrations and concentration ratios. Biochemical markers, such as lipid peroxidation (LPO) and antioxidant enzymes, are widely used to assess the toxic stress, integrity of the immune system, and tissue damage in different organisms [14].

Although there is a considerable amount of information available on toxicity of individual herbicides to fish and aquatic invertebrates, there is less information on toxicity of herbicide mixtures to these organisms. Furthermore, the impacts of Stomp in fish have so far undergone little research, and there is still a great need to properly assess the impact of Stomp on fish. Therefore, the present work was conducted to shed some light on the hazardous effects of Roundup- and Stomp-based herbicides and their combination on Nile catfish (*Clarias gariepinus*).

Materials and Methods

Ethical approval

All animal-related procedures were carried out in accordance with the Ethical Committee of Zagazig University.

Fish and experimental design

A total number of 120 Nile catfish (*C. gariepinus*) with a body weight ranged from 90 to 115 g were used. Fish were obtained from the ponds of the Central Laboratory of Aquaculture Research, Abbassa, Abou-Hammad, Sharkia, Egypt. Fish were apparently healthy and free from skin lesions or external parasites; they were maintained in glass aquaria (50x40x150 cm capacity) having 180 L of dechlorinated tap water. Each aquarium provided with aerator, thermostatically controlled with heater and thermometer. Fish were acclimatized for 2 weeks to the laboratory environment. Fish were fed 3 times daily on a basal diet contained 35.4% crude protein (from Hendrix Co.) The amount of food per day was 3% of fish body weight. The experiment was conducted for 2 weeks.

The fish were divided into four equal groups: The first group kept as control, the second group exposed to 1/2 96 h lethal concentration 50 (LC_{50}) of Roundup (14.5 mg/L) [15], whereas the third one exposed to 1/2 96 h LC_{50} of Stomp (420 µg/L) [16]. The fourth group exposed to a combination of 1/2 96 h LC_{50} of both of Roundup and Stomp.

Tested compounds

Roundup (glyphosate-based herbicide)

It was obtained in a commercial form Roundup. It is containing 48% emulsion concentration (EC), obtained from Monsanto Agriculture Company, USA.

Empirical Formula: $C_3H_8NO_5P$

Chemical Formula: N- (phosphonomethyl) glycine.

State: Clear, viscous amber-colored solution.

Stomp (pendimethalin-based herbicide)

Stomp®, it is containing 50% EC (BASF PLC), an orange-yellow liquid emulsive herbicide of the dinitroaniline type [17]. It contains the inert components (50%), as petroleum solvents (naphthalene and ethylene dichloride).

Empirical formula: $C_{13}H_{19}N_3O$.

Chemical formula: [n-(1-ethylpropyl)-3,4dimethyl-2,6-dinitrobenzenamine].

State: Orange-yellow solution.

Sampling and measurements

Blood samples were obtained at 1st, 8th, and 15th days of treatment; blood samples were collected from the caudal blood vessel [18] using sterile syringes, which was left to be clotted at room temperature followed by centrifugation at 3000 rpm, for 15 min for serum separation for biochemical studies, another part of blood at 15th day of exposure was collected in glass tubes containing 10% ethylenediaminetetraacetic acid (EDTA) solution and centrifuged at 3000 rpm for 30 min. The plasma was removed completely followed by separation of leukocytes for evaluation of phagocytic activity, and then fish were sacrificed by decapitation and dissected. Specimens from livers of the treated and control groups were obtained and preserved in 10% neutral-buffered formalin for histopathological examination.

Immunotoxic study

Chemicals used for studying the phagocytic activity

1. Microbial strain: *Candida albicans* was kindly supplied by the Department of Bacteriology, Mycology and Immunity, Faculty of Veterinary Medicine, Zagazig University. It was used in a concentration of 5×10^6 CFU/ml.

2. Culture media:
    A. Sabouraud's dextrose agar
        Media used for isolation and cultivation of *C. albicans*. This media was prepared according to the method described by Cruickshank *et al.* [19]. The ingredients were dissolved in distilled water at 121°C for 15 min. after being autoclaved and cooled to 45°C, chloramphenicol was added at concentration of 100 mg/L to the medium, pH was adjusted to be around 5.
    B. Roswell Park Memorial Institute 1640 medium (RPMI 1640) with l-glutamine
        The medium was obtained from GIBCO limited, UK, in a sterile patent preparation. The pH was adjusted to 7.2 by adding 2 g/L sodium bicarbonate. This medium was used for leukocytes cultivation.

3. Buffers
    A. Phosphate-buffered saline (PBS)
        PBS was prepared according to the method described by Cruickshank *et al.* [19]. The PBS pH was adjusted to 7.0 and the sterilized by autoclaving at 121°C for 15 min. This buffer was used for anticoagulant preparation, cell washing, and for serial dilution in killing assay.
    B. Anticoagulant buffer
        EDTA solution (10%) in distilled water; it was used as 1:5 volumes of blood.

Evaluation of phagocytic activity by Wilkinson [20], Lucy and Lary [21]

1. Preparation of Hank's balanced salt solution (HBSS) [19].
2. Preparation of *C. albicans* for determining the phagocytic activity

   C. albicans was grown on Sabouraud's 2% dextrose broth for 48 h at 37°C to obtain the organism in the yeast phase only. The cultures were spinned at 1500 rpm for 10 min and the deposit washed twice with PBS, and filtered through sterile gauze. The yeasts were resuspended in HBSS so as to give a concentration of 5×10^6 CFU/ml.

   The yeasts were killed by heating at 100°C in water bath for 30 min. A large batch was prepared and divided into small aliquots sufficient for each test. These were stored at −20°C until needed.
3. Preparation of leukocytes suspension for phagocytosis assay [20,21].
   a. Peripheral blood leukocytes suspension was prepared by sterile procedures
   b. 2.5 ml of blood were collected after 15 days of exposure and carefully layered on surface of Ficoll hypaque solution 1.077 density gradient equal volumes in sterile plastic tube
   c. Centrifugation at 2400 rpm for 30 min at 18-20°C. The mononuclear cells form a white opaque band at Ficoll plasma interface. This layer was aspirated by sterile Pasteur pipette and placed in sterile plastic tube containing HBSS
   d. The separated cells washed 3 times in HBSS at 2500, 1500, and 1000 rpm, respectively, each for 10 min
   e. Sedimented cells were suspended in 1 ml of the RPMI media containing 1% fetal calf serum.
4. Preparation for phagocytosis assay

   In sterile plastic tubes, put 0.25 ml leukocyte suspension, 0.25 ml heat-killed *C. albicans*, 0.25 ml pooled serum, and 0.25 ml HBSS. The tubes were incubated at 37°C for 30 min. They were centrifuged at 2500 rpm for 5 min, and the supernatant was removed with Pasteur pipette leaving a drop into which the sediment was resuspended. Smears were prepared from the deposit, dried in air, and stained with Leishman's stain.

Evaluation of phagocytic activity

Under a light microscope using oil immersion lens, 10 fields, each containing about 20 phagocytes, were examined. The total number of phagocytic cells and the number of phagocytes with ingested yeast cells in individual phagocytes were determined to calculate the percentage of phagocytosis and the phagocytic index (PI). The mean particle number associated with each cell represents the PI.

$$PI = \frac{\text{Total number of ingested yeast cells}}{\text{Total number of infected phagocytes}}$$

The number of cells ingesting *Candida* represents the phagocytic percentage (P%).

$$P\% = \frac{\text{Number of phagocytes with ingested yeast cells}}{\text{Total number of phagocytes}} \times 100$$

Biochemical studies

Determination of superoxide dismutase (SOD) activity according to the method described by Misra and Fridivich [22] and modified by Packer and Glazer [23], catalase (CAT) activity according to the method described by Sinha [24], reduced glutathione (GSH) according to the method described by Beutler [25] and modified by Beutler *et al.* [26], glutathione-S-transferase activity (GST) according to Habig *et al.* [27], and glutathine peroxidase activity (GPx) according to Puertas *et al.* [28].

Histopathological study

Histopathological examination of livers of control and treated groups that were collected and fixed in 10% buffered neutral formalin solution, dehydrated in gradual ethanol (70-100%), cleared in xylene, and embedded in paraffin. 5 µ thick paraffin sections were prepared, and then routinely stained with hematoxylin and eosin dyes according to Suvarna *et al.* [29], and then examined microscopically.

Statistical analysis

The obtained data were analyzed using the SPSS software, version 16 (SPSS Inc., Chicago, IL, USA). Groups' data were compared by one-way analysis of variance. The statistical significance was accepted at ($p<0.05$).

Results

Effect of Roundup and Stomp on phagocytic activity

The data illustrated in Table-1 and Figure-1 indicated the effect of Roundup and/or Stomp treatment on phagocytic activity of *C. gariepinus* leukocytes against

Table-1: Changes in phagocytic percent (p%) and PI in *C. gariepinus* exposed to Roundup, Stomp, and both after 15 days of exposure (mean±SE) (n=30).

Group	Treatment	Phagocytic percent (p%)	PI
1	Control	33.46±3.51ᵃ	1.35±0.05ᵃ
2	1/2 LC₅₀ Roundup	20.16±1.03ᵇ	0.964±0.03ᵇ
3	1/2 LC₅₀ Stomp	27.08±1.53ᵃ	1.01±0.03ᵇ
4	1/2 LC₅₀ Roundup and 1/2 LC₅₀ Stomp	13.5±1.55ᶜ	0.936±0.06ᵇ

Means within the same column having the different superscripts are significantly different at (p<0.05). PI=Phagocytic index, SE=Standard error, LC₅₀=Lethal concentration 50

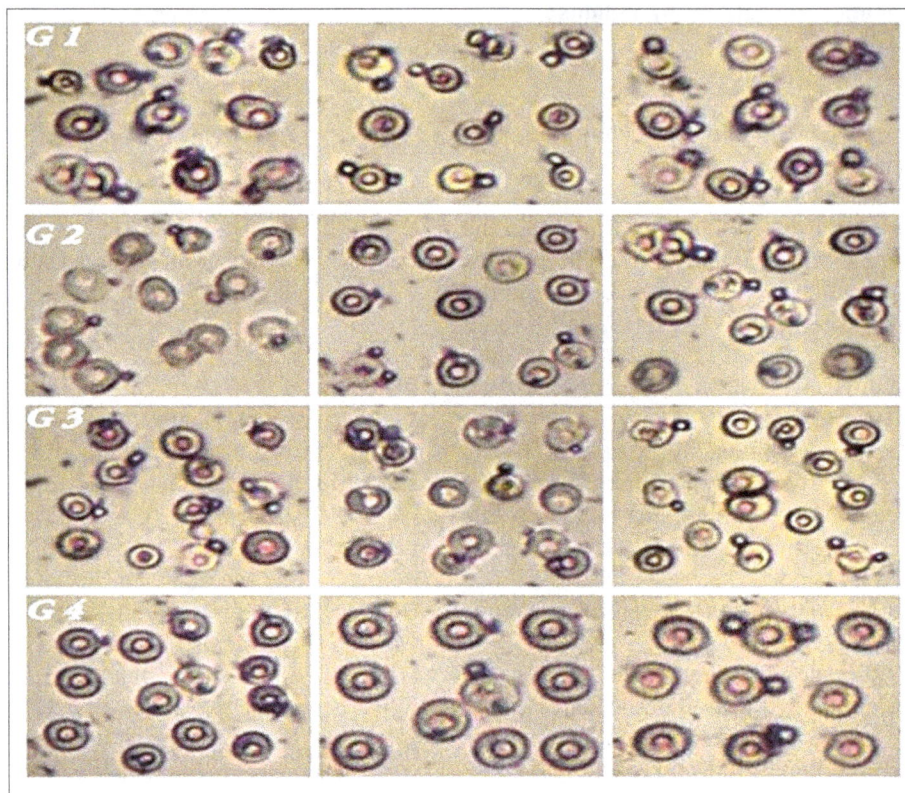

Figure-1: Photograph of phagocyte cells showing the effect of Roundup, Stomp, and both on phagocytic activity of *Clarias gariepinus* after 15 days of exposure. (G1) Phagocyte cells engulfing yeast cells in *C. gariepinus* of control group. (G2) Phagocyte cells showing destruction and inhibition of phagocytosis in group exposed to Roundup. (G3) Phagocyte cells showing destruction and inhibition of phagocytosis in group exposed to Stomp. (G4) Phagocyte cells showing severe destruction and inhibition of phagocytosis in group exposed to combination of Roundup and Stomp.

yeast cells at 15th day of exposure. The phagocytic percent (P%) was significantly reduced in the Roundup-treated group compared to the control one, while there was a non-significant decrease of the phagocytic percent in group treated with Stomp when compared with the control group. On the other hand, the phagocytic percent in group treated with both Roundup and Stomp showed an obvious significant decrease comparing with control group. In addition, the data illustrated clear significance difference between all treated groups when compared with each other. Regarding the PI, there was a significant decrease in all treated groups when compared to the control one.

Effect of Roundup and Stomp on SOD and CAT activities

Concerning the SOD activity in serum of *C. gariepinus,* our study showed a significant increase in fish exposed to the combination of both Roundup and Stomp at 1st day of exposure. While there was no significant increase in fish exposed to Roundup or Stomp separately compared with the control group. At 8th day of exposure, SOD activity increased significantly in fish exposed to Roundup, but there was no significant increase in the Stomp-treated group, while the increase in SOD activity was highly obvious in the combined treated group. Furthermore, the three treated groups depicted significance difference when compared with each other. Meanwhile, at 15th day of

exposure, the SOD activity elevated significantly in all treated groups compared to the control one (Table-2).

Regarding the CAT activity, the present study showed a significant elevation in fish exposed to Stomp while the elevation was obviously significant in groups exposed to Roundup and the combination of both herbicides comparing with the control group at 1st day of exposure.

At 8th day of exposure, fish exposed to Roundup or Stomp separately showed a significant increase in CAT activity, while the elevation was highly obvious in groups exposed to the combination of both herbicides comparing with the control group and also when comparing with Roundup and Stomp-treated groups. At 15th day of exposure, the elevation in CAT activity was significant only in fish exposed to the combination of Roundup and Stomp, but there was no significant increase at other treated groups comparing with the control group (Table-2).

Effect of Roundup and Stomp on the activities of reduced GSH, GST, and GPx

Regarding the GSH level in serum of *C. gariepinus,* the current study demonstrated a significant decrease in Roundup exposed group and obviously significant decrease in the combined treated group at 1st day of exposure compared to the control group, and also, there was significance difference in GSH level when comparing the treated groups with each other.

While at 8th and 15th day of exposure the decrease in GSH level was significant in all treated groups when compared to the control one (Table-3).

Concerning the GST activity, no significant variations versus control were observed in all treated groups at 1st day of exposure. At 8th day of exposure, fish exposed to the combination of both Roundup and Stomp showed a significant reduction in GST activity, but there was no significant alteration in other treated groups comparing with control one. While at 15th day of exposure, the reduction in GST activity was obvious in Roundup-treated group and highly obvious in group treated with the combination of both herbicides, besides, our data revealed that there was significance difference in GST level when comparing the three treated groups with each other, but no significant reduction was observed in Stomp-treated group compared to the control one (Table-3).

Regarding the GPx activity, fish exposed to Roundup showed a significant increase at all durations of exposure compared to the control one. In Stomp-treated group, the GPx activity showed a significant elevation at the 8th day of exposure but did not show any significant elevation at other durations of exposure when compared with the control group. Fish exposed to the combination of both herbicides showed an obviously significant elevation compared to the control group in all durations of exposure (Table-3).

Histopathological findings

The liver of the control revealed normal hepatocytes and sinusoidal architectures (Figure-2a).

However, the liver of Roundup showed severe congestion in hepatoportal blood vessels (Figure-2b). Multifocal areas of coagulative necrosis invaded with numerous leukocytes and erythrocytes were visualized (Figure-2c). Severe hydropic degeneration and macrovesicular steatosis were detected (Figure-2d). The liver of Stomp showed moderate congestion, severe hydropic degeneration, and vacuolation in the hepatocytes (Figure-2e). The portal areas revealed periductal fibrosis and round cells infiltration besides hyalinization in the wall of blood vessels (Figure-2f). The reported lesions in both exposures to Roundup and Stomp were severe and represented by extensive coagulative necrosis and perivascular edema (Figure-2g). Intense interstitial and portal aggregations of round cells were noticed (Figure-2h).

Discussion

Aquatic environments are commonly impacted by various pesticides (including herbicides, fungicides, and insecticides) from different sources. Fish species are described as suitable monitors for the effects of noxious compounds because of their ecological and economical relevance [9]. In addition, changes at cellular and biochemical levels are among the most sensitive biological responses reported after fish exposure to aquatic pollutants [30].

The immune system of vertebrates, including that of fish, reacts with a particular sensitivity to xenobiotic exposure [31]. Phagocytic activity is a primitive defense mechanism and an important component of

Table-2: Changes in SOD and CAT activities of *C. gariepinus* exposed to Roundup, Stomp, and both at 1st, 8th, and 15th days of exposure (mean±SE) (n=30).

Parameters	SOD (unit/mg protein)			CAT (μmol H$_2$O$_2$ decomposed/ml)		
	1st	8th	15th	1st	8th	15th
Control	40.26±1.16[a]	42.50±0.78[a]	44.35±2.85[a]	28.38±2.75[a]	31.89±0.55[a]	44.63±1.20[a]
1/2 LC$_{50}$ Roundup	47.89±3.03[a]	52.60±1.65[b]	51.57±1.54[b]	67.37±3.77[c]	49.16±3.60[b]	48.16±1.8[ab]
1/2 LC$_{50}$ Stomp	46.28±1.29[ab]	43.74±3.60[a]	51.22±1.82[b]	47.03±0.31[b]	44.71±1.83[b]	46.91±2.6[ab]
1/2 LC$_{50}$ Roundup and 1/2 LC$_{50}$ Stomp	52.03±3.60[b]	60.44±0.25[c]	56.52±2.33[b]	69.50±1.46[c]	56.26±1.00[c]	51.98±1.3[b]

Means within the same column having the different superscripts were significantly different (p<0.05). SOD=Superoxide dismutase, CAT=Catalase, *C. gariepinus=Clarias gariepinus*, SE=Standard error, LC$_{50}$=Lethal concentration 50

Table-3: Changes in GSH, GST, and GPx activities of *C. gariepinus* exposed to Roundup, Stomp, and both at 1st, 8th, and 15th days of exposure (Mean±SE) (n=30).

Parameters	GSH (mg/ml)			GST (U/l)			GPx (mU/ml)		
	1st	8th	15th	1st	8th	15th	1st	8th	15th
Control	4.73±0.05[a]	4.44±0.25[a]	4.53±0.38[a]	0.39±0.017[a]	0.46±0.036[a]	0.45±0.02[a]	19.42±0.73[c]	13.65±0.89[c]	11.39±0.53[c]
1/2 LC$_{50}$ Roundup	3.28±0.50[b]	2.75±0.33[b]	2.83±0.24[b]	0.31±0.012[a]	0.35±0.03[a]	0.27±0.06[b]	23.19±0.53[b]	21.28±0.64[b]	21.89±0.86[b]
1/2 LC$_{50}$ Stomp	4.39±0.31[a]	2.84±0.30[b]	2.88±0.24[b]	0.35±0.08[a]	0.38±0.03[a]	0.38±0.02[a]	20.97±0.49[bc]	20.80±0.87[b]	13.44±1.07[c]
1/2 LC$_{50}$ Roundup and 1/2 LC$_{50}$ Stomp	1.43±0.19[c]	2.06±0.36[b]	2.53±0.28[b]	0.30±0.017[a]	0.22±0.04[b]	0.14±0.03[c]	28.34±1.52[a]	24.32±0.65[a]	28.23±2.55[a]

Means within the same column having the different superscripts were significantly different (p<0.05). LC$_{50}$=Lethal concentration 50, GSH=Reduced glutathione, GST=Glutathione-S-transferase activity, GPx=Glutathione peroxidase, *C. gariepinus=Clarias gariepinus*, SE=Standard error

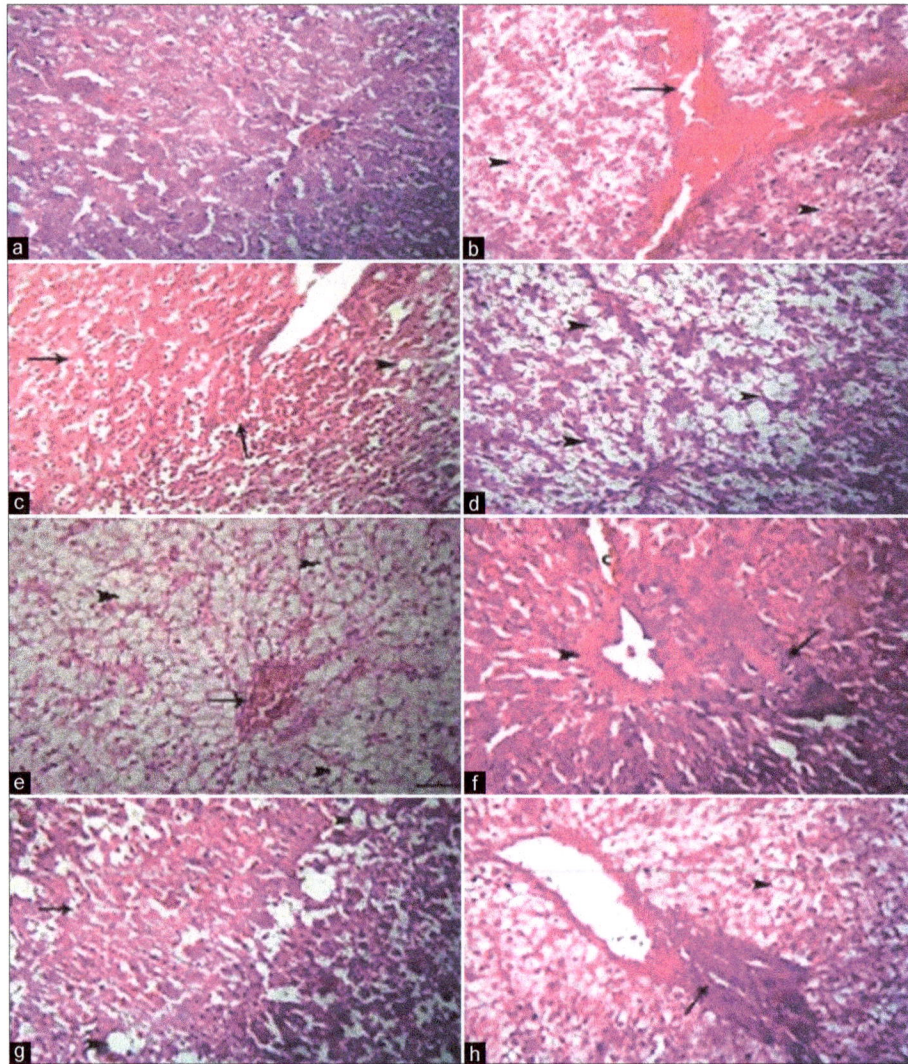

Figure-2: Liver from different groups: Control shows normal hepatocytes and sinusoidal architectures (a), Roundup shows severe congestion in hepatoportal blood vessels (arrow) (b), area of necrosis invaded with numerous leukocytes and erythrocytes (arrows) (c), and macrovesicular steatosis (d). Stomp shows congestion and severe hydropic degeneration and vacuolation in the hepatocytes (arrowheads) (e) and portal area with periductal fibrosis and round cells infiltration (arrow), and hyalinization in the wall of blood vessel (arrowhead) (f). Both Roundup and Stomp shows extensive coagulative necrosis (arrow) and perivascular edema (g) and aggregation of round cells in the portal area (arrow) (h). Hematoxylin and eosin × Scale bar = 25 μm.

the non-specific immune system [32]. Phagocytosis is a response helpful to assess the immunological impact of environmental pollutants [33]. The obtained results revealed that the phagocytic activity was decreased significantly in Roundup and/or Stomp-treated fish. Our results concurred with those obtained by Kreutz *et al.* [34] in silver catfish exposed to 10% of the 96 h-LC$_{50}$ glyphosate. A similar result was also observed in rainbow trout exposed to pendimethalin [35]. This decrease in phagocytic activity may be attributed to high soluble concentrations of herbicide disturb cell phagocytic activity. In fact, the membrane integrity of cells could be impaired by uptake of chemical compounds in organisms, which could interfere with the fluidity of cell membranes restricting the deformation of the membrane essential to the phagocytic endocytosis process [36] On the contrary of our result, Mohamed [37] studied the effect of the herbicide

Roundup on *Biomphalaria alexandrina* hemocytes and revealed a highly significant increase in the phagocytic activity that may lead to cytotoxic effects.

Matricon-Gondran and Letocart [38] speculated that these cytotoxic effects may be due to the changes in the sensitivity of intercellular adhesion molecules involved in the ingestion of foreign materials, resulting in increase of phagocytic activity.

Herbicides have the potential to introduce ROSs into biological systems, leading to oxidative stress on non-target organisms [39]. Fish, as many other vertebrates, are endowed with defensive mechanisms to counteract the harmful effects of ROS resulting from the metabolism of various chemicals or xenobiotics [40].

ROSs are naturally produced during several cellular pathways of the aerobic metabolism, including oxidative phosphorylation, electron transport chains in mitochondria and microsomes, the activity of oxidoreductase enzymes, which produce ROS as intermediates or final products, and even immunological reactions, such as active phagocytosis [41].

SOD and CAT enzymes have related functions [42]. SOD is a group of metalloenzymes that plays a crucial antioxidant role and constitutes the primary defense against the toxic effects of superoxide radicals in aerobic organisms. SOD catalyzes the transformation of superoxide radicals to hydrogen peroxide and water and is the first enzyme to cope with oxyradicals [43]. CAT is an enzyme that is located in the peroxisomes and facilitates the removal of hydrogen peroxide, which is metabolized to molecular oxygen and water [44]. Nwani *et al.* [45] assessed the alteration in LPO and antioxidant enzymes activities. They found that induction of oxidative stress in the blood and gill cells were evidenced by increased LPO level while antioxidants, namely, SOD and CAT responded in a concentration-dependent manner.

In the present work, the SOD and CAT activities increased after exposure of *C. gariepinus* to Roundup and/or Stomp. The increase in these enzyme activities is most likely a response to the increased ROS generation induced by pesticide toxicity [46]. This hypothesis was corroborated by Monteiro *et al.* [42], who described the simultaneous induction of SOD and CAT activities in *Brycon cephalus* exposed to methyl parathion and Pieniazek *et al.* [47], who found an increment in CAT levels in human erythrocytes after exposure to glyphosate and Roundup. The increases in the serum SOD and CAT activities that were observed in this study may be meant to neutralize the overproduction of superoxide anions and hydrogen peroxides due to the oxidative stress induced by herbicides. Our findings supported by a previous observation of Noori [48], who mentioned that the failure in the neutralization events of oxidative status results in oxidative stress which leads to the cell death by LPO.

Reduced GSH is a main non-protein thiol and is a primary reductant in cells [49]. The main role of GSH is based on its ability to protect cells against oxidative damage caused by free radicals by providing a reduced medium to cells; GSH also serves as an important substrate for the reductive detoxification of reactive intermediates such as hydrogen peroxide or hydroperoxides. Consequently, estimation of the level of this compound should provide essential data describing the processes which happen in cells [50]. In the current study, the GSH level was significantly decreased in the Roundup and/or Stomp exposed fish. This result was in accordance with those obtained by Danion *et al.* [51] in *Oncorhynchus mykiss* exposed to pendimethalin and also with previous studies, which reported a GSH depletion with other pesticides and herbicides in different cellular populations *in vitro* [50,52] and *in vivo* [53] but were opposed to others [54,55]. The decrease in GSH content may be related to utilization of this antioxidant in the

metabolism of herbicides through GSH-Px activity. The action of this enzyme was strictly linked with the GSH concentration because it catalyzed the reaction between GSH and hydrogen peroxide, resulting in the formation of GSH disulfide. Thus, it could be assumed that herbicides, by lowering the level of GSH and decreasing the GSSG-Red activity, led to an oxidative imbalance and induced oxidative processes.

GSTs are a group of enzymes that catalyze the conjugation of reduced GSH with a variety of electrophilic metabolites and are involved in the detoxification of both reactive intermediates and oxygen radicals [44]. It has been demonstrated that the activity of these enzymes may be enhanced in the liver of fish exposed to a variety of pollutants, and even low-level organic contamination can lead to increased hepatic GST activity in fish [56]. However, in the present work, *C. gariepinus* exposed to the herbicides Roundup and Stomp showed decrease in GST activity.

This decrease may reinforce the idea of the presence of oxidants that would lead to the inactivation of the enzymatic activity [57] considering that GST is sensitive to products of the Haber–Weiss reaction [58]. The inhibition of GST was also observed in the liver of goldfish after 96 h exposure to Roundup [6]. Conversely, when *Prochilodus lineatus* was exposed to Roundup [59] found a significant increase in liver GST after 24 and 96 h exposure.

GPx catalyzes the reduction of hydrogen peroxide and lipid peroxides and is considered an efficient protective enzyme against LPO at the expense of GSH [60]. In this work, our result revealed a significant elevation in GPX activity in serum of *C. gariepinus* exposed to Roundup and/or Stomp. This increase is in consistence with that result obtained by Gehin *et al.* [61] in HaCaT cultured cells exposed to glyphosate or Roundup. This increase may indicate that the antioxidant pathway was stimulated, probably due to the increased production of peroxides. Although this enzyme acts principally in the removal of organic peroxides, it is also involved in the metabolization of hydrogen peroxide [62]. The aforementioned results of our study concerning immunotoxicity and oxidative stress came in harmony with histopathological changes in the liver after exposure to Roundup, which revealed severe congestion in hepatoportal blood vessels, multifocal areas of coagulative necrosis invaded with numerous leukocytes and erythrocytes and severe hydropic degeneration and macrovesicular steatosis were detected. This result was nearly similar to that found in *Piaractus mesopotamicus* [63] and *P. lineatus* [64]. In this work, the most frequent encountered types of degenerative changes are those of hydropic degeneration, cloudy swelling, vacuolization, and focal necrosis. The liver of the exposed fish had slightly vacuolated cells showing evidence of fatty degeneration. Necrosis of some portions of the liver tissue that were observed probably resulted from the excessive work required by the fish to get rid of the toxicant from its body during the process of detoxification by the liver. The inability of fish to regenerate new liver cells may also have led to necrosis [65].

While the liver of *C. gariepinus* exposed to Stomp showed moderate congestion, severe hydropic degeneration, and vacuolation in the hepatocytes. The portal areas revealed periductal fibrosis and round cells infiltration besides hyalinization in the wall of blood vessels. This result parallel to findings of Nabela *et al.* [66], who reported that these changes may be attributed by the enterohepatic pathway of the Stomp (pendimethalin-based herbicide).

Conclusion

The current study implicated that using Roundup and Stomp separately caused significant deleterious effects on aquatic vertebrates. However, the use of their combination exaggerated their obvious toxic effects. In turn, their toxicity can end up in humans through the food chain. The suitable controlled and regular use of herbicides is recommended, to obtain the beneficial effects of these resources without polluting the environment and without leaving their residues in food and water sources with potentially negative effects on human health.

Authors' Contributions

GGM, FES, and AHAH generated the concept and designed the study. GGM and WME carried out the practical part and drafted the manuscript. GGM revised and approved the final manuscript.

Acknowledgments

This work is supported by the Department of Forensic Medicine and Toxicology, Faculty of Veterinary Medicine, Zagazig University, Egypt. Furthermore, authors thank Professor Dr. Mohammed Hamed Mohammed, Professor of Pathology, Faculty of Veterinary Medicine, Zagazig University, for his help in examining the histopathological study. This work was done on authors' expense without funding from any organization.

Competing Interests

The authors declare that they have no competing interests.

References

1. Diez, M.C. (2010) Biological aspects involved in the degradation of organic pollutants. *J. Soil Sci. Plant Nutr.,* 10: 244-267.

2. Glusczak, L., Loro, V.L., Pretto, A., Moraes, B.S., Raabe, A., Duarte, M.F., da Fonseca, M.B., de Menezes, C.C. and Valladao, D.M.D. (2011) Acute exposure to glyphosate herbicide affects oxidative parameters in Piava (*Leporinus obtusidens*). *Arch. Environ. Contam. Toxicol.,* 61: 624-630.

3. Rossi, S.C., da Silva, M.D., Piancini, L.D.S., Ribeiro, C.A.O., Cestari, M.M. and de Assis, H.C.S. (2011) Sublethal effects of waterborne herbicides in tropical freshwater fish. *Bull. Environ. Contam. Toxicol.,* 87: 603-607.

4. Stara, A., Kristan, J., Zuskova, E. and Velisek, J. (2013) Effect of chronic exposure to prometryne on oxidative stress and antioxidant response in common carp (*Cyprinus carpio* L.). *Pestic. Biochem. Physiol.,* 105: 18-23.

5. Wagenhoff, A., Townsend, C.R., Phillips, N. and Matthaei, C.D. (2011) Subsidy-stress and multiple-stressor effects along gradients of deposited fine sediment and dissolved nutrients in a regional set of streams and rivers. *Freshw. Biol.,* 56: 1916-1936.

6. Lushchak, O.V., Kubrak, O.I., Storey, J.M., Storey, K.B. and Lushchak, O.I. (2009) Low toxic herbicide Roundup induces mild oxidative stress in goldfish tissues. *Chemosphere,* 76: 932-937.

7. EPA, (Environmental Protection Agency). (2011) Pesticides industry sales and usage: 2006 and 2007 market estimates. In: Grube, A., Donaldson, D., Kiely, T. and Wu, L., editors. Biological and Economic Analysis Division, Office of Pesticide Programs, Office of Chemical Safety and Pollution Prevention. U.S. Environmental Protection Agency, Washington, DC, USA.

8. Romero, D.M., de Molina, M.C.R. and Juarez, A.B. (2011) Oxidative stress induced by a commercial glyphosate formulation in a tolerant strain of *Chlorella kessleri*. *Ecotoxicol. Environ. Saf.,* 74: 741-747.

9. Jiraungkoorskul, W., Upatham, E.S., Kruatrachue, M., Sahaphong, S., Vichasri-Grams, S. and Pokethitiyook, P. (2002) Histopathological effects of Roundup, a glyphosate herbicide, on Nile tilapia (*Oreochromis niloticus*). *ScienceAsia,* 28: 121-127.

10. Fetvadjieva, N., Straka, F., Michailova, P., Balinov, I., Lubenov, I., Balinova, A., Pelov, V., Karsova, V. and Tsvetkov, D. (1994) In: Fetvadjieva, N., editor. Handbook of Pesticides. 2nd Revised. Zemizdat Inc., Sofia. p330.

11. Meister, R.T., editor. (1992) Farm Chemicals Handbook '92. Meister Publishing Company, Willoughby, Ohio, USA. p197-202.

12. Lushchak, V.I. (2011) Environmentally induced oxidative stress in aquatic animals. *Aquat. Toxicol.,* 101: 13-30.

13. Perez, J., Domingues, I., Monteiro, M., Soares, A.M. and Loureiro, S. (3013) Synergistic effects caused by atrazine and terbuthylazine on chlorpyrifos toxicity to early - Life stages of the zebrafish *Danio rario. Environ. Sci. Pollut. Res.,* 20: 4671-4680.

14. Dabas, A., Nagpure, N.S., Kumar, R., Kushwaha, B., Kumar, P. and Lakra W. (2012) Assemment of tissue-specific effect of cadmium on antioxidant defense system and lipid peroxidation in freshwater murrel, *Channa punctatus. Fish Physiol. Biochem.,* 38: 468-482.

15. Abdelghani, A.A., Tchounwou, P.B., Anderson, A.C., Sujono, H., Heyer, L.R. and Monkiedje, A. (1997) Toxicity evaluation of single and chemical mixtures of Roundup, Garlon-3A, 2,4-D, and synthetic detergent surfactant to channel catfish (*Ictalurus punctatus*), bluegill sunfish (*Lepomis microchirus*), and crawfish (*Procambarus* spp.). *Environ. Toxicol. Water,* 12: 237-243.

16. Kidd, H. and James, D.R. (1991) The Agrochemicals Handbook. 3rd ed. Royal Society of Chemistry Information Services, Cambridge, UK. p3-11.

17. USEPA, (United State Environmental Protection Agency). (1987) Pesticide Tolerance for Pendimethalin. Fed. Regist. 52: 47734.5. Dec. 16-1987. USEPA, Washington, DC, USA. p10-117.

18. Lucky, Z. (1977) Methods for the Diagnosis of Fish Diseases. 1st ed. Amerind Publishing Co., Pvt., Ltd., New Delhi, Bombay, Calcutta and New York. p140.

19. Cruickshank, R., Duguid, R., Marmion, B.P. and Swain, R.A. (1975) Natural and acquired immunity in: Medical microbiology. In: Cruickshank, R. and Swain, R.A., editors. Microbiology; Infection and Immunology. Vol. 1. Part 1. Churchill Livingstone, Edinburgh and London. p137.

20. Wilkinson, P.C. (1977) In: Thompson, R.A., editor. Techniques in Clinical Immunology. Oxford Blackwell Publication, USA. p201-212.

21. Lucy, F.I. and Larry, D.B. (1982) Ontageny and line differences in mitogenic responces of chicken lymphocyte. *Poult. Sci.*, 62: 579-584.

22. Misra, H. and Fridivich, I. (1972) Role of superoxide anion in autooxidation of epinephrine, simple assay for SOD. *J. Biochem.*, 247: 3170-3175.

23. Packer, L. and Glazer, A.N. (1990) Method in enzymology. Oxygen Radicals in Biological Systems, Part B; Oxygen Radicals and Antioxidants. Vol. 186. Academic Press Inc., New York. p355-367.

24. Sinha, A.K. (1972) Colorimetric assay of catalase. Analytical Biochemistry, 47, 389 p251.

25. Beutler, E. (1957) Glutathione instability of drug - Sensitive red cells; A new method for the *in vitro* detection of drug sensitivity. *J. Lab. Clin. Med.*, 49: 84-95.

26. Beutler, E., Duron, O. and Kelly, B.M. (1963) Improved method for the determination of blood glutathione. *J. Lab. Clin. Med.*, 61: 822-888.

27. Habig, W.H., Pabst, M.J. and Jacoby, W.B. (1974) Glutathione S-transferases. The first enzymatic step in mercapturic acid formation. *J. Biol. Chem.* 249: 7130-7139.

28. Puertas, M.C., Martos, J.M.M., Cobo, M.P., Carrera, M.D. and Exposito, M.J.R. (2012) Plasma oxidative stress parameters in men and women with early stage Alzheimer type dementia. *Exp. Gerontol.*, 47: 625-630.

29. Suvarna, S.K., Layton, C. and Bancroft, J.D. (2013) Bancroft's Theory and Practice of Histological Techniques. 7th ed. Churchill Livingstone, Elsevier, England.

30. Sandrini, J.Z., Rola, R.C., Lopes, F.M., Buffon, H.F., Freitas, M.M., Martins, C.M.G. and Rosa, C.E. (2013) Effects of glyphosate on cholinesterase activity of the mussel Pernaperna and the fish *Danio rerio* and *Jenynsia multidentata*: *In vitro* studies. *Aquat. Toxicol.*, 130: 171-173.

31. Betoulle, S., Duchiron, C. and Deschaux, P. (2000) Lindane differently modulates intracellular calcium levels in two populations of rainbow trout (*Oncorhynchus mykiss*) immune cells: Head kidney phagocytes and peripheral blood leucocytes. *Toxicology*, 145: 203-215.

32. Harikrishnan, R., Balasundaram, C., Kim, M.C., Kim, J.S., Han, Y.J. and Heo, M.S. (2009) Innate immune response and disease resistance in *Carassius auratus* by triherbal solvent extracts. *Fish Shellfish Immunol.*, 27: 508-515.

33. Galloway, T.S. and Depledge, M.H. (2001) Immunotoxicity in invertebrates, measurement and ecotoxicological relevance. *Ecotoxicology*, 10: 5-23.

34. Kreutz, L.C., Barcellos, L.J.G., Valle, S.F., Silva, T.O., Anziliero, D., Santos, E.D., Pivato, M. and Zanatta, R. (2011) Altered hematological and immunological parameters in silver catfish (*Rhamdia quelen)* following short term exposure to sublethal concentration of glyphosate. *Fish Shellfish Immunol.*, 30: 51-57.

35. Danion, M., Le Floch, S., Kanan, R., Lamour, F. and Quentel, C. (2012) Effects of *in vivo* chronic exposure to pendimethalin/Prowl 400® on sanitary status and the immune system in rainbow trout (*Oncorhynchus mykiss*). *Sci. Total Environ.*, 424: 143-152.

36. Camus, L., Jones, M., Børseth, J., Grøsvik, B., Regoli, F. and Depledge, M. (2002) Total oxyradical scavenging capacity and cell membrane stability of haemocytes of the *Arctic scallop, Chlamys islandicus*, following benzo(a)pyrene exposure. *Mar. Environ. Res.*, 54: 425-430.

37. Mohamed, A.H. (2011) Sublethal toxicity of Roundup to immunological and molecular aspects of *Biomphalaria alexandrina* to *Schistosoma mansoni* infection. *Ecotoxicol. Environ. Saf.*, 74: 754-760.

38. Matricon-Gondran, M. and Letocart, M. (1999) Internal defenses of the snail *Biompha-laria glabrata* I. Characterization of hemocytes and fixed phagocytosis. *J. Invertebr. Pathol.*, 74: 224-234.

39. Ortiz-Ordonez, E., Uria-Galicia, E., Ruiz-Picos, R.A., Duran, A.G.S., Trejo, Y.H., Sedeno-Diaz, J.E. and Lopez-Lopez, E. (2011) Effect of Yerbimat herbicide on lipid

40. Blahová, J., Plhalová, L., Hostovský, M., Divišov, L., Dobšíková, R., Mikulíková, I., Štěpánová, S. and Svobodová, Z. (2013) Oxidative stress responses in zebrafish *Danio rerio* after subchronic exposure to atrazine. *Food Chem. Toxicol.*, 61: 82-85.

41. Regoli, F. and Giuliani, M.E. (2014) Oxidative pathways of chemical toxicity and oxidative stress biomarkers in marine organisms. *Mar. Environ. Res.*, 93: 106-117.

42. Monteiro, D.A., de Almeida, J.A., Rantin, F.T. and Kalinin, A.L. (2006) Oxidative stress biomarkers in the freshwater characid fish, *Brycon cephalus*, exposed to organophosphorus insecticide Folisuper 600 (methyl parathion). *Comp. Biochem. Phys. C.*, 143: 141-149.

43. Kohen, R. and Nyska, A. (2002) Oxidation of biological systems: Oxidative stress phenomena, antioxidants, redox reactions, and methods for their quantification. *Toxicol. Pathol.*, 30: 620-650.

44. Van der Oost, R., Beyer, J. and Vermeulen, N.P. (2003) Fish bioaccumulation and biomarkers in environmental risk assessment: A review. *Environ. Toxicol. Pharmacol.*, 13: 57-149.

45. Nwani, C.D., Nagpure, N.S., Kumar, R., Kushwaha, B. and Lakra, W.S. (2013) DNA damage and oxidative stress modulatory effects of glyphosate-based herbicide in freshwater fish, *Channa punctatus. Environ. Toxicol. Pharmacol.*, 36: 539-547.

46. John, S., Kale, M., Rathore, N. and Bhatnagar, D. (2001) Protective effect of vitamin E in dimethoate and malathion induced oxidative stress in rat erythrocytes. *J. Nutr. Biochem.*, 12: 500-504.

47. Pieniazek, D., Bukowska, B. and Duda, W. (2004) Comparison of the effect of Roundup Ultra 360 SL pesticide and its active compound glyphosate on human erythrocytes. *Pestic. Biochem. Physiol.*, 79: 27-34.

48. Noori, S. (2012) An overview of oxidative stress and antioxidant defensive system. *Scientific Reports,* 1:413.

49. Yilmaz, S., Atessahin, A., Sahna, E., Karahan, I. and Ozer, S. (2006) Protective effect of lycopene on adriamycin-induced cardiotoxicity and nephrotoxicity. *Toxicology*, 218: 164-171.

50. Bukowska, B. (2003) Effects of 2,4-d and its metabolite 2,4-dichlorophenol on antioxidant enzymes and level of glutathione in human erythrocytes. *Comp. Biochem. Physiol. C.*, 135: 435-441.

51. Danion, M., Le Floch, S., Lamour, F. and Quentel, C. (2014) Effects of *in vivo* chronic exposure to pendimethalin on EROD activity and antioxidant defenses in rainbow trout (*Oncorhynchus mykiss*). *Ecotoxicol. Environ. Saf.*, 99: 21-27.

52. Cereser, C., Boget, S., Parvaz, P. and Revol, A. (2001) Thiram-induced cytotoxic-ity is accompanied by a rapid and drastic oxidation of reduced glutathione with consecutive lipid peroxidation and cell death. *Toxicology*, 163: 153-162.

53. Banerjee, B.D., Seth, V., Bhattacharya, A., Pasha, S.T. and Chakraborty, A.K. (1999) Biochemical effects of some pesticides on lipid peroxidation and free-radical scavengers. *Toxicol. Lett.*, 107: 33-47.

54. Slaughter, M.R., Thakkar, H. and O'Brien, P.J. (2002) Effect of diquat on the antioxidant system and cell growth in human neuroblastoma cells. *Toxicol. Appl. Pharmacol.*, 178: 63-70.

55. Tsukamoto, M., Tampo, Y., Sawada, M. and Yonaha, M. (2002) Paraquat induced oxidative stress and dysfunction of the glutathione redox cycle in pulmonary microvascular endothelial cells. *Toxicol. Appl. Pharmacol.*, 178: 82-92.

56. Machala, M., Petřivalský, M., Nezveda, K., Ulrico, R., Dušek, L., Piačka, V. and Svobodová, Z. (1997) Responses of carp hepatopancreatic 7-ethoxyresorufin-O-deethylase and glutathione-dependent enzymes to organic pollutants - A

field study. *Environ. Toxicol. Chem.,* 16: 1410-1416.

57. Bagnyukova, T.V., Chahrak, O.I. and Lushchak, V.I. (2006) Coordinated response of goldfish antioxidant defenses to environmental stress. *Aquat. Toxicol.,* 78: 325-331.

58. Hermes-Lima, M. and Storey, K.B. (1993) *In vitro* oxidative inactivation of glutathione S-transferase from a freeze tolerant reptile. *Mol. Cell. Biochem.,* 124: 149-158.

59. Modesto, K.A. and Martinez, C.B.R. (2010) Roundup causes oxidative stress in liver and inhibits acetylcholinesterase in muscle and brain of the fish *Prochilodus lineatus. Chemosphere,* 78: 294-299.

60. Moreno, I., Pichardo, S., Góomez-Amores, L., Mate, A., Vazquez, C.M. and Ameán, A.M. (2005) Antioxidant enzyme activity and lipid peroxidation in liver and kidney of rats exposed to microcystin-*LR* administered intraperitoneally. *Toxicon,* 45: 395-402.

61. Gehin, A., Guyon, C. and Nicod, L. (2006) Glyphosate-induced antioxidant imbalance in HaCaT: The protective effect of vitamins C and E. *Environ. Toxicol. Pharmacol.,* 22: 27-34.

62. Maran, E., Fernández, M., Barbieri, P., Font, G. and Ruiz, M.J. (2009) Effects of four carbamate compounds on antioxidant parameters. *Ecotoxicol. Environ. Saf.,* 72: 922-930.

63. Shiogiri, N.S., Paulino, M.G., Carraschi, S.P., Baraldi, F.G., Cruz, C. and Fernandes, M.N. (2012) Acute exposure of a glyphosate-based herbicide affects the gills and liver of the neotropical fish, *Piaractus mesopotamicus. Environ. Toxicol. Pharmacol.,* 2: 388-496.

64. Langiano, V.C. and Martinez, C.B. (2008) Toxicity and effects of a glyphosate-based herbicide on the neotropical fish *Prochilodus lineatus. Comp. Biochem. Physiol. C.,* 147: 222-231.

65. Abd-Algadir, M.I., Elkhier, M.K.S. and Idris, O.F. (2011) Changes of fish liver (*Tilapia nilotica*) made by herbicide (Pendimethalin). *J. Appl. Biosci.,* 43: 2942-2946.

66. Nabela, I.E., Reda, R.M. and El-Araby, I.E. (2011) Assessment of Stomp® (Pendimethalin) toxicity on *Oreochromis niloticus. J. Am. Sci.,* 7: 568-576.

Permissions

All chapters in this book were first published in VW, by Veterinary World; hereby published with permission under the Creative Commons Attribution License or equivalent. Every chapter published in this book has been scrutinized by our experts. Their significance has been extensively debated. The topics covered herein carry significant findings which will fuel the growth of the discipline. They may even be implemented as practical applications or may be referred to as a beginning point for another development.

The contributors of this book come from diverse backgrounds, making this book a truly international effort. This book will bring forth new frontiers with its revolutionizing research information and detailed analysis of the nascent developments around the world.

We would like to thank all the contributing authors for lending their expertise to make the book truly unique. They have played a crucial role in the development of this book. Without their invaluable contributions this book wouldn't have been possible. They have made vital efforts to compile up to date information on the varied aspects of this subject to make this book a valuable addition to the collection of many professionals and students.

This book was conceptualized with the vision of imparting up-to-date information and advanced data in this field. To ensure the same, a matchless editorial board was set up. Every individual on the board went through rigorous rounds of assessment to prove their worth. After which they invested a large part of their time researching and compiling the most relevant data for our readers.

The editorial board has been involved in producing this book since its inception. They have spent rigorous hours researching and exploring the diverse topics which have resulted in the successful publishing of this book. They have passed on their knowledge of decades through this book. To expedite this challenging task, the publisher supported the team at every step. A small team of assistant editors was also appointed to further simplify the editing procedure and attain best results for the readers.

Apart from the editorial board, the designing team has also invested a significant amount of their time in understanding the subject and creating the most relevant covers. They scrutinized every image to scout for the most suitable representation of the subject and create an appropriate cover for the book.

The publishing team has been an ardent support to the editorial, designing and production team. Their endless efforts to recruit the best for this project, has resulted in the accomplishment of this book. They are a veteran in the field of academics and their pool of knowledge is as vast as their experience in printing. Their expertise and guidance has proved useful at every step. Their uncompromising quality standards have made this book an exceptional effort. Their encouragement from time to time has been an inspiration for everyone.

The publisher and the editorial board hope that this book will prove to be a valuable piece of knowledge for researchers, students, practitioners and scholars across the globe.

List of Contributors

Biswa Ranjan Maharana
Department of Veterinary Parasitology, College of Veterinary Science and Animal Husbandry, Junagadh Agricultural University, Junagadh, Gujarat, India

Anup Kumar Tewari, Buddhi Chandrasekaran Saravanan and Naduvanahalli Rajanna Sudhakar
Division of Parasitology, Indian Veterinary Research Institute, Izatnagar, Uttar Pradesh, India

R. G. Shrimali, M. D. Patel and R. M. Patel
Department of Veterinary Medicine, College of Veterinary Science & Animal Husbandry, Navsari Agricultural University, Navsari - 396 450, Gujarat, India

Vijayata Choudhary, Mukesh Choudhary, Sunanda Pandey, Vandip D. Chauhan and J. J. Hasnani
Department of Veterinary Parasitology, Veterinary College, Anand Agricultural University, Anand, Gujarat, India

Narender Kumar, A. Kumaresan, L. Sreela, Shiwani Tiwari and Subhash Chandra
Theriogenology Laboratory, Livestock Production Management Section, ICAR - National Dairy Research Institute (NDRI), Karnal - 132 001, Haryana, India

A. Manimaran
Southern Regional Station, ICAR - National Dairy Research Institute, Adugodi, Hosur road, Bengaluru - 560 030, Karnataka, India

Tapas Kumar Patbandha
Polytechnic in Animal Husbandry, College of Veterinary Science and A.H., Junagadh Agricultural University, Junagadh - 362 001, Gujarat, India

Taruna Bhati, Prerna Nathawat, Rahul Yadav, Jyoti Bishnoi and Anil Kumar Kataria
Department of Veterinary Microbiology and Biotechnology, College of Veterinary and Animal Science, Rajasthan University of Veterinary and Animals Sciences, Bikaner, Rajasthan, India

Sandeep Kumar Sharma
Department of Veterinary Microbiology and Biotechnology, Post Graduate Institute of Veterinary Education and Research, Rajasthan University of Veterinary and Animals Sciences, Bikaner, Rajasthan, India

N. Kumar and S. A. Lone
Division of Animal Reproduction, Gynecology & Obstetrics, NDRI, Karnal, Haryana, India

J. K. Prasad and S. K. Ghosh
Germ Plasm Centre, Division of Animal Reproduction, Indian Veterinary Research Institute, Izatnagar, Bareilly, Uttar Pradesh, India

M. H. Jan
Central Institute for Research on Buffalo, Hisar, Haryana, India

Ritu Agrawal, S. D. Hirpurkar, C. Sannat and Amit Kumar Gupta
Department of Veterinary Microbiology, College of Veterinary Science & Animal Husbandry, Anjora, Durg, Chhattisgarh, India

M. H. Khan
ICAR-National Research Centre on Mithun, Jharnapani, Medziphema - 797 106, Nagaland, India

K. Manoj
ICAR Research Complex for NEH Region, Umiam - 793 103, Meghalaya, India

S. Pramod
Central Institute for Research on Cattle, Meerut - 255 001, Uttar Pradesh, India

A. Manimaran, S. Jeyakumar, V. Sejian, Narender Kumar, A. Anantharaj and D. N. Das
Southern Regional Station, ICAR - National Dairy Research Institute, Adugodi, Bengaluru - 560 030, Karnataka, India

A. Kumaresan and T. K. Mohanty
Theriogenology Laboratory, ICAR - National Dairy Research Institute, Karnal-132 001, Haryana, Uttar Pradesh, India

L. Sreela, M. Arul Prakash and P. Mooventhan
ICAR - National Dairy Research Institute, Karnal - 132 001, Haryana, India

Raghavendra Prasad Mishra, Udit Jain and Basanti Bist
Department of Veterinary Public Health, College of Veterinary Sciences and Animal Husbandry, Pandit Deen Dayal Upadhayay Pashu Chikitsa Vigyan Vishvidhyalaya Ewam Go-Anusandhan Sansthan, Mathura - 281 001, Uttar Pradesh, India

Amit Kumar Verma
Department of Veterinary Epidemiology and Preventive Medicine, College of Veterinary Sciences and Animal Husbandry, Pandit Deen Dayal Upadhayay Pashu Chikitsa Vigyan Vishvidhyalaya Ewam Go-Anusandhan Sansthan, Mathura - 281 001, Uttar Pradesh, India

Ashok Kumar
Division of Veterinary Public Health, Indian Veterinary Research Institute, Izatnagar, Bareilly, Uttar Pradesh, India

Anshul Kumar Khare, Robinson J. J. Abraham, V. Appa Rao and R. Narendra Babu
Department of Livestock Products Technology (Meat Science), Madras Veterinary College, Tamil Nadu Veterinary and Animal Sciences University, Chennai - 600 007, Tamil Nadu, India

A. P. Patel, S. R. Bhagwat and M. M. Pawar
Department of Animal Nutrition, College of Veterinary Science and Animal Husbandry, Sardarkrushinagar Dantiwada Agricultural University, Banaskantha, Gujarat, India

K. B. Prajapati
Livestock Research Station, Sardarkrushinagar Dantiwada Agricultural University, Banaskantha, Gujarat, India

H. D. Chauhan and R. B. Makwana
Department of Livestock Production and Management, College of Veterinary Science and Animal Husbandry, Sardarkrushinagar Dantiwada Agricultural University, Banaskantha, Gujarat, India

Shailesh Kumar Gupta, Kumaresh Behera, C. R. Pradhan and Dayanidhi Behera
Department of Livestock Production and Management, College of Veterinary Sciences and Animal Husbandry, Bhubaneswar - 751 003, Odisha, India

Arun Kumar Mandal
Department of Veterinary Anatomy and Histology, College of Veterinary Sciences and Animal Husbandry, Bhubaneswar - 751 003, Odisha, India

Kamdev Sethy
Department of Animal Nutrition, College of Veterinary Sciences and Animal Husbandry, Bhubaneswar - 751 003, Odisha, India

Kuladip Prakash Shinde
Livestock Production Management Section, ICAR - National Dairy Research Institute (NDRI), Karnal - 132 001, Haryana, India

D. G. Kalambhe, N. N. Zade, S. P. Chaudhari, S. V. Shinde, W. Khan and A. R. Patil
Department of Veterinary Public Health, Nagpur Veterinary College, Nagpur, Maharashtra, India

Touqeer Ahmed, Rafiqul Islam, Farooz Ahmad Lone and Asloob Ahmad Malik
Division of Animal Reproduction, Gynaecology and Obstetrics, Faculty of Veterinary Sciences and Animal Husbandry, Sher-e-Kashmir University of Agricultural Sciences & Technology of Kashmir, Shuhama, Alusteng, Srinagar, Jammu & Kashmir, India

Muhammad Mustapha, Yachilla Maryam Bukar-Kolo, Yaqub Ahmed Geidam and Isa Adamu Gulani
Department of Veterinary Medicine, Faculty of Veterinary Medicine, University of Maiduguri, PMB 1069 Maiduguri, Borno State, Nigeria

A. D. Singh and Opinder Singh
Department of Veterinary Anatomy, Guru Angad Dev Veterinary and Animal Sciences University, Ludhiana - 141 004, Punjab, India

R. Lakshmi and K. K. Jayavardhanan
Department of Veterinary Biochemistry, College of Veterinary and Animal Sciences, Thrissur, Kerala, India

T. V. Aravindakshan
Centre for Advanced Studies in Animal Genetics and Breeding, College of Veterinary and Animal Sciences, Thrissur, Kerala, India

P. Patric Joshua
Department of Pharmacology, Sri Muthukumaran Medical College Hospital and Research Institute, Dr. M.G.R. Medical University, Chennai, Tamil Nadu, India

C. Valli
Department of Animal Nutrition, Institute of Animal Nutrition, Tamil Nadu Veterinary and Animal Sciences University, Chennai, Tamil Nadu, India

V. Balakrishnan
Department of Animal Nutrition, Madras Veterinary College, Tamil Nadu Veterinary and Animal Sciences University, Chennai, Tamil Nadu, India

Jaspal Singh Hundal, Simrinder Singh Sodhi, Jaswinder Singh and Udeybir Singh Chahal
Department of Veterinary and Animal Husbandry Extension Education, Guru Angad Dev Veterinary and Animal Sciences University, Ludhiana, Punjab, India

Aparna Gupta
Krishi Vigyan Kendra, Ropar, Punjab Agricultural University, Ludhiana, Punjab, India

Murugaiyah Marimuthu
Department of Veterinary Clinical Studies, Faculty of Veterinary Medicine, Universiti Putra Malaysia, 43400 UPM Serdang, Selangor, Malaysia
Department of Veterinary Pathology and Microbiology, Faculty of Veterinary Medicine, Universiti Putra Malaysia, 43400 UPM Serdang, Selangor, Malaysia

Norisal Binti Nasai, Konto Mohammed and Eric Lim Teik Chung
Department of Veterinary Clinical Studies, Faculty of Veterinary Medicine, Universiti Putra Malaysia, 43400 UPM Serdang, Selangor, Malaysia

Abdulnasir Tijjani, Muhammad Abubakar Sadiq and Yusuf Abba
Department of Veterinary Pathology and Microbiology, Faculty of Veterinary Medicine, Universiti Putra Malaysia, 43400 UPM Serdang, Selangor, Malaysia

Mohammed Ariff Bin Omar and Faez Firdaus Jesse Abdullah
Department of Veterinary Clinical Studies, Faculty of Veterinary Medicine, Universiti Putra Malaysia, 43400 UPM Serdang, Selangor, Malaysia
Research Centre for Ruminant Disease, Faculty of Veterinary Medicine, Universiti Putra Malaysia, 43400 UPM Serdang, Selangor, Malaysia

Ajaz Ahmad and C. K. Singh
Department of Veterinary Pathology, College of Veterinary Science, Guru Angad Dev Veterinary and Animal Sciences University, Ludhiana - 141 004, Punjab, India

Mukul Anand and Sarvajeet Yadav
Department of Veterinary Physiology, College of Veterinary Sciences and Animal Husbandry, Uttar Pradesh Pandit Deen Dayal Upadhayaya Pashu Chikitsa Vigyan Vishwavidyalaya Evam Go Anusandhan Sansthan, Mathura - 281 001, Uttar Pradesh, India

B. Sampath Kumar, Vasili Ashok, P. Kalyani and G. Remya Nair
Department of Veterinary Biochemistry, College of Veterinary Science, Sri Venkateswara Veterinary University, Korutla, Karimnagar, Telangana, Andhra Pradesh, India

Simona Di Pietro and Chiara Crinò
Department of Veterinary Science, University of Messina, Polo Universitario Annunziata, 98168 Messina, Italy

Valentina Rita Francesca Bosco
DVM, Veterinary Medical Centre S. Chiara, Viale Vittorio Veneto, 96014 Floridia (SR), Italy

Francesco Francaviglia
DVM, Local Public Health Unit (ASP) of Palermo, Via G. Cusmano 24, 90141, Palermo, Italy

Elisabetta Giudice
Department of Chemical, Biological, Pharmaceutical and Environmental Sciences, University of Messina, Viale F. Stagno d'Alcontres 31, 98168 Messina, Italy

Manoj Kumar, Poonam Ratwan, Jamuna Valsalan and A. K. Chakravarty
Division of Dairy Cattle Breeding, ICAR-National Dairy Research Institute, Karnal - 132 001, Haryana, India

Vikas Vohra
Department of Animal Genetic Resources, ICAR-National Bureau of Animal Genetic Resources, Karnal - 132 001, Haryana, India

C. S. Patil
Department of Animal Genetics and Breeding, Lala Lajpat Rai University of Veterinary & Animal Sciences, Hisar, Haryana, India

K. Puhle Japheth, R. K. Mehla, Pranay Bharti and T. Chandrasekar
Division of Livestock Production Management, ICAR-National Dairy Research Institute, Karnal - 132 001, Haryana, India

Mahendra Singh
Division of Dairy Cattle Physiology, ICAR-National Dairy Research Institute, Karnal - 132 001, Haryana, India

A. K. Gupta and Ramendra Das
Division of Dairy Cattle Breeding, ICAR-National Dairy Research Institute, Karnal - 132 001, Haryana, India

Khan Idrees Mohd, Meena Mrigesh, Balwinder Singh and Ishwar Singh
Department of Veterinary Anatomy, College of Veterinary & Animal Sciences, G.B. Pant University of Agriculture and Technology, Pantnagar, Uttarakhand, India

Anil Gattani and Ajeet Kumar
Department of Veterinary Biochemistry, Bihar Veterinary College, Patna, Bihar, India

Arti Pathak, Vaibhav Mishra and Jitendra Singh Bhatia
Department of Veterinary Physiology & Biochemistry, Apollo College of Veterinary Medicine, Jaipur, Rajasthan, India

Ashwani Kumar Roy, Mahendra Singh, Parveen Kumar and B. S. Bharath Kumar
Division of Dairy Cattle Physiology, National Dairy Research Institute, Karnal, Haryana, India

S. Parthasarathy
Division of Veterinary Public Health, Indian Veterinary Research Institute, Izatnagar, Bareilly - 243 122, Uttar Pradesh, India

Suresh Chandra Das
Veterinary Public Health Laboratory, Indian Veterinary Research Institute, Eastern Regional Station, Kolkata - 700 037, West Bengal, India

Ashok Kumar
Assistant Director General (Animal Health), Indian Council of Agricultural Research, Krishi Bhawan, New Delhi, India

Hemanta Nath, Mousumi Hazorika, Mrinmoy Datta and Avijit Haldar
Animal Reproduction Division, ICAR Research Complex for North Eastern Hill Region, Tripura Centre, Agartala,Lembucherra, West Tripura, India

Dipjyoti Rajkhowa
ICAR Research Complex for NEH Region, Barapani, Umiam, Meghalaya, India

Gihan G. Moustafa, F. E. Shaaban, A. H. Abo Hadeed and Walaa M. Elhady
Department of Forensic Medicine and Toxicology, Faculty of Veterinary Medicine, Zagazig University, Alzeraa Street Postal Code 44511, Zagazig City, Sharkia Province, Egypt

Index